Emergency Imaging
Case Review Series

T0195225

SECOND EDITION

JAMLIK-OMARI JOHNSON, MD, FASER

Associate Professor
Radiology and Imaging Sciences
Chief of Radiology and Imaging Sciences, Emory University Hospital Midtown
Director of Emergency and Trauma Imaging, Emory Healthcare
Atlanta, Georgia

ELSEVIER

ELSEVIER

1600 John F. Kennedy Blvd.
Ste 1600
Philadelphia, PA 19103-2899

EMERGENCY IMAGING: CASE REVIEW SERIES, SECOND EDITION

ISBN: 978-0-323-42875-0

Library of Congress Control Number: 2018961458

Content Strategist: Kayla Wolfe
Content Development Specialist: Angie Breckon
Content Development Manager: Kathryn DeFrancesco
Publishing Services Manager: Deepthi Unni
Project Manager: Haritha Dharmarajan

Printed in China

Last digit is the print number: 9 8 7 6 5 4 3 2 1

Working together
to grow libraries in
developing countries

www.elsevier.com • www.bookaid.org

Emergency Imaging

Case Review Series

Series Editor
David M. Yousem, MD, MBA
Associate Dean for Professional Development
Johns Hopkins University School of Medicine
Vice Chairman of Program Development
Department of Radiology
Johns Hopkins Medical Institution
Baltimore, Maryland

Volumes in the CASE REVIEW Series
Brain Imaging
Breast Imaging
Cardiac Imaging
Duke Review of MRI Physics
Emergency Radiology
Gastrointestinal Imaging
General and Vascular Ultrasound
Genitourinary Imaging
Head and Neck Imaging
Imaging Physics
Musculoskeletal Imaging
Neuroradiology
Non-Interpretive Skills for Radiology
Nuclear Medicine and Molecular Imaging
Obstetric and Gynecologic Ultrasound
Pediatric Radiology
Spine Imaging
Thoracic Imaging
Vascular and Interventional Imaging

List of Contributors

Farhan Ahmed
Medical Student
St. George's University School of Medicine
Grenada, West Indies

Maher Ahmed
Windsor University School of Medicine
St. Kitts, West Indies

Rizwan Ahmed, DO
Resident
Department of Diagnostic and Interventional Radiology
Advocate Illinois Masonic Medical Center
Chicago, Illinois

Amanda Batten, DO, Capt USAF
Assistant Professor
Division of Emergency and Trauma Imaging
San Antonio Uniformed Services Health Education Consortium
San Antonio, Texas

Ferdia Bolster, MBBCh, BAO
UW Medicine Harborview Medical Center
Seattle, Washington

Naga Ramesh Chinapuvvula, MD
Assistant Professor
Emergency and Trauma Radiology
UTHealth
The University of Texas Health Science Center, Houston/McGovern Medical School
Houston, Texas

Aprile Gibson, MD
Teleradiologist
Virtual Radiologics
Eden Prairie, Minnesota

Ibad Haider
CEO, BWell Pharmacy
CFO, Autism & Behavioral Spectrum
Autism and Behavioral Spectrum
St. Louis, Missouri

Tarek Hanna, MD
Associate Director, Division of Emergency and Trauma Imaging
Program Director, Emergency Radiology Fellowship
Assistant Professor, Department of Radiology and Imaging Sciences
Emory University School of Medicine
Atlanta, Georgia

Gayatri Joshi, MD
Assistant Professor, Division of Emergency Radiology
Emory University School of Medicine
Atlanta, Georgia

Iqra Khan, BA, MD
Department of Emergency Medicine
Saint Louis University School of Medicine
St. Louis, Missouri

Taleef R. Khan, MBA, MD
Resident
Department of Orthopaedics and Sports Medicine
University of Washington
Seattle, Washington

Tahuriah Khan, DO
Instructor
Department of Emergency Medicine
Western Michigan University
Homer Stryker, MD School of Medicine
Kalamazoo, Michigan

Marshall Kong, MD
Assistant Professor
Department of Radiology
University of Cincinnati Medical Center
Cincinnati, Ohio

Kiran Maddu, MBBS
Emory University School of Medicine
Atlanta, Georgia

Braham Malghani

Faroukh Mehkri, DO
Resident
Department of Emergency Medicine
University of Connecticut
Hartford Hospital
Hartford, Connecticut

Sarah McCord
Medical Student
Emory University School of Medicine
Atlanta, Georgia

Leonora Mui, MD
Assistant Professor of Clinical Radiology
Zucker School of Medicine at Hofstra/Northwell
Manhasset, New York

Nabeel Mumtaz
Alabama College of Osteopathic Medicine
Class of 2021 Candidate
Dothan, Alabama
Columbia University IHN Class of 2015
New York, New York
Illinois Wesleyan Class of 2014
Bloomington, Illinois

Justin Rafael, MD
Associate Radiologist
Radiology Associates of South Florida
Baptist Health South Florida
Florida International University Herbert

Wertheim College of Medicine
Miami, Florida

Meir Scheinfeld, MD, PhD
Director of Emergency Radiology
Montefiore Medical Center
Associate Professor
Albert Einstein College of Medicine
Bronx, New York

Shoaib Shariff, MBBS
Baqai Medical University
Karachi, Pakistan

Haris Shekhani, MD, MBID
Clinical Research Associate
Interventional Radiology,
Emergency Radiology, MR Imaging
Emory University
Atlanta, Georgia

Frank Taddeo, MD
Resident, Family Medicine
Piedmont Columbus Regional
Columbus, Georgia

Darren Transue, MD
Attending Radiologist
Radiology Specialists of Florida
Florida Hospital Department of Radiology
Assistant Professor
University of Central Florida College of Medicine
Orlando, Florida

Nupur Verma, MD
Assistant Professor
Abdominal and Cardiac Imaging
Director of Abdominal CT
Director or Critical Care Imaging
University of Florida
Gainsville, Florida

Brianna Vey, MD
Resident Physician
Emory University School of Medicine
Atlanta, Georgia

Jason D. Weiden, MD
Assistant Program Director, Emergency Radiology Fellowship Program
Assistant Professor, Division of Emergency and Trauma Imaging
Department of Radiology and Imaging Sciences
Emory University School of Medicine
Atlanta, Georgia

Yara Younan, MD
Resident, Diagnostic Radiology
Department of Radiology
University of Massachusetts Medical School
Worcester, Massachusetts

Foreword

I am very happy to see the latest edition of Emergency Radiology Case Review edited by Dr. Jamlik-Omari Johnson with cases written by a number of talented radiologists. This is a burgeoning field with ever increasing demand. Some of that demand has been assumed by NightHawk services, which provides off-hours imaging review for many practices. I have seen several of my Johns Hopkins residents and neuroradiology fellows take advantage of this entrepreneurial opportunity, as a permanent commitment, as a moonlighting opportunity, or as a transition between jobs.

Emergency department (ED) radiology is not like other fields of radiology which may be dominated by oncologic imaging. Obviously, there are more vascular, traumatic, and infectious disease that are represented. However, the real challenge is the need to master all organ systems, something that is daunting to a "narrow" subspecialist such as myself. In fact, I always say that I admire the "jack-of-all-trades" generalist much more so than the specialist. Keeping up with all branches of the radiology literature is an enormous task—I only have to know my tiny field of neuroradiology. I do very few things very well. I also recognize that, in this branch of radiology, communication skills are paramount. Emergency radiologists are our voice.

For those of us who read within our specialty, the ED cases are often challenging and foreboding. Lots of images, lots of reconstructions, lots of nuances. All of us could learn from this well-written book.

With this philosophical bent and admiration for those who choose this field, I congratulate Dr. Johnson on this edition of the Case Review Series in Emergency Radiology. I know that it will be quite popular and well read. Best of luck and many thanks to those people who specialize in this arena: thank you for allowing many of us to sleep safely and securely at night!

Welcome Emergency Radiology, 2nd edition to our Case Review Series.

David M. Yousem, MD, MBA
Case Review Series
Associate Dean for Professional Development
Johns Hopkins University School of Medicine
Vice Chairman of Program Development
Department of Radiology
Johns Hopkins Medical Institution
Baltimore, Maryland

Preface

Across the United States, 260 patients present to an emergency department (ED) every minute. Taken in aggregate, 137 million patients were seen in EDs in 2015 according to the CDC.[1] These numbers reflect a trend of sustained growth in ED visits year after year. Imaging patients, as a vital tool not only to triage, but also to plan treatment, is now commonplace. An estimated 70% of ED patients receive imaging during their encounter.[2] The sustained growth within the ED setting and the importance of imaging have fostered not only the growth of Emergency Radiology or, as I now refer to it, Emergency and Trauma Imaging, but also the Emergency Radiologist.

But who is the Emergency Radiologist? The question begs an answer. Although the answers may vary slightly, a common core exists. At Emory University our dedicated team of radiologists provide around-the-clock coverage for some of our sickest and most vulnerable patients as they pass through the ED gateways. We also partner with our Emergency, Trauma, Medicine, Obstetrical and Gynecological, and Oncologic colleagues to quickly, comprehensively, and appropriately evaluate patients answering the emergent clinical queries and helping to triage patients to the next station. The breadth and scope of our practice spans multiple modalities (radiography, ultrasound, computed tomography, magnetic resonance, nuclear medicine), multiple disciplines, and multiple body regions. We provide a one-stop shop for emergent imaging and interpretation. We operate in the chaos and the quickly paced emergency setting. Often times as a first responder, a gatekeeper, a consultant, or a clinician—and always—as an advocate for patients. As the field of Emergency and Trauma Imaging continues to grow and mature, we hope the understanding and appreciation for the role of the Emergency Radiologist keeps pace.

My colleagues from around the country and I have compiled this series of cases, not as an exhaustive compendium of every possible ED clinical scenario, but as a reflection of our broad daily practices. It is intended not just for the Emergency Radiologist, but for individuals who may find themselves in the unfamiliar territory of providing imaging support for the ED. We have highlighted pertinent clinical and background information, imaging findings, management consideration, and reference material. We hope that the entities you will encounter will rekindle and augment your knowledge and reignite or spark a passion for this exciting, growing, and dynamic subspeciality.

Jamlik-Omari Johnson, MD

---

[1]National Hospital Ambulatory Medical Care Survey: 2015 Emergency Department Summary Tables, tables 1, 4, 15, 25, 26 (https://www.cdc.gov/nchs/data/nhamcs/web_tables/2015_ed_web_tables.pdf).

[2]National Hospital Ambulatory Medical Care Survey: 2010 Emergency Department Summary Tables. http://www.cdc.gov/nchs/data/ahcd/nhamcs_emergency/2010_ed_web_tables.pdf.

To ACH—Thank you for the love and support during not only this journey but over all these many happy years.

To my colleagues-in-arms—Every day and through the night, we fight the good fight. We strengthen our discipline and make a difference at every level. I could not be prouder of the work we do.
—Jamlik-Omari Johnson, MD

Contents

Case 1

History: 22-year-old female patient presents with right lower quadrant pain.

1. Which of the following would be included in the differential diagnosis for the images presented? (Choose all that apply.)
   A. Pelvic inflammatory disease (PID)
   B. Acute cholecystitis
   C. Acute appendicitis
   D. Irritable bowel syndrome (IBD)
2. Which of the following is a common symptom in acute appendicitis?
   A. Pain in the right upper quadrant
   B. Inability to pass gas
   C. Abdominal swelling
   D. Increased appetite
3. What is the most common tool to diagnose acute appendicitis in the adult population?
   A. Computed tomography (CT)
   B. Ultrasonography (US)
   C. Exploratory laparotomy
   D. Radiography
4. Which of the following statements regarding the pathogenesis of acute appendicitis is *false*?
   A. Increased pressure and distention of the appendix can be caused by luminal obstruction.
   B. Lumen obstruction is always the cause of acute appendicitis.
   C. Viral or bacterial infections can occur after an appendectomy.
   D. Obstruction of venous outflow and then arterial inflow can result in gangrene.

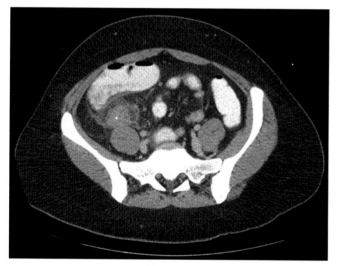

Fig. 1.1

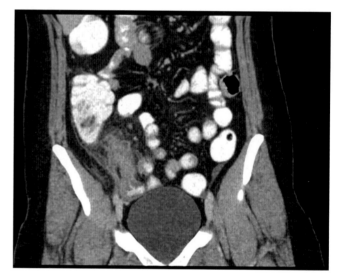

Fig. 1.2

Case 2

History: 72-year-old male with acute right-sided hemiparesis.

1. Which of the following would be included in the differential diagnosis for the images presented? (Choose all that apply.)
   A. Transient ischemic attack (TIA)
   B. Meningitis
   C. Acute middle cerebral artery (MCA) infarction
   D. Hypertensive intracranial hemorrhage

2. Which of the following is the most likely cause of the salient finding in Fig. 2.1?
   A. Hemoconcentration
   B. Intravascular thrombus
   C. Atherosclerotic calcification
   D. Contrast material

3. On CT perfusion imaging, which combination describes the characteristic blood flow within the penumbra?
   A. Decreased mean transit time (MTT), decreased cerebral blood volume (CBV), increased cerebral blood flow (CBF)
   B. Increased MTT, decreased CBV, increased CBF
   C. Decreased MTT, increased CBV, decreased CBF
   D. Increased MTT, normal CBV, decreased CBF

4. What time frame and percentage of MCA territory involvement pair is desired for a patient to receive intravenous (IV) tissue plasminogen activator (tPA) therapy?
   A. 4.5 hours or less; <33%
   B. 8 hours or less; <66%
   C. 4.5 hours or less; >33%
   D. 8 hours or less; >66%

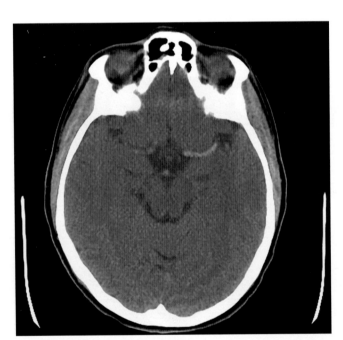

Fig. 2.1

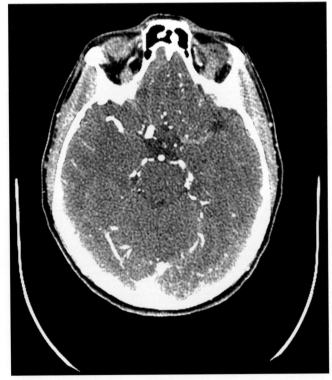

Fig. 2.2

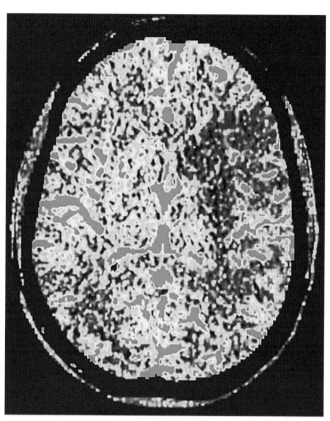

Fig. 2.3

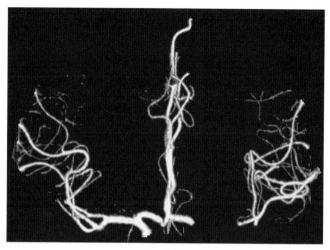

Fig. 2.4

Case 3

History: 69-year-old female presenting with right lower extremity pain.

1. Which of the following differential diagnoses is *rarely* associated with the imaging presented? (Choose all that apply.)
   A. Baker's cyst
   B. Cellulitis
   C. Lymphedema
   D. Chronic venous insufficiency
   E. Superficial thrombosis
2. Which of the following can be a symptom seen in patients with deep venous thrombosis (DVT)?
   A. Deep pain and swelling in both arms
   B. Frequent redness and swelling in left hand
   C. Leg pain on right side of calf
   D. Leg pain on the back of the calf

3. Which of the following treatments should be considered for patients with a DVT if anticoagulation is contraindicated?
   A. Low-molecular-weight heparin
   B. Warfarin
   C. Inferior vena cava filter
   D. tPA
4. Which of these patients with DVT is the best candidate for an inferior vena cava (IVC) filter?
   A. 32-year-old with second occurrence of DVT and protein S deficiency
   B. 45-year-old with DVT and pulmonary embolism (PE)
   C. 22-year-old pregnant women with first-time DVT
   D. 76-year-old on warfarin develops atrial fibrillation, pulmonary embolus, and DVT

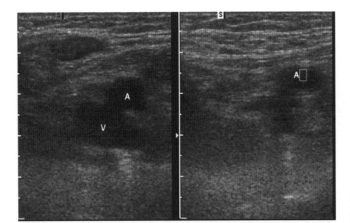

Fig. 3.1

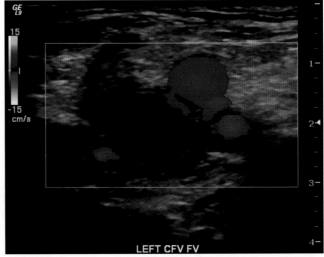

Fig. 3.2

Case 4

History: 30-year-old male presenting with dull chest pain and dyspnea.

1. Which of the following would be included in the differential diagnosis for the imaging presented? (Choose all that apply.)
   A. Pulmonary embolism (PE)
   B. Intrinsic intraluminal tumor
   C. Esophagitis
   D. Angina
2. Which of the following symptoms is most commonly associated with PE?
   A. Cyanosis
   B. Mastalgia
   C. Cephalgia
   D. Delusional disorders
3. What is the most appropriate examination to evaluate a 30-week pregnant patient with suspected PE?
   A. Lung scintigraphy
   B. Transthoracic echocardiography (TTE)
   C. Pulmonary angiography
   D. CT pulmonary angiography (CTPA)
   E. Venous duplex ultrasound

4. How would the CT finding of right ventricular strain alter immediate clinical management?
   A. Shock and death are a risk; patient should receive intense monitoring.
   B. Shock and death are a risk; patient should receive thrombolytic therapy.
   C. There is a high risk for recurrent PE; patient should receive heparin rather than warfarin.
   D. There is a high risk for ongoing embolization; patient should receive an IVC filter.

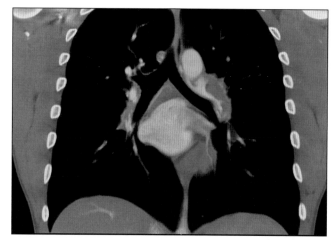

Fig. 4.2

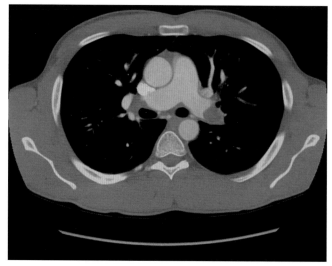

Fig. 4.1

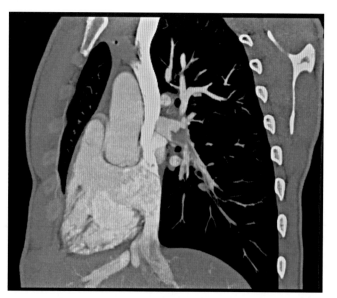

Fig. 4.3

Case 5

History: 43-year-old male presenting with left lower quadrant abdominal pain.

1. Which of the following would be included in the differential diagnosis for the imaging findings presented? (Choose all that apply.)
   A. Colon adenocarcinoma
   B. Epiploic appendagitis
   C. Acute diverticulitis
   D. Acute appendicitis
2. Which of the following is a risk factor for developing acute diverticulitis?
   A. Increasing age
   B. Low body mass index
   C. Dietary nuts and corn
   D. High-fiber diet

3. Which imaging finding is more consistent with colon adenocarcinoma than with diverticulitis?
   A. Gradual increase in colonic wall thickness
   B. Presence of free fluid
   C. Lymphadenopathy
   D. Long (5–10 cm) segment of affected colon
4. Which complication is *not* commonly associated with acute diverticulitis?
   A. Fistula formation
   B. Small bowel obstruction
   C. Perforation
   D. Infectious colitis

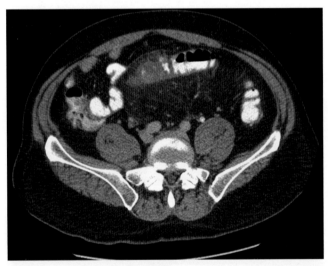

Fig. 5.1

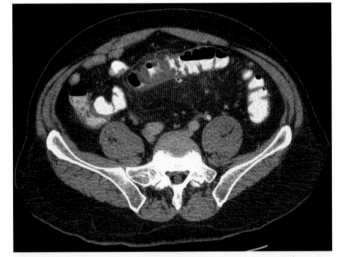

Fig. 5.2

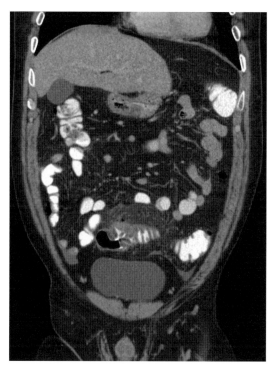

Fig. 5.3

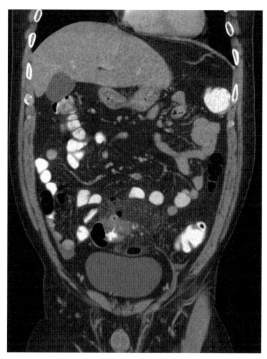

Fig. 5.4

Case 6

History: 83-year-old male presenting after fall on concrete with bruising to face and head.

1. Which of the following would be included in the differential diagnosis for the imaging findings presented? (Choose all that apply.)
   A. Subdural hemorrhage
   B. Cerebral atrophy
   C. Epidural hemorrhage
   D. Subdural empyema
2. Which of the following is often associated with a "lucid interval" prior to losing consciousness?
   A. Subdural hemorrhage
   B. Arteriovenous malformation
   C. Subarachnoid hemorrhage
   D. Epidural hemorrhage
3. Which imaging finding on head CT typically suggests subdural hemorrhage rather than epidural hemorrhage?
   A. Lentiform (biconcave) shape
   B. Crescentic shape
   C. "Bag of worm" appearance
   D. "Ring enhancing" lesion
4. Patients most commonly develop subdural empyema as a result of which of the following?
   A. Orbital cellulitis
   B. Mastoiditis
   C. Frontal sinusitis
   D. Meningitis

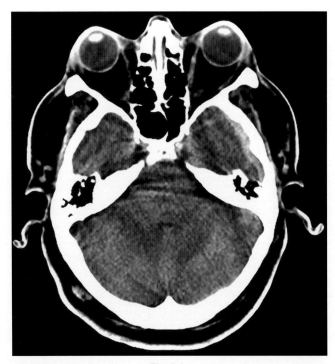

Fig. 6.1

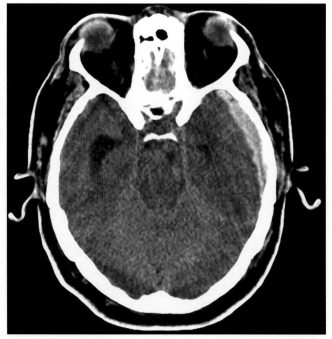

Fig. 6.2

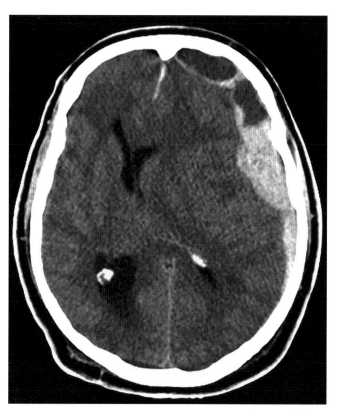

Fig. 6.3

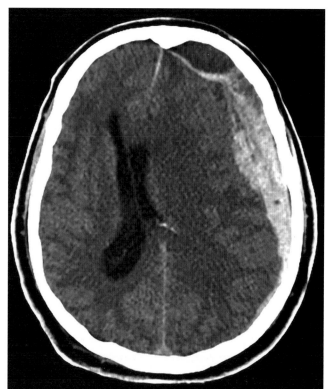

Fig. 6.4

Case 7

History: 31-year-old male presenting with decreasing consciousness after a motor vehicle accident.

1. Which of the following would be included in the differential diagnosis for the imaging findings presented? (Choose all that apply.)
   A. Epidural hemorrhage
   B. Subdural hemorrhage
   C. Epidural infection
   D. Meningioma
2. What is the "classic" shape of an epidural hemorrhage on head CT?
   A. Biconvex/lentiform
   B. Crescentic
   C. Square/rhomboid
   D. Blood will not appear on head CT

3. What is the most common cause of epidural hemorrhage in young adults?
   A. Rupture of preexisting arteriovenous malformation
   B. Vascular damage secondary to cerebral infection
   C. Medication-induced vasospasm
   D. Trauma
4. What is the best initial treatment for symptomatic/severe epidural hemorrhage?
   A. Immediate neurosurgery consult and surgery
   B. Observation and serial CT examinations
   C. Elevation of head and IV fluid administration
   D. Treatment not indicated if hemorrhage suspected to be severe

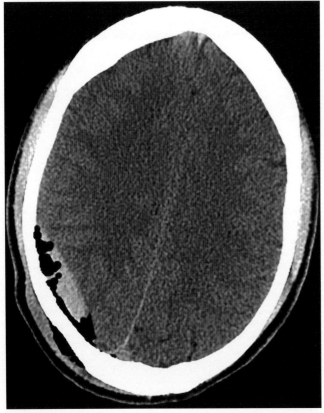

Fig. 7.1

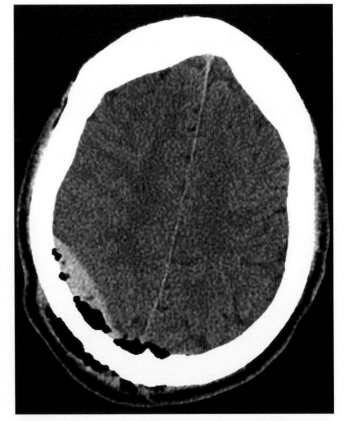

Fig. 7.2

Case 8

History: 60-year-old man presenting with a harsh, productive cough he had for the last few days.

1. Which of the following would be included in the differential diagnosis for the imaging presented? (Choose all that apply.)
   A. Pulmonary malignancy
   B. Foreign body airway obstruction
   C. Myocarditis
   D. Gastroesophageal reflux disease (GERD)
2. The patient is human immunodeficiency virus (HIV)-positive. Which of the following is the most common organism responsible for this patient's presentation?
   A. Cytomegalovirus
   B. *Pneumocystis jiroveci*
   C. *Streptococcus pneumoniae*
   D. *Mycobacterium tuberculosis*
   E. *Klebsiella pneumoniae*
3. Which diagnostic test is recommended for patients presenting with community-acquired pneumonia?
   A. Chest CT scan
   B. Blood culture
   C. Pulse oximetry
   D. Gram staining the sputum
4. If the patient is type 1 penicillin allergic, what is an appropriate treatment?
   A. Cephalosporin
   B. Carbapenem
   C. Cefazolin
   D. Clarithromycin

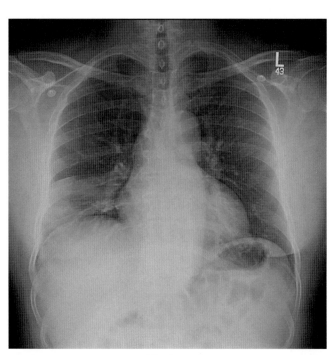

Fig. 8.1

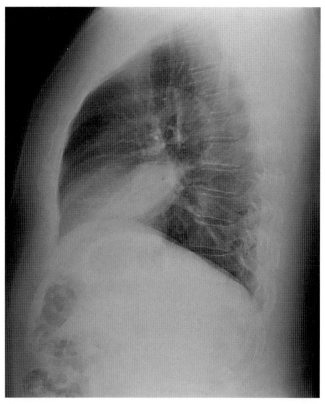

Fig. 8.2

Case 9

History: 44-year-old woman presents with acute abdominal pain localized to the right upper quadrant, fever, and vomiting.

1. Which of the following would be included in the differential diagnosis for the imaging findings presented? (Choose all that apply.)
   A. Gallbladder polyps
   B. Acute cholecystitis
   C. Choledocholithiasis
   D. Adenomyomatosis
2. Which of the following is most commonly associated with the correct diagnosis in question 1?
   A. Gastroparesis
   B. Alcohol use
   C. Smoking
   D. Gallstones

3. Major criteria for CT diagnosis include:
   A. Gallstones
   B. Pericholecystic fluid collections
   C. Gallbladder thickening/edema
   D. Sludge
4. Which imaging modalities are diagnostic for this condition?
   A. US
   B. CT
   C. Radiography
   D. Nuclear medicine

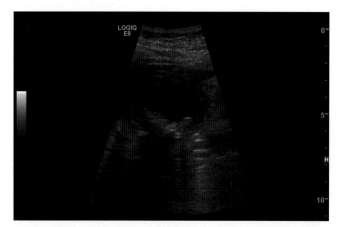

Fig. 9.1

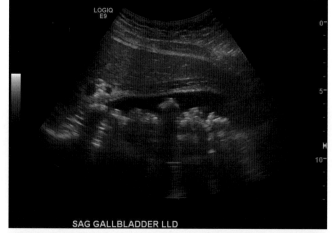

Fig. 9.2

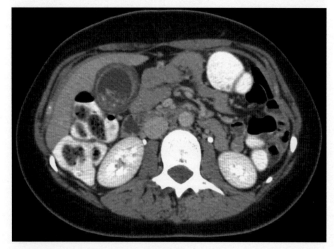

Fig. 9.3

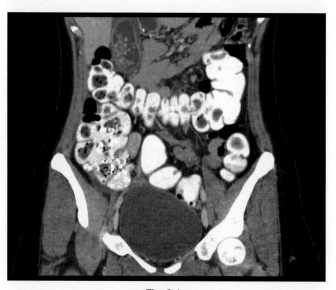

Fig. 9.4

Case 10

History: 26-year-old man presenting with wrist pain following a fall on an outstretched hand while playing soccer.

1. Which of the following would be included in the differential diagnosis for the imaging findings presented? (Choose all that apply.)
   A. Scapholunate ligament injury
   B. Scaphoid fracture
   C. Kienbock's disease
   D. Hook of hamate fracture
2. Regarding anatomic distribution and prognosis of scaphoid fractures, which of the following is true?
   A. Proximal pole scaphoid fractures are most common and have the highest rates of nonunion.
   B. Scaphoid wrist fractures are least common and have the lowest rates of nonunion.
   C. Distal pole scaphoid fractures most common and have the highest rates of nonunion.
   D. Distal pole scaphoid fractures are least common and have the lowest rates of nonunion.

3. A known complication of scaphoid waist fractures is:
   A. Avascular necrosis of the distal pole
   B. Nonunion of the fracture
   C. Avascular necrosis of the proximal pole
   D. Progression to scapholunate advanced collapse (SLAC) wrist in a majority of cases
4. Immediately following injury, what percent of scaphoid fractures may be occult on radiographs?
   A. 5%
   B. 10%
   C. 20%
   D. 65%

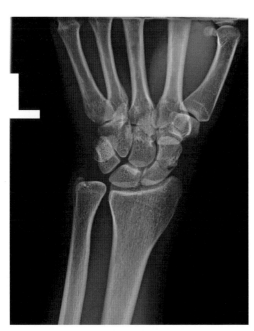

Fig. 10.1

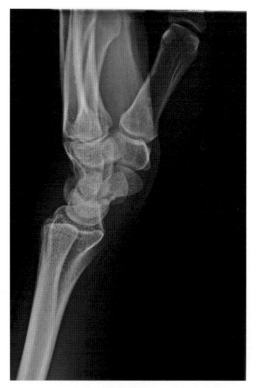

Fig. 10.2

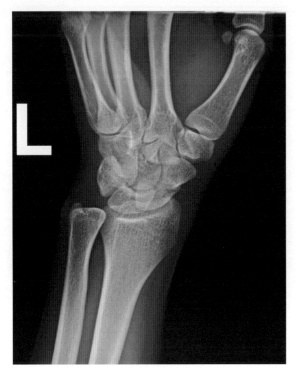

Fig. 10.3

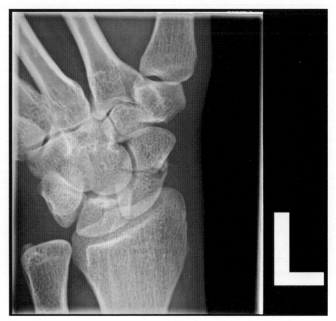

Fig. 10.4

Case 11

History: 35-year-old electrician presenting with right shoulder pain and numbness.

1. Which of the following would be included in the differential diagnosis for the imaging findings presented? (Choose all that apply.)
   A. Anterior shoulder dislocation
   B. Posterior shoulder dislocation
   C. Inferior shoulder dislocation
   D. Humoral head fracture

2. Posterior shoulder dislocations can result from which of the following?
   A. Seizures
   B. Fall on an outstretched arm
   C. Electrocution
   D. All of the above

3. Posterior shoulder dislocation accounts for what percent of all shoulder dislocations?
   A. 95% to 97%
   B. 2% to 5%
   C. 0.5%
   D. 30% to 32%

4. Patient with a posterior shoulder dislocation will present with their arm positioned:
   A. Internally rotated and adducted
   B. Externally rotated and slightly abducted
   C. Hyperabducted
   D. Hyperadducted

5. Posterior shoulder dislocation is most associated with which characteristic injury?
   A. Fracture of the clavicle
   B. Hills-Sachs lesion
   C. Reverse Hill-Sachs
   D. Rotator cuff tear

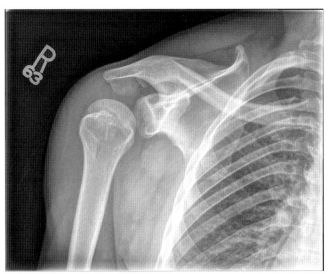

Fig. 11.1

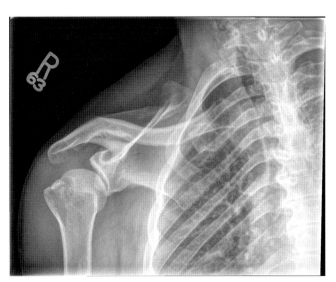

Fig. 11.2

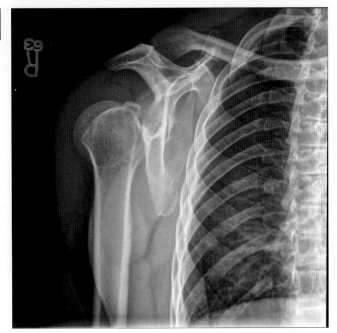

Fig. 11.3

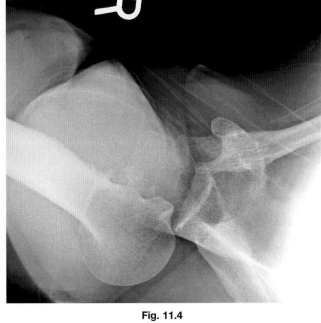

Fig. 11.4

Case 12

History: 46-year-old woman presenting with diarrhea for 4 days after recent treatment for community-acquired pneumonia.

1. Which of the following would be included in the differential diagnosis for the imaging findings presented? (Choose all that apply.)
   A. Pseudomembranous colitis
   B. Ischemic colitis
   C. Portal hypertensive colopathy
   D. Cytomegalovirus
2. What is the name given to the radiologic finding where enteric contrast is seen trapped between the thickened haustral folds?
   A. Accordion sign
   B. Ring sign
   C. Target sign
   D. Halo sign
3. What is the most common cause of toxic megacolon?
   A. Ulcerative colitis
   B. Crohn's disease
   C. *Clostridium difficile* (pseudomembranous colitis)
   D. Cytomegalovirus
4. What is the appropriate management of pseudomembranous colitis?
   A. Amoxicillin
   B. Clindamycin
   C. Metronidazole
   D. Vancomycin

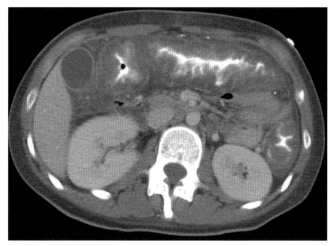

Fig. 12.1

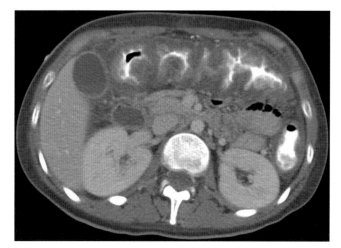

Fig. 12.2

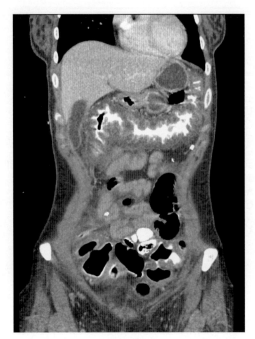

Fig. 12.3

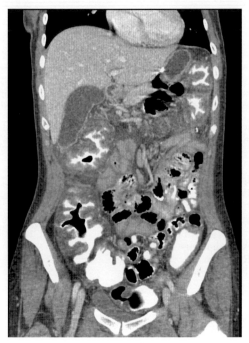

Fig. 12.4

Case 13

History: 28-year-old female with sickle cell anemia and 5 months of atraumatic hip pain.

1. Which of the following would be included in the differential diagnosis for the imaging findings presented? (Choose all that apply.)
   A. Septic arthritis
   B. Subchondral fracture
   C. Transient osteoporosis of the femoral head
   D. Avascular necrosis (AVN)
2. Which of the following are risk factors for AVN of the femoral head?
   A. Steroid use
   B. Trauma
   C. Sickle cell anemia
   D. Gaucher's disease
   E. All of the above

3. In early AVN, what would be the expected radiographic appearance?
   A. Subchondral crescent
   B. Normal radiographs or possibly mild localized osteopenia
   C. Hazy sclerosis
   D. Subchondral collapse
4. Regarding the treatment of AVN, which of the following is true?
   A. Advanced AVN with collapse and secondary osteoarthritis often requires total hip replacement.
   B. Early AVN can be treated with core decompression, a drilling process that relieves pressure and increases local blood supply.
   C. Early detection of AVN is of utmost importance, particularly if caused by medications.
   D. All of the above.

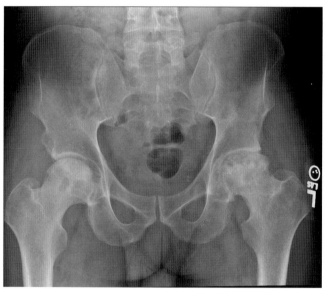

Fig. 13.1

Case 14

History: 57-year-old woman with tearing chest pain.

1. Which of the following would be included in the differential diagnosis for the imaging findings presented? (Choose all that apply.)
   A. Abdominal aortic aneurysm
   B. PE
   C. Aortic dissection
   D. Aortitis
2. Which situation may require only medical management rather than surgery?
   A. Aortic rupture
   B. Organ malperfusion
   C. Ascending aortic dissection
   D. Descending aortic dissection

3. Which DeBakey category involves a tear only in the ascending aorta?
   A. I
   B. II
   C. III
   D. IV
4. Which is *not* a known contributing factor for aortic dissection?
   A. Marfan's syndrome
   B. Smoking
   C. Chronic hypertension
   D. Diabetes

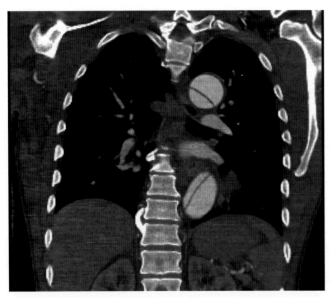

Fig. 14.1

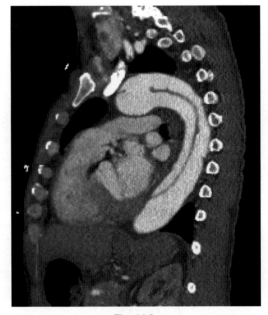

Fig. 14.2

Case 15

History: 34-year-old male with acute wrist pain following an injury during a tennis match.

1. Which of the following would be included in the differential diagnosis for the imaging findings presented? (Choose all that apply.)
   A. Scaphoid fracture
   B. Capitate fracture
   C. Synovial osteochondromatosis
   D. Triquetral fracture
2. Which of the following is true regarding this type of fracture?
   A. They often involve the triquetral body.
   B. They have a high association with capitate injuries.
   C. They most commonly involve the dorsal ridge of the triquetrum.
   D. They are often treated surgically.
3. Which radiographic view of the wrist best demonstrates this finding?
   A. Anteroposterior (AP)
   B. Lateral
   C. Oblique
   D. Reverse oblique
   E. B, C, and D

4. Mechanistically, dorsal triquetral fractures can:
   A. Occur during forced hyperflexion, resulting in ulnar styloid impaction on the dorsal triquetrum
   B. Occur during forced hyperextension, resulting in avulsion of the dorsal radiotriquetral ligament
   C. Occur during forced hyperflexion, resulting in avulsion of the dorsal radiotriquetral ligament
   D. Occur during forced hyperextension, resulting in ulnar styloid impaction on the dorsal triquetrum
   E. C and D

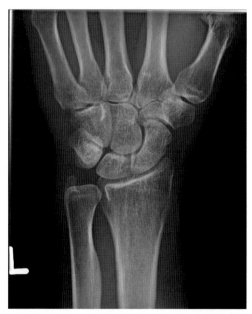

Fig. 15.1

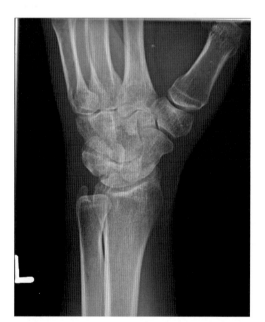

Fig. 15.2

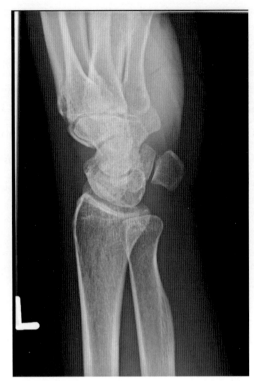

Fig. 15.3

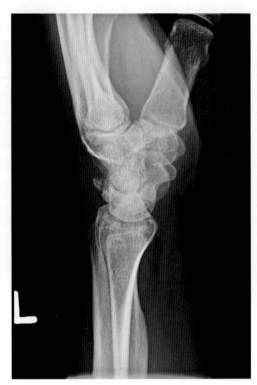

Fig. 15.4

Case 16

History: 24-year-old woman presents with abdominal pain.

1. Which of the following would be included in the differential diagnosis for the imaging findings presented? (Choose all that apply.)
   A. Failed intrauterine pregnancy (IUP)
   B. Ovarian torsion
   C. Bicornuate uterus with a normal IUP
   D. Ectopic pregnancy
2. Which of the following is the most common location for the diagnosis in question 1?
   A. Ampullary
   B. Cornual/interstitial
   C. Ovarian
   D. Intraabdominal
3. At what discriminatory value of the β-hCG should an IUP be visualized by transvaginal ultrasound?
   A. 500 mIU/mL
   B. 1000 mIU/mL
   C. 2000 mIU/mL
   D. 6500 mIU/mL
4. Which of the following is the preferred method of treatment for a stable patient without evidence of hemoperitoneum on sonography, especially if she desires preserved fertility?
   A. Expectant management
   B. Laparotomy/laparoscopy
   C. Ultrasound-guided, percutaneous injection of potassium chloride
   D. Intramuscular methotrexate injection

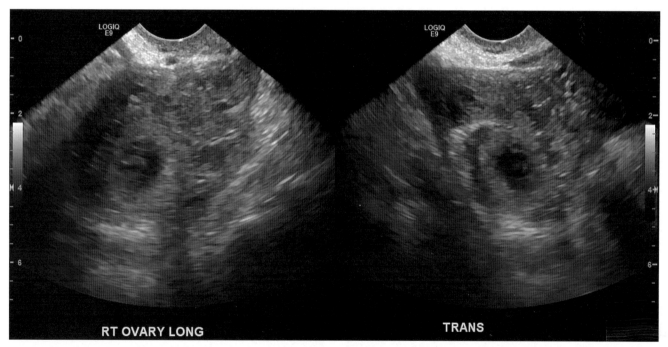

Fig. 16.1

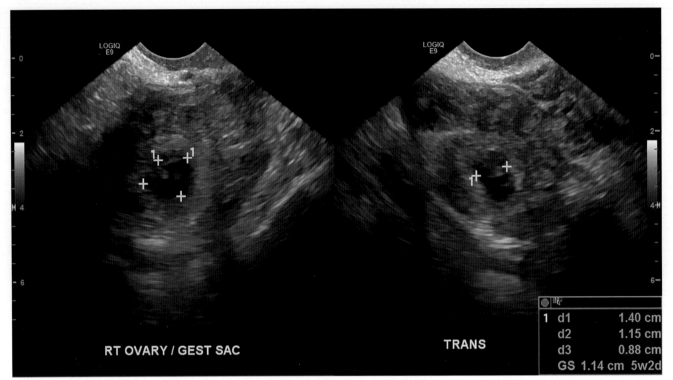

Fig. 16.2

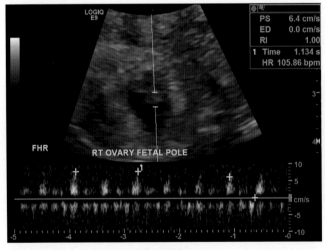

Fig. 16.3

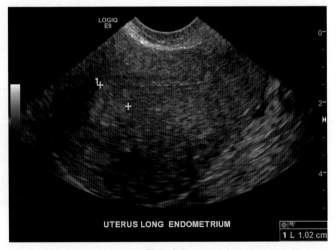

Fig. 16.4

Case 17

History: 25-year-old male presents with acute right scrotal pain.

1. Which of the following would be included in the differential diagnosis for the imaging findings presented? (Choose all that apply.)
   A. Testicular torsion
   B. Epididymitis/epididymoorchitis
   C. Testicular tumor
   D. Torsion of the testicular appendage
2. Which of the following is ideal for sonographic (US) evaluation of acute scrotal pain?
   A. Low-frequency transducer (3–5 MHz), curvilinear probe, gray-scale imaging alone
   B. Low-frequency transducer (3–5 MHz), curvilinear probe, gray-scale, and color Doppler
   C. High-frequency transducer (9–15 MHz), linear probe, gray-scale alone
   D. High-frequency transducer (9–15 MHz), linear probe, gray-scale, and color Doppler

3. Which of the following best defines the US imaging findings of epididymoorchitis?
   A. Small testis and epididymis; increased echogenicity; decreased vascular flow
   B. Enlarged testis and epididymis; decreased echogenicity or heterogeneous echogenicity; decreased vascular flow; associated hydrocele and scrotal wall edema/thickening
   C. Enlarged testis and epididymis; decreased echogenicity or heterogeneous echogenicity; increased vascular flow; associated hydrocele and scrotal wall edema/thickening
   D. Enlarged testis and epididymis; increased echogenicity; decreased vascular flow; associated hydrocele and scrotal wall edema/thickening
4. Which of the following is not true regarding epididymoorchitis?
   A. Relief of pain when the testes are elevated over the symphysis pubis, a maneuver called Prehn sign
   B. In adolescents the cause is most often a sexually transmitted infection.
   C. Surgical intervention is often warranted, especially in the adolescent population.
   D. Color Doppler examination reveals increased blood flow to the epididymis and/or testis.

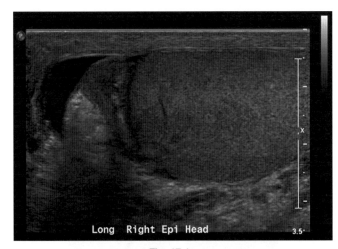

Fig. 17.1

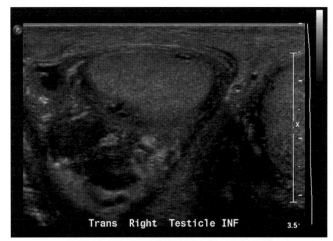

Fig. 17.2

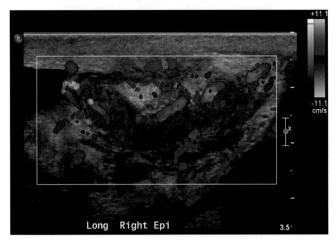

Fig. 17.3

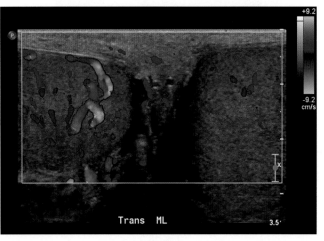

Fig. 17.4

Case 18

History: 26-year-old male African-American presents with right-sided abdominal pain.

1. Which of the following would be included in the differential diagnosis for the findings presented? (Choose all that apply.)
   A. Constipation
   B. Diverticulitis
   C. Urinary tract infection (UTI)
   D. Pyelonephritis
   E. All of the above
2. In addition to dysuria and white blood cells in the urine, what supplementary symptoms would support the diagnosis of pyelonephritis?
   A. Inguinal pain and lymphadenopathy
   B. Flank pain and tenderness
   C. Lower quadrant pain with rebound tenderness
   D. Periumbilical pain and bruising around umbilicus

3. What imaging modality would be most helpful in determining the etiology of this type of UTI?
   A. CT of abdomen/pelvis with and without contrast
   B. CT of abdomen/pelvis with IV contrast only
   C. CT of abdomen/pelvis with oral contrast only
   D. CT of abdomen/pelvis without contrast
   E. US of the abdomen
4. What is the best imaging modality to assess recurrent pyelonephritis in the pediatric patient?
   A. 99m-technetium-dimercaptosuccinic acid (DMSA) renal scintigraphy
   B. CT
   C. US
   D. Radiography

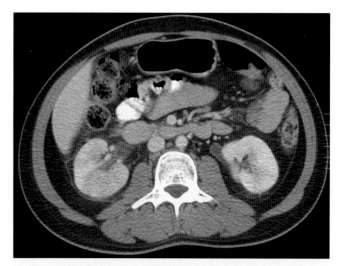

Fig. 18.1

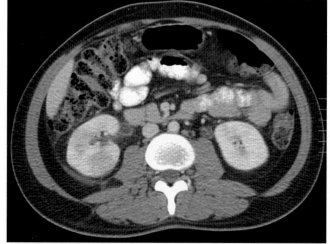

Fig. 18.2

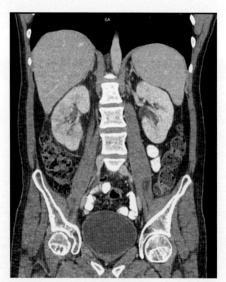

Fig. 18.3

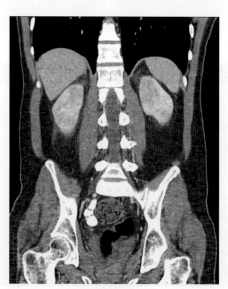

Fig. 18.4

Case 19

History: 32-year-old female with chronic diarrhea and right lower quadrant pain.

1. Which of the following would be included in the differential diagnosis for the imaging findings presented? (Choose all that apply.)
   A. Shigellosis
   B. Celiac disease
   C. Crohn's disease
   D. Traveler's diarrhea
   E. Appendicitis
2. Which imaging findings indicate Crohn's disease is the most likely cause of this patient's diarrhea?
   A. Bowel wall thickening
   B. Comb sign
   C. Strictures or fistulas
   D. All of the above

3. Which imaging finding is pathognomonic for inflammatory bowel disease?
   A. Submucosal fat halo sign
   B. Bowel wall thickening
   C. Phlegmon formation
   D. Small bowel obstruction
4. Which are potential complications of Crohn's disease?
   A. Strictures
   B. Fistula formation
   C. Small bowel obstruction
   D. Need for bowel resection
   E. All of the above

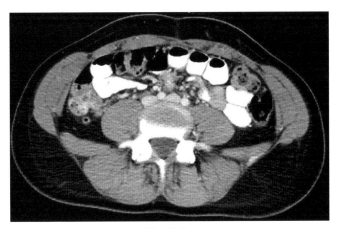

Fig. 19.1

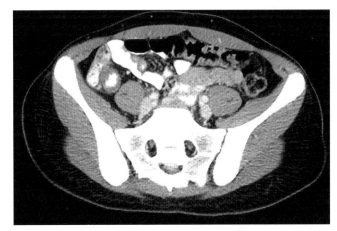

Fig. 19.2

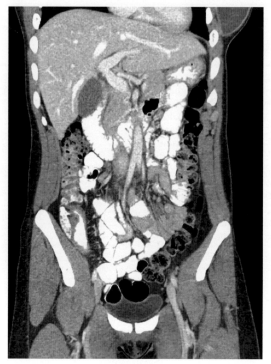

Fig. 19.3

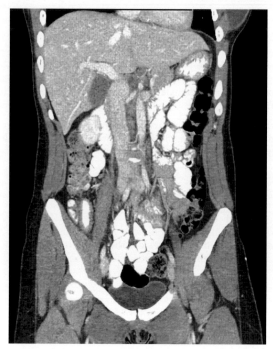

Fig. 19.4

Case 20

History: 24-year-old female status post fall on out-stretched hand (FOOSH) presents with elbow pain.

1. Which of the following would be included in the differential diagnosis for the imaging findings presented? (Choose all that apply.)
   A. Elbow joint effusion
   B. Septic arthritis
   C. Olecranon bursitis
   D. Radial head fracture

2. With regard to normal radiographic findings, which of the following is true?
   A. An anterior fat pad is normally hidden in the coronoid fossa, and not visible.
   B. A posterior fat pad can be partially visible in a normal adult if there is elbow flexion.
   C. An anterior fat pad can be partially visible in a normal adult if there is elbow flexion.
   D. A posterior fat pad is normally hidden in the coronoid fossa, and not visible.

3. The most common elbow fracture in the pediatric and adult populations respectively are:

   A. Supracondylar fractures in children; radial head/neck fractures in adults
   B. Olecranon fractures in children; radial head/neck fractures in adults
   C. Radial head/neck fractures in children; supracondylar fractures in adults
   D. Radial head fractures are the most common fractures in both children and adults.

4. Regarding patient management in posttraumatic radiographs demonstrating elevated fat pads but no definite fracture, which of the following is true?
   A. Patients often go on to CT, which provides increased sensitivity for detection of nondisplaced fractures.
   B. Patients often go on to magnetic resonance imaging (MRI), which provides nearly 100% sensitivity for detection of nondisplaced fractures and can aid in characterization of ligamentous injury.
   C. In the presence of an elbow joint effusion without identifiable fracture, a nondisplaced radial head fracture is assumed, and the patient is treated presumptively with immobilization.
   D. Stress radiograph AP and oblique views are obtained with the patient making a fist to elicit fracture displacement.

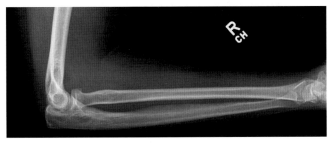

Fig. 20.1

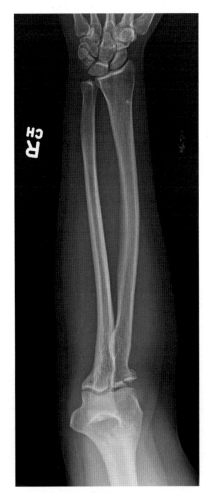

Fig. 20.2

Case 21

History: 55-year-old with nausea and vomiting.

1. Which of the following would be included in the differential diagnosis for the imaging findings presented? (Choose all that apply.)
   A. Small bowel obstruction
   B. Adynamic ileus
   C. Enteritis
   D. None of the above

2. What is the most common cause of the nausea and vomiting?
   A. Adhesions
   B. Hernias
   C. Tumor
   D. Volvulus

3. Computed tomography may be helpful with small bowel obstruction in determining which of the below?
   A. Complications
   B. Transition point
   C. Possible etiology
   D. All of the above

4. Which of the following is true about closed loop small bowel obstruction?
   A. Occurs when there is a loop of small bowel with a proximal and distal transition point
   B. Closed loop small bowel may rotate around its mesenteric axis causing a volvulus.
   C. May appear as a U or S shape converging at the site of obstruction
   D. All of the above
   E. None of the above

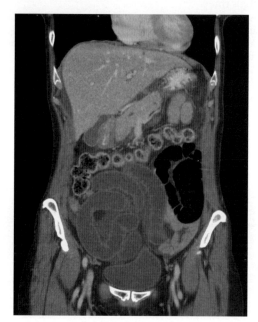

Fig. 21.3

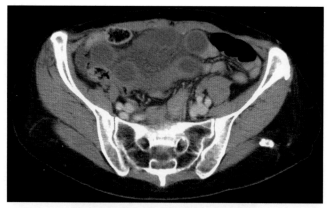

Fig. 21.1

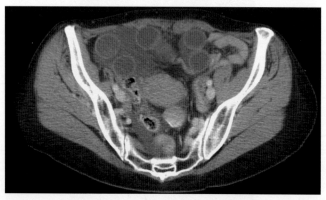

Fig. 21.2

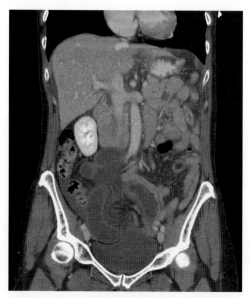

Fig. 21.4

Case 22

History: 53-year-old female status post trauma with hypoxia and altered mental status after being admitted to the intensive care unit (ICU).

1. Which of the following would be included in the differential diagnosis of the imaging findings presented? (Choose all that apply.)
   A. Unilateral bronchial intubation
   B. Pneumothorax
   C. Pleural effusion
   D. Mucus plug development
2. What is the best way to identify unilateral mainstem intubation?
   A. CO_2 capnography verification
   B. Radiographic verification
   C. CT confirmation of tube placement
   D. Auscultation of lungs and epigastrium

3. What is the ideal location for the tip of the endotracheal tube (ETT)?
   A. Past the carina on either side of the midline for stable positioning
   B. Below the clavicular line and approximately 2 cm above the carina
   C. Above the clavicular line and approximately 2 cm below the carina
   D. The ideal location for the ETT varies person to person.
4. What is a common radiologic finding of endobronchial intubation on chest radiograph?
   A. Collapse of lobe and obstructed segments
   B. Pericardial fluid development and jugular venous distention
   C. Pulmonary edema and Kerley B lines
   D. Collapse of the inferior vena cava

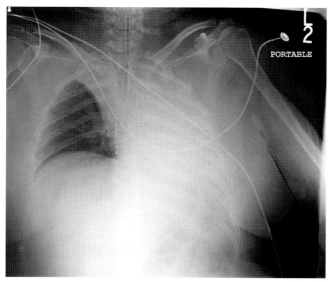

Fig. 22.1

Case 23

History: 53-year-old female presents with shortness of breath, chest pain, and cough.

1. Which of the following would be included in the differential diagnosis for the imaging findings presented? (Choose all that apply.)
   A. Mannitol toxicity
   B. Pulmonary edema
   C. Hypersensitivity reaction
   D. Toxic inhalation
2. Which imaging finding suggests pulmonary edema? (Choose all that apply.)

A. Bilateral alveolar opacification
B. Loss of the left hemidiaphragm
C. Fibrosis of the bronchi
D. Enlargement of the cardiac silhouette

3. Which of the following is specific to cardiogenic pulmonary edema?
   A. Kerley B lines
   B. Bronchial calcification
   C. Lines of Zahn
   D. Barrel-shaped chest

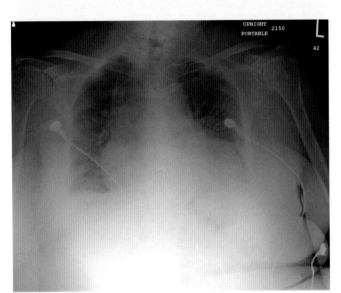

Fig. 23.1

Case 24

History: 29-year-old male presents with chest pain, tachycardia, hypotension.

1. Which of the following would be included in the differential diagnosis for the imaging findings presented? (Choose all that apply.)
   A. Pleural effusion
   B. Right upper lobe collapse secondary to endobronchial intubation
   C. Pneumothorax
   D. Bilateral tension pneumothorax
2. What is the best image finding that suggests a tension pneumothorax is present rather than a spontaneous pneumothorax?
   A. Visible translucency and absence of vascular markings on left side
   B. Presence of a small bleb along the visceral pleural margin
   C. A shift of the mediastinum has occurred to the contralateral side.
   D. Marked depression of left diaphragm

3. Which of the following would differentiate between a flail chest and a pneumothorax?
   A. Dysphasia
   B. Decreased diaphragmatic excursion
   C. Paradoxic chest movement
   D. Tachycardia
4. Which of following best describes a secondary spontaneous pneumothorax?
   A. Pneumothorax secondary to lung disease weakening the alveolar-pleural barrier
   B. Pneumothorax caused by trauma or a wound
   C. Pneumothorax secondary to air trapped in pleural space creating positive pressure on mediastinum
   D. Pneumothorax caused by a rupture of a subpleural bleb

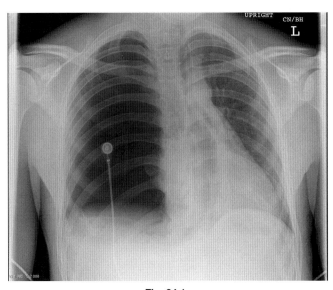

Fig. 24.1

Case 25

History: 73-year-old male awoke with severe left parietal headache and vomiting.

1. Which of the following would be included in the differential diagnosis for the imaging findings presented? (Choose all that apply.)
   A. Asymmetric dural sinus anatomy
   B. Arachnoid granulation
   C. Dural venous thrombosis
   D. Venous infarct
2. All of the following are risk factors for this condition, except:
   A. Trauma
   B. Infection
   C. Pregnancy
   D. Hypertension
   E. Malignancy

3. Which of the following regarding dural venous thrombosis is most correct?
   A. Is more common in males than females
   B. Most commonly occurs in the sigmoid sinus
   C. Most common symptom is headache
   D. Rarely seen in neonates
4. The "empty delta sign":
   A. May occur in any dural venous sinus
   B. May be seen on Non-enhanced CT (NECT) or noncontrast MRI
   C. May be seen on contrast-enhanced CT or MRI
   D. Is observed in the acute phase only (0–5 days)

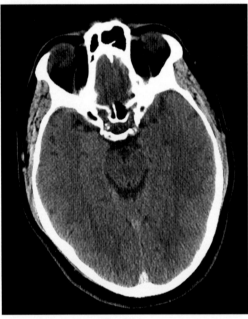

Fig. 25.1

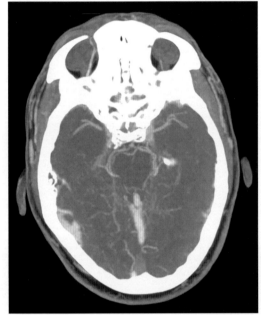

Fig. 25.2

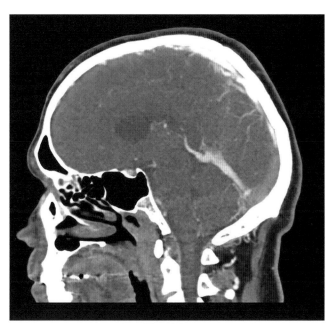

Fig. 25.3

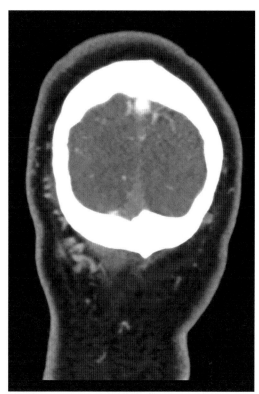

Fig. 25.4

Case 26

History: 56-year-old male presents with the worst headache of his life.

1. Which of the following would be included in the differential for the imaging findings presented? (Choose all that apply.)
   A. Subarachnoid hemorrhage
   B. Subdural hematoma
   C. Epidural hematoma
   D. Intraparenchymal hemorrhage
2. What is the likely etiology of this CT finding?
   A. Hypertensive emergency
   B. Ruptured aneurysm
   C. Arteriovenous malformation
   D. Brain tumor
3. What type of imaging would you initially order for a patient presenting with the worst headache of their life?
   A. Noncontrast MRI
   B. Radiographs
   C. Noncontrast CT
   D. No imaging indicated
4. A common complication associated with this bleed is hydrocephalus. What type of hydrocephalus is likely in this patient?
   A. Communicating
   B. Noncommunicating
   C. Normal-pressure hydrocephalus
   D. Ex vacuo hydrocephalus

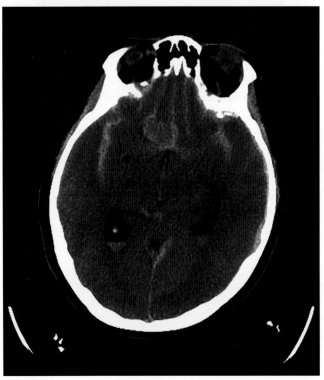

Fig. 26.1

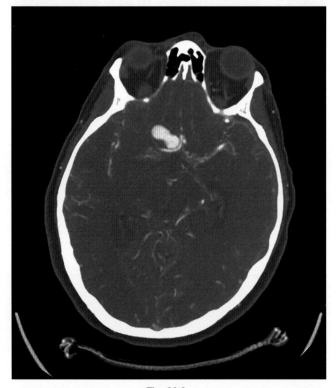

Fig. 26.2

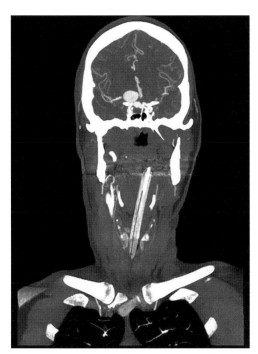

Fig. 26.3

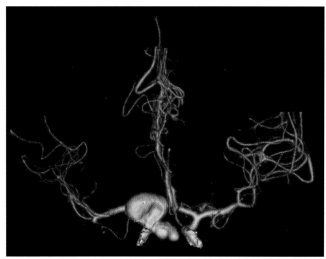

Fig. 26.4

Case 27

History: 23-year-old male comes to the emergency department (ED) following blunt trauma to the eye.

1. Which of the following would be included in the differential for the imaging findings presented? (Choose all that apply.)
   A. Zygomatic fracture
   B. Orbital floor fracture
   C. Retinal detachment
   D. Mandible fracture
2. What might be an additional presenting sign?
   A. Restricted vertical movement of the eyes
   B. Difficulty opening jaw
   C. Shortness of breath
   D. Bell's palsy

3. When might surgery be indicated for this patient?
   A. Score of 10 on pain scale
   B. Enophthalmos greater than 2 mm on imaging
   C. Age greater than 55
   D. Pretrauma vision deficits
4. What is the weakest point of the orbit?
   A. Orbital floor
   B. Superior orbital rim
   C. Zygomatic inferolateral orbital rim
   D. Lateral orbital wall

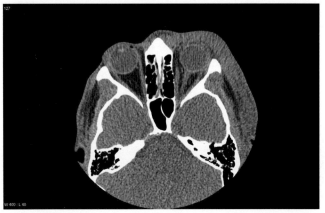

Fig. 27.1

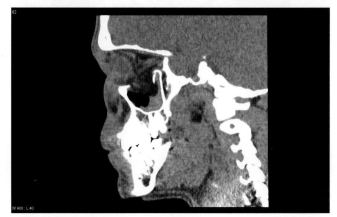

Fig. 27.2

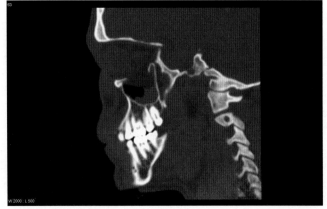

Fig. 27.3

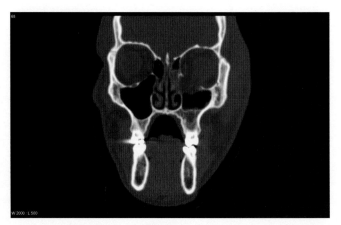

Fig. 27.4

Case 28

History: 23-year-old male presents to the ED following a fistfight with "troublemakers" at a nearby bar.

1. Which of the following would be included in the differential for the imaging finding presented? (Choose all that apply.)
   A. Mandible fracture
   B. Le Fort fractures
   C. Right orbital fracture
   D. Zygomatic fracture
2. Which one of the following bones does not articulate the zygoma?
   A. Temporal
   B. Maxillary
   C. Mandible
   D. Sphenoid

3. What do all Le Fort fractures have in common?
   A. Fracture of the pterygoid plates
   B. Occur along the same suture lines
   C. Involvement of the orbit
   D. Sparing of the nasal bones
4. What is the management of a zygomatic fracture?
   A. Zygomatic reduction and fixation
   B. Nonsteroidal antiinflammatory drugs (NSAIDs) and follow-up
   C. Opioid pain medication
   D. Stabilize patient with airway, breathing and circulation (ABCs)

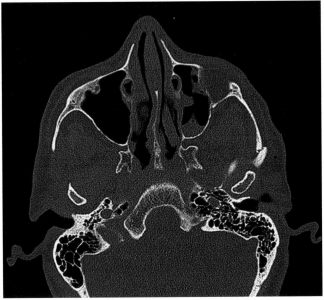

Fig. 28.1

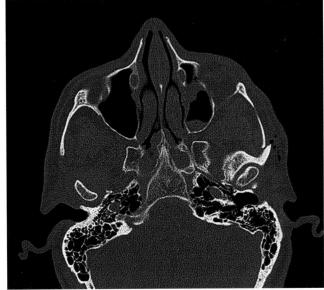

Fig. 28.2

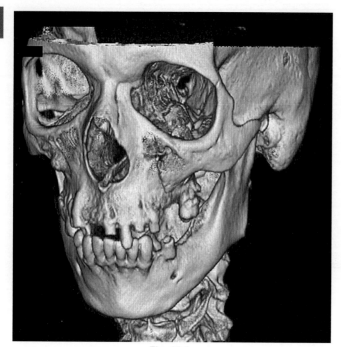

Fig. 28.3

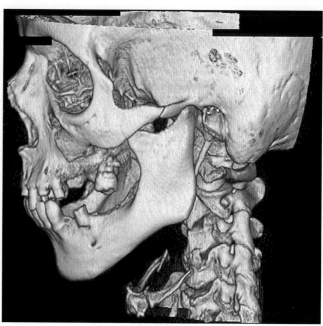

Fig. 28.4

Case 29

History: 28-year-old male presents to the ED following blunt trauma to his face.

1. Which of the following would be included in the differential for the imaging finding presented? (Choose all that apply.)
   A. Mandible fracture
   B. Le Fort fractures
   C. Right orbital fracture
   D. Zygomatic fracture
2. Which of the following imaging modalities has the lowest sensitivities for diagnosing a mandibular fracture?
   A. Panorex imaging
   B. CT
   C. Face radiography
   D. MRI

3. What is the appropriate treatment for this patient?
   A. NSAIDs and follow-up
   B. Opioid pain medicine
   C. Surgery
   D. Splint
4. Which part of the mandible is most likely to be injured in a fracture?
   A. Mental
   B. Body
   C. Angle
   D. Condyle

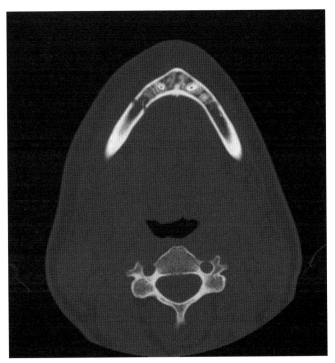

Fig. 29.1

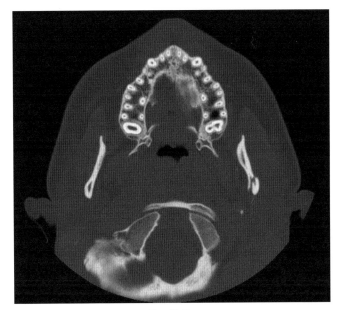

Fig. 29.2

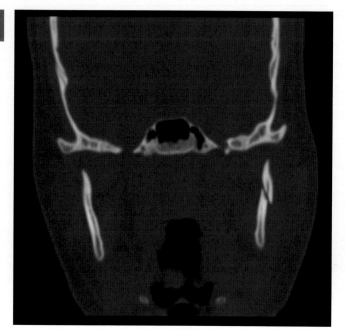

Fig. 29.3

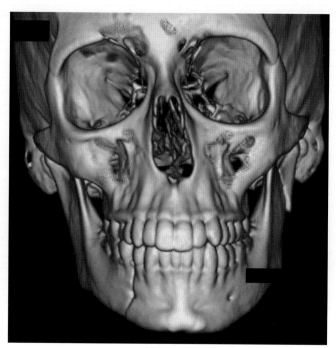

Fig. 29.4

Case 30

History: 26-year-old female presents to the clinic with facial pain that is worse when bending forward.

1. Which of the following would be included in the differential for the imaging finding presented? (Choose all that apply.)
   A. Trigeminal neuralgia
   B. Migraines
   C. Acute maxillary sinusitis
   D. Orbital fracture
2. How is this condition diagnosed in practice?
   A. CT scan
   B. Clinically based on symptoms
   C. MRI
   D. Single-photon emission CT (SPECT)

3. Which of the following symptoms would this patient NOT present with?
   A. Purulent nasal discharge
   B. Headache
   C. Halitosis
   D. Dysphagia
4. What percentage of cases result from bacterial causes?
   A. 5%
   B. 15%
   C. 75%
   D. 90%

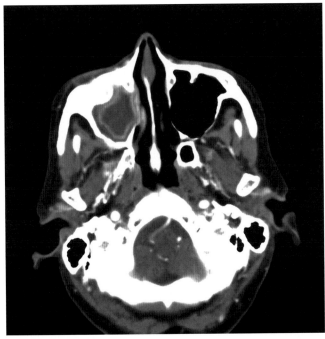

Fig. 30.1

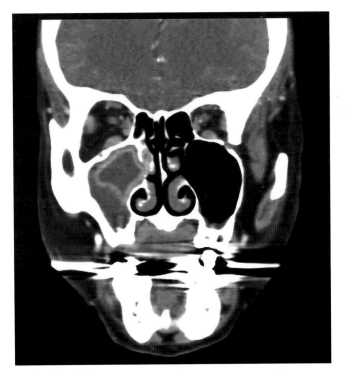

Fig. 30.2

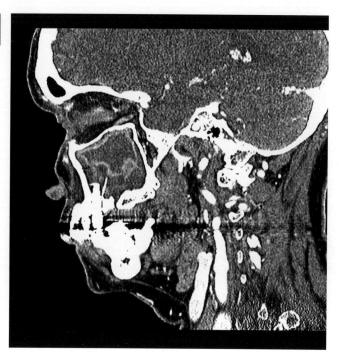

Fig. 30.3

Case 31

History: 16-year-old adolescent with complaints of sore throat and fever.

1. Which of the following would be included in the differential for the imaging finding presented? (Choose all that apply.)
   A. Sinusitis
   B. Tonsillitis
   C. Foreign body
   D. Orbital cellulitis
2. Which one of the following infectious etiologies is most likely to cause this condition?
   A. Viral
   B. Bacterial
   C. Fungal
   D. Parasites

3. Which of the following would be appropriate treatment for this patient?
   A. Antibiotics and drainage
   B. Pain relief and antiinflammatory meds
   C. Salt water gargle
   D. Aspirin
4. Given a bacterial etiology, what long-term sequel may result from a failure to treat?
   A. Encephalopathy
   B. Rheumatic fever
   C. Neoplasm
   D. Autoimmunity

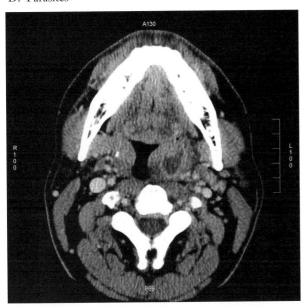

Fig. 31.1

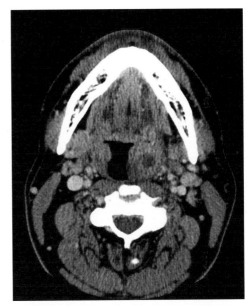

Fig. 31.2

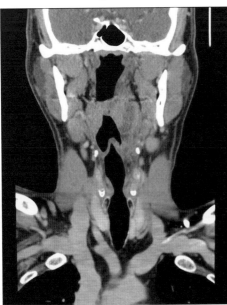

Fig. 31.3

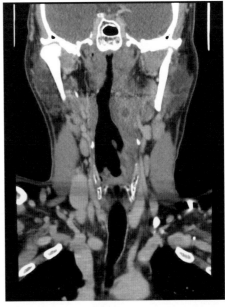

Fig. 31.4

Case 32

History: 5-year-old boy presents with sore throat.

1. Which of the following would be included in the differential diagnosis for the following images? (Choose all that apply.)
   A. Bacterial tracheitis
   B. Epiglottitis
   C. Retropharyngeal abscess
   D. Laryngocele
2. Which organism is the most common cause of epiglottitis?
   A. *Haemophilus influenza* type B (Hib)
   B. *Streptococcus pneumoniae*
   C. *Staphylococcus aureus*
   D. *Pseudomonas aeruginosa*

3. Which finding on imaging distinguishes laryngocele from epiglottitis?
   A. Soft-tissue neck x-ray showing epiglottic enlargement
   B. Lateral neck x-ray showing supraglottic narrowing
   C. CT contrast of neck showing nonenhancing fluid collection at level of arytenoid cartilage
   D. Unremarkable MRI
4. What clinical features are distinctive of epiglottitis in children?
   A. Sore throat, difficulty breathing, fever
   B. Dysphagia, difficulty breathing, fever
   C. Respiratory distress, drooling, and "tripod" or "sniffing" position
   D. Sore throat, ear pain, and vomiting

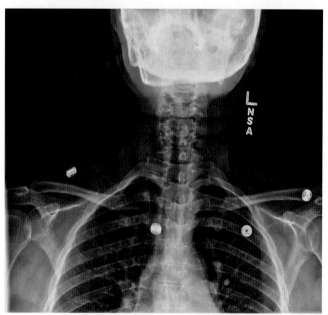

Fig. 32.1

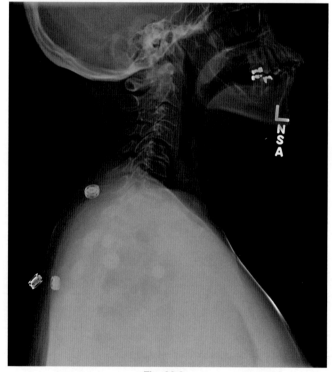

Fig. 32.2

Case 33

History: 5-year-old boy presents with sudden visual loss, limited eye movement, and fever.

1. Which of the following would be included in the differential for the imaging findings presented? (Choose all that apply.)
   A. Neoplasm
   B. Orbital cellulitis
   C. Retinal detachment
   D. Acute angle-closure glaucoma
2. What is the first-line imaging modality for this presentation?
   A. CT without contrast
   B. CT with contrast
   C. MRI without contrast
   D. MRI with contrast

3. Which of the following bacteria would *not* cause this presentation?
   A. *Streptococcus pneumonia*
   B. *Staphylococcus aureus*
   C. *Streptococcus pyogenes*
   D. *Klebsiella pneumonia*
4. What is the initial treatment for this patient?
   A. IV antibiotics
   B. Endoscopic drainage
   C. External drainage
   D. NSAIDs and follow-up

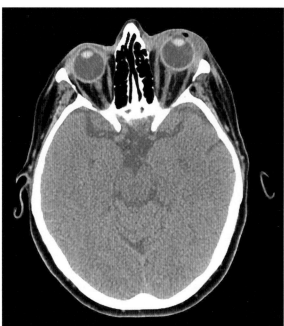

Fig. 33.1

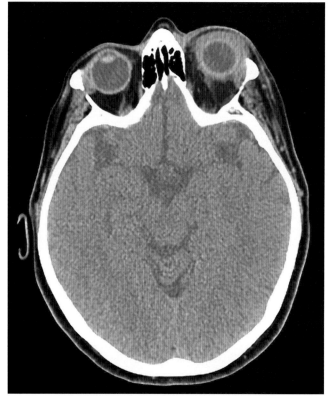

Fig. 33.2

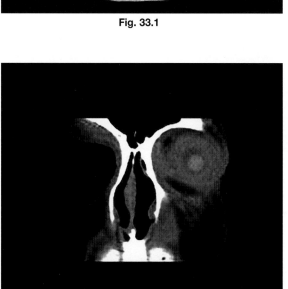

Fig. 33.3

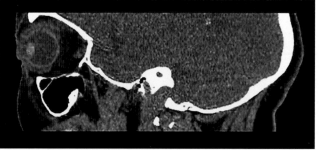

Fig. 33.4

Case 34

History: 32-year-old male presents with excruciating neck pain following a diving incident.

1. Which of the following would be included in the differential for the imaging findings presented? (Choose all that apply.)
   A. Hangman fracture
   B. Jefferson fracture
   C. Teardrop fracture
   D. Spinal stenosis
2. Which neurologic findings are associated with this condition?
   A. Truncal ataxia
   B. Vertical nystagmus
   C. Horner's syndrome
   D. None

3. What is the mechanism by which this injury occurs?
   A. Hyperextension of the spine
   B. Hyperflexion of the spine
   C. Axial loading onto the spine
   D. Blunt trauma to the posterior spinal column
4. Which of the following would be an appropriate treatment for a patient with this condition?
   A. Surgical fusion
   B. Immobilization and discharge
   C. Opioid pain medications
   D. Rest, ice, compression, and elevation (RICE)

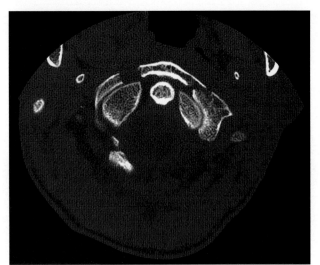

Fig. 34.1

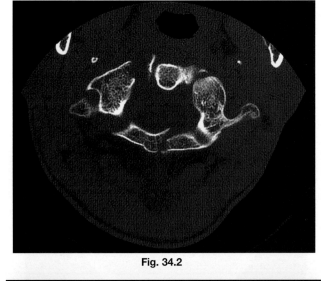

Fig. 34.2

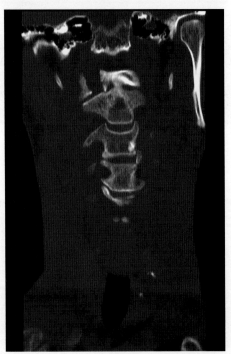

Fig. 34.3

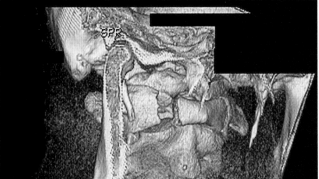

Fig. 34.4

Case 35

History: 66-year-old female presents to the ED following a motor vehicle accident.

1. Which of the following would be included in the differential for the imaging findings presented? (Choose all that apply.)
   A. Hangman's fracture
   B. Osteophytes
   C. Dens fracture
   D. Teardrop fracture
2. Which type of dens fracture is present?
   A. Type I
   B. Type II
   C. Type III
   D. Type IV

3. Given the fracture type, what would be the appropriate treatment?
   A. Surgical fusion
   B. Stabilize the neck and discharge patient
   C. CT follow-up in 6 months
   D. Opioid pain medications
4. Dens fractures most often occur by which mechanism?
   A. Hyperextension of the neck
   B. Hyperflexion of the neck
   C. Compression of the spine
   D. Blunt trauma

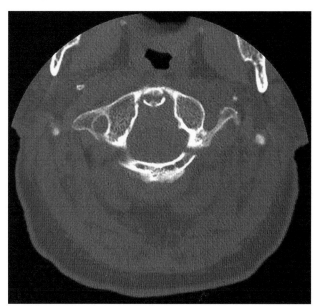

Fig. 35.1

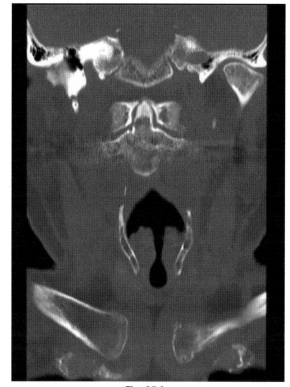

Fig. 35.2

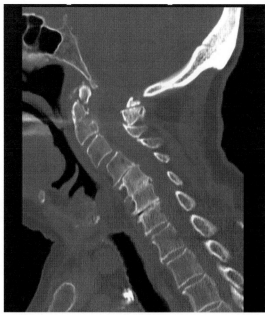

Fig. 35.3

Case 36

History: 25-year-old female presents with acute abdominal pain.

1. Which of the following would be included in the differential diagnosis for the imaging findings presented? (Choose all that apply.)
   A. Hiatal hernia
   B. Gastric ulcer
   C. Distended stomach
   D. Outlet obstruction
2. Coronal CT images demonstrate:
   A. Paraesophageal hiatal hernia
   B. Sliding hiatal hernia
   C. Midgut volvulus
   D. Gastric volvulus

3. The following statements about gastric volvulus are true, except:
   A. Mesenteroaxial volvulus is more common than organoaxial volvulus in adults.
   B. Organoaxial volvulus occurs along the long axis of the stomach.
   C. Mesenteroaxial volvulus occurs along the short axis of the stomach.
   D. Organoaxial occurs in the setting of trauma or paraeso-phageal hernia.
4. Borchardt triad includes all except:
   A. Sudden epigastric pain
   B. Intractable retching
   C. Inability to pass a nasogastric tube
   D. Vomiting

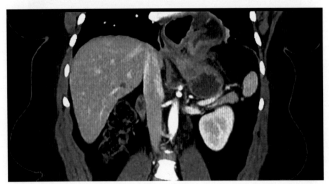

Fig. 36.1

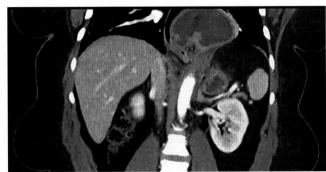

Fig. 36.3

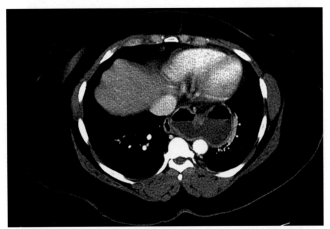

Fig. 36.2

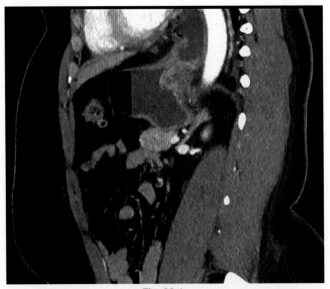

Fig. 36.4

Case 37

History: 30-year-old male jumped from the third floor of a burning building.

1. Which of the following would be included in the differential diagnosis for the imaging findings presented? (Choose all that apply.)
   A. Perched facet joint
   B. Listhesis
   C. Burst fracture
   D. Herniated disk
2. A burst fracture is a type of:
   A. Chalk stick fracture
   B. Compression fracture
   C. Listhesis
   D. Crush fracture

3. Which type of burst fracture do we see in this case?
   A. Type A dual retropulsion
   B. Type B classic burst
   C. Type C posteroinferior retropulsion
   D. Type D2 burst-sagittal translation
4. Which one the following describes a classic spinal burst fracture fragment retropulsion?
   A. Fragments are retropulsed from the posterosuperior corner with the inferior endplates remaining intact.
   B. Fragments originating from both the posterosuperior and posteroinferior margins of the involved vertebral body are retropulsed in the spinal canal.
   C. Fragments are retropulsed posteroinferiorly with intact superior endplates.
   D. Fragments are retropulsed unilaterally.

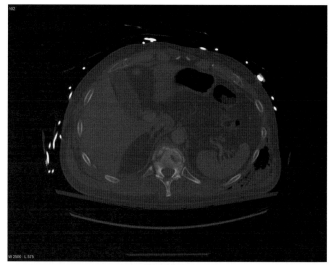

Fig. 37.1

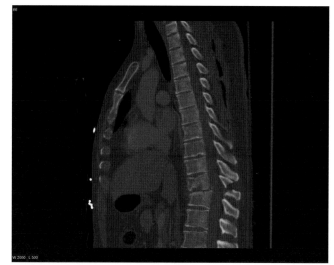

Fig. 37.3

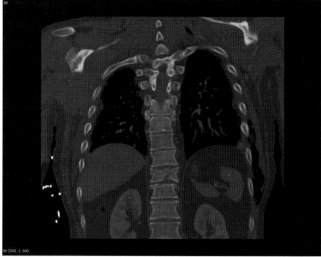

Fig. 37.2

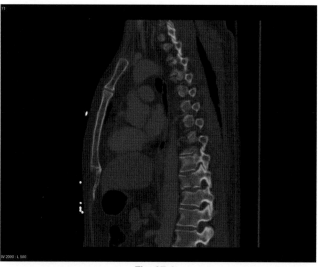

Fig. 37.4

Case 38

History: 67-year-old male comes in to the ED with sharp chest pain after having the wind knocked out of him during a mugging.

1. Which of the following would be included in the differential diagnosis for the imaging findings presented? (Choose all that apply.)
   A. Sternal fracture
   B. Traumatic aortic injury
   C. Costochondritis
   D. Paget's disease
2. Patients with sternal fractures can present with all of the following, except:
   A. Crepitus
   B. Bronchitis
   C. Localized tenderness
   D. Hypoxemia
   E. Respiratory insufficiency
3. Which of the following is true when it comes to sternal fractures?
   A. Low mortality rate at 5% of isolated sternal fractures
   B. Sternal fractures are quite uncommon in the United States.
   C. Sternal fractures occur 20% of the time in car accidents.
   D. Of sternal fractures, two-thirds have a concomitant injury with higher mortality.
4. Which entity will not be well evaluated by this examination?
   A. Detect myocardial contusions
   B. Detect rib fractures
   C. Detect pulmonary contusions
   D. Detect pneumothorax

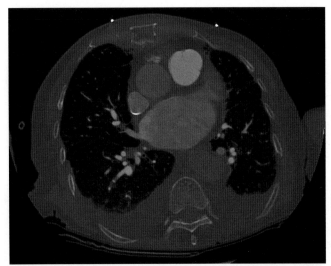

Fig. 38.1

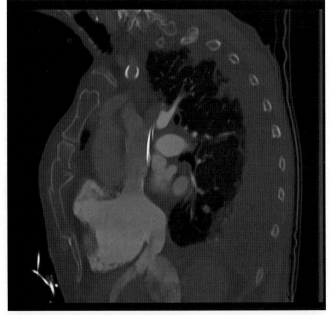

Fig. 38.2

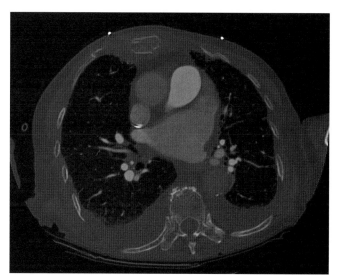

Fig. 38.3

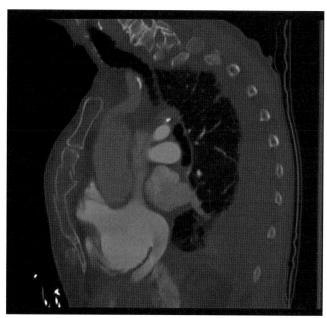

Fig. 38.4

Case 39

History: 47-year-old male is complaining of epigastric pain.

1. Which of the following would be included in the differential diagnosis for the imaging findings presented? (Choose all that apply.)
   A. Duodenal ulcer
   B. Gastric ulcer
   C. Gastritis
   D. Pancreatitis
   E. Peritonitis
2. Which would be the next best step in management?
   A. CT of the abdomen
   B. Fluid resuscitation and pain management
   C. Immediate laparotomy
   D. Serum amylase and lipase
   E. US of the abdomen

3. Which would be the best imaging choice for diagnosis in the ED setting?
   A. CT of the abdomen
   B. Endoscopic retrograde cholangiopancreatography (ERCP)
   C. MRI of the abdomen
   D. US
   E. X-ray of the abdomen
4. Which would be the most likely complication for the above diagnosis?
   A. Abscess
   B. Cancer
   C. Infarction of the spleen
   D. Pneumothorax
   E. Volvulus

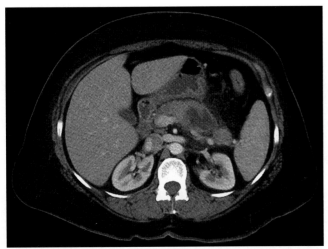

Fig. 39.1

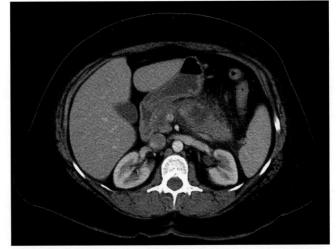

Fig. 39.2

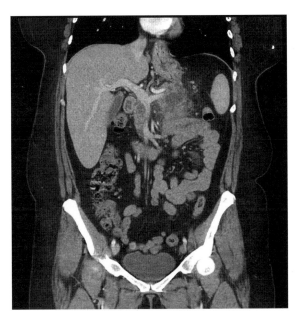

Fig. 39.3

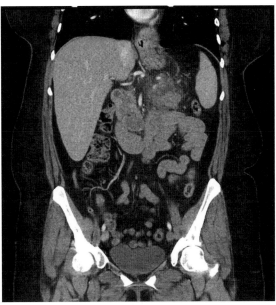

Fig. 39.4

Case 40

History: 43-year-old male presenting with left flank pain and hematuria.

1. Which of the following would be included in the differential diagnosis for the imaging findings presented? (Choose all that apply.)
   A. Congenital megaureter
   B. Chronic ureteropelvic junction (UPJ) obstruction
   C. Obstructing ureterovesicular junction (UVJ) calculus
   D. Bladder outlet obstruction
2. All of the following statements regarding this condition are true, except:
   A. Approximately 77% of ureteral stones are surrounded by a rim of soft tissue known as the "soft tissue rim sign," which assists in differentiation from phleboliths.
   B. Approximately 50% of stones are not visible on abdominal radiographs.
   C. Size of stone is an important predictor of spontaneous passage.
   D. Forniceal rupture may lead to further kidney damage secondary to increased intrapelvic pressure.
3. Which of the following statements regarding renal stones is most correct?
   A. Calcium stones account for 75% of renal calculi.
   B. Cystine stones account for 25% of renal calculi.
   C. Most patients with uric acid stones suffer from gout.
   D. Chronic *S. aureus* infection is the most common organism associated with struvite stones.
4. All of the following are risk factors for renal stone formation, except:
   A. Horseshoe kidney
   B. Primary hyperparathyroidism
   C. Milk-alkali syndrome
   D. High dietary intake of calcium
   E. Renal tubular acidosis (type 1)

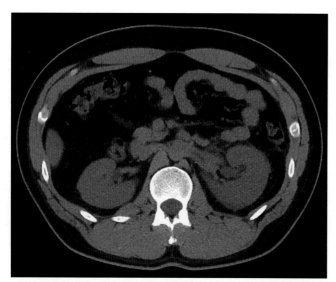

Fig. 40.1

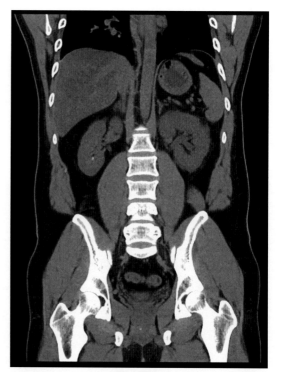

Fig. 40.2

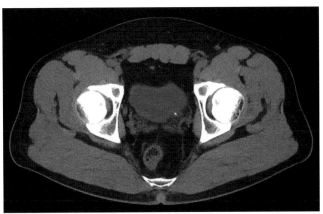

Fig. 40.4

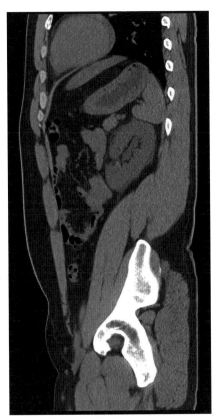

Fig. 40.3

Case 41

History: 33-year-old female presents with severe abdominal pain of 1.5 hours duration. Pain was initially in the epigastric area but now has generalized to abdominal pain with rigidity. No prior surgical history.

1. Which of the following would be included in the differential diagnosis for the imaging findings presented? (Choose all that apply.)
   A. Appendicolith
   B. Bowel perforation
   C. Subcutaneous emphysema
   D. Recent abdominal surgery
2. Which is the most common site for intestinal perforation?
   A. Duodenum
   B. Appendix
   C. Diverticuli of the sigmoid colon
   D. Diverticuli of the descending colon
   E. Ileocecal junction

3. Where does air tend to collect in the most common perforation site?
   A. Paramesenteric gutters
   B. Right subhepatic space
   C. Along the fissure of ligamentum teres
   D. Morison's pouch
   E. Paracolic gutter
4. What is a sonographic sign of free intraperitoneal air?
   A. Increased lucency in the right upper quadrant
   B. Periportal free gas sign
   C. Cupola sign
   D. Comet-shaped artifact

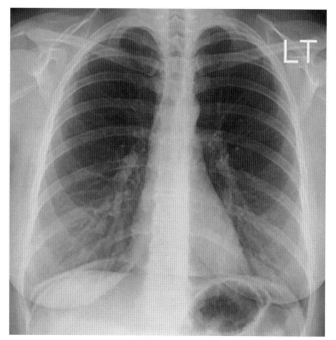

Fig. 41.1

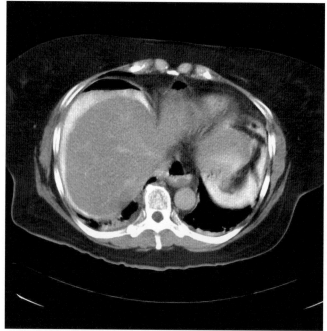

Fig. 41.2

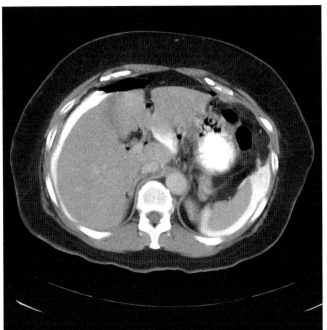

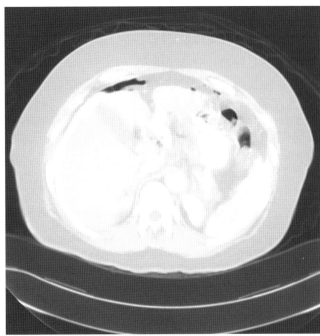

Fig. 41.3   **Fig. 41.4**

Case 42

History: 18-year-old female with acute onset pelvic pain.

1. Which of the following would be included in the differential diagnosis based on the imaging findings presented? (Choose all that apply.)
   A. Tuboovarian abscess
   B. Ovarian cyst
   C. Pyelonephritis
   D. Ovarian torsion
   E. Ovarian endometrioma

2. Which radiographic findings indicate ovarian torsion is the most likely cause of this patient's pain?
   A. Ovarian enlargement with possible free pelvic fluid
   B. Decreased or absent intraovarian venous flow on Doppler
   C. Whirlpool sign
   D. All of the above

3. Which imaging modality is first line when working up a patient for ovarian torsion?
   A. Pelvic x-ray
   B. CT abdomen pelvis with contrast
   C. US
   D. MRI

4. At what size will an ovarian mass most likely evolve into a torsion?
   A. 2 cm
   B. 3 cm
   C. 4 cm
   D. 5 cm

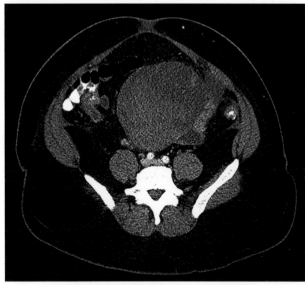

Fig. 42.1

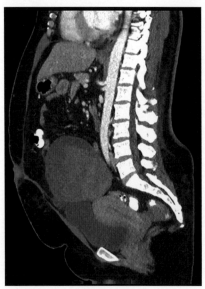

Fig. 42.2

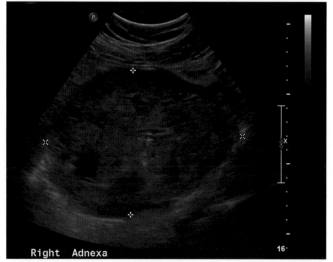

Fig. 42.3

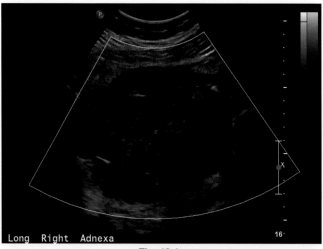

Fig. 42.4

Case 43

History: 27-year-old pregnant female presents with vaginal bleeding.

1. Which of the following would be included in the differential diagnosis for the imaging findings presented? (Choose all that apply.)
   A. Viable IUP
   B. Ectopic pregnancy
   C. Perigestational hemorrhage
   D. Intrauterine fetal demise
2. Which structure is first visualized in the gestational sac at approximately 5 to 6 weeks?
   A. Fetal pole
   B. Yolk sac
   C. Crown-rump length
   D. Placenta

3. At what crown-rump length should a fetal heartbeat be visualized on ultrasound?
   A. 3 mm
   B. 5 mm
   C. 7 mm
   D. 9 mm
4. A gestational sac is present measuring 18 mm, but no fetal pole is visualized. What should be the next step in management?
   A. Dilation and curettage
   B. Methotrexate administration
   C. Laparoscopy
   D. Repeat ultrasound in 14 days.

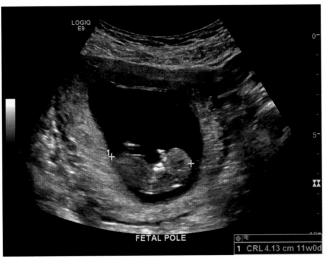

Fig. 43.1

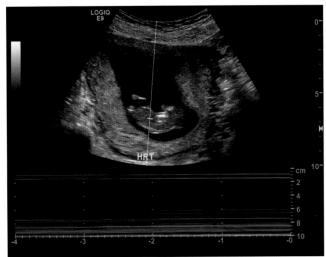

Fig. 43.3

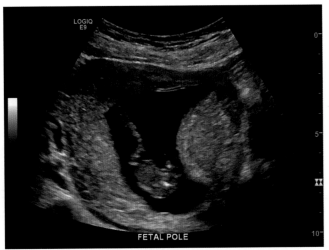

Fig. 43.2

Case 44

History: 19-year-old male with severe, left scrotal pain.

1. Which of the following would be included in the differential diagnosis for the imaging findings presented? (Choose all that apply.)
   A. Torsion of the testicular appendage
   B. Testicular malignancy
   C. Epididymoorchitis
   D. Testicular torsion
2. Which of the following is the first and most specific finding for the diagnosis in question 1?
   A. Hydrocele formation
   B. Loss of venous Doppler flow
   C. Heterogeneity of the testicular parenchyma
   D. Loss of arterial Doppler flow

3. Which of these represents the correct time and salvage rate percentage pair?
   A. 6 hours – 20%
   B. 12 to 24 hours – 40%
   C. 6 hours – 100%
   D. 12 to 24 hours – 70%
4. Which is the preferred treatment option?
   A. Manual detorsion
   B. Surgical detorsion and orchiopexy
   C. IV antibiotics
   D. Conservative therapy with NSAIDs

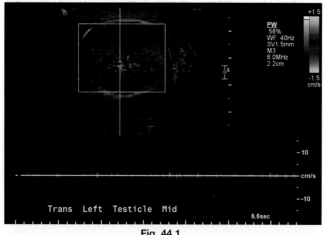

Fig. 44.1

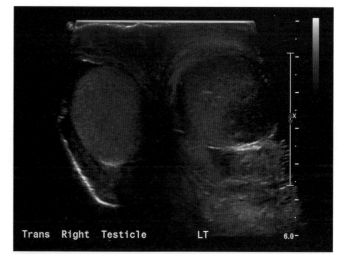

Fig. 44.3

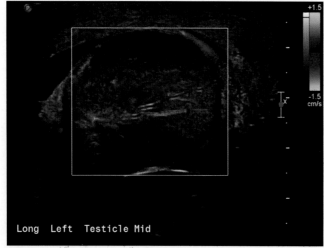

Fig. 44.2

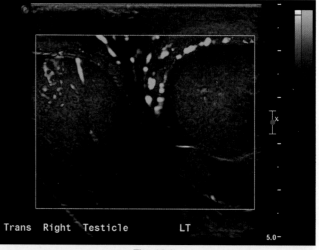

Fig. 44.4

Case 45

History: 9-year-old boy presents holding his right forearm and wrist in pain.

1. Which of the following would be included in the differential diagnosis for the imaging findings presented? (Choose all that apply.)
   A. Galeazzi fracture
   B. Colles' fracture
   C. Smith fracture
   D. Barton fracture
2. Which of the following is a type II fracture in this category?
   A. Occurs as a result of axial loading of the forearm in supination, which causes dorsal displacement of the radius and volar dislocation of the distal ulna
   B. Occurs as a result of axial loading of the forearm in supination, which causes dorsal displacement of the radius and dorsal dislocation of the distal ulna
   C. Occurs as a result of axial loading of the forearm in pronation, which causes anterior displacement of the radius and dorsal dislocation of the distal ulna
   D. Occurs as a result of axial loading of the forearm in pronation, which causes anterior displacement of the radius and volar dislocation of the distal ulna

3. What is the next step in management in a child presenting with this type of fracture?
   A. Open reduction and internal fixation and immobilization in supination in an above-elbow cast for 4 to 6 weeks
   B. Closed reduction and immobilization in supination in an above-elbow cast for 4 to 6 weeks
   C. Open reduction and internal fixation of the radius
   D. Kirschner wire fixation of ulna to radius
4. The distal radioulnar joint is primarily stabilized by which of the following?
   A. Palmar radioulnar ligament
   B. Triangular fibrocartilage complex (TFCC)
   C. Dorsoradioulnar ligament
   D. Interosseous membrane (IOM)

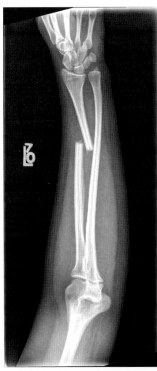

Fig. 45.1

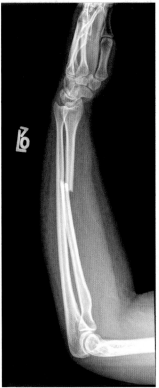

Fig. 45.2

Case 46

History: 19-year-old male street fighter presents with right hand swelling and pain for 1 day.

1. Which of the following would be included in the differential diagnosis for the imaging findings presented? (Choose all that apply.)
   A. Bennett's fracture
   B. Galeazzi fracture
   C. Boxers fracture
   D. 5th metacarpal neck fracture
2. This fracture type accounts for what percent of all hand fractures?
   A. 5%
   B. 20%
   C. 10%
   D. 30%
3. Which antibiotics would you give to the patient in the setting of an open fracture?
   A. Cefazolin (or a first-generation cephalosporin) every 8 hours for three doses
   B. Piperacillin/tazobactam or cephalosporin (cefazolin) and tobramycin. Continue for 24 hours after wound closure.
   C. Piperacillin/tazobactam or cefazolin and tobramycin plus penicillin for anaerobic bacteria, if needed, for 3 days.
   D. Piperacillin/tazobactam or cefazolin and tobramycin plus penicillin for anaerobic bacteria if needed. Continue for 3 days after wound closure.

4. Patient presents with a closed fracture of the fifth metacarpal neck without rotational deformity and without associated injury. On radiograph, palmar angulation of 50 degrees is noted. What is the next step in management?
   A. Apply neighbor strapping for 1 week; apply high arm sling and follow protection, rest, ice, compression, elevation instructions.
   B. Apply metacarpal block, reduce fracture, apply ulnar gutter back slab, and apply high arm sling.
   C. Consult on-call plastics team.
   D. Discharge patient with boxer's fracture education sheet with a follow-up appointment in 7 days.

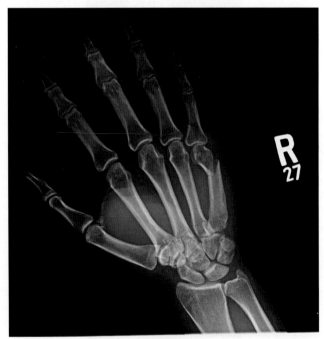

Fig. 46.1

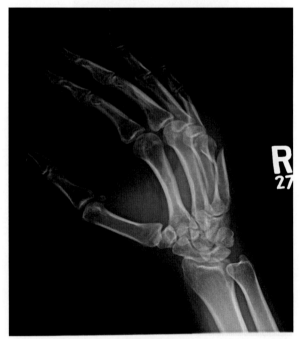

Fig. 46.2

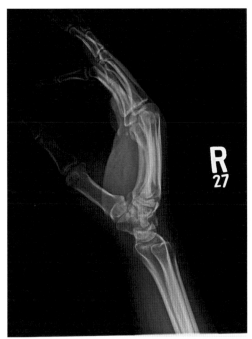

Fig. 46.3

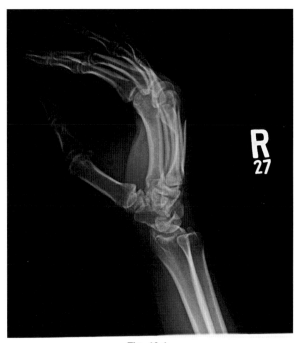

Fig. 46.4

Case 47

History: 32-year-old male presents to the ED with severe pain in hip and upper leg, following a motor vehicle accident.

1. Which of the following would be included in the differential diagnosis for the imaging findings presented? (Choose all that apply.)
   A. Pelvic fracture
   B. Slipped capital femoral epiphysis (SCFE)
   C. Hip dislocation
   D. Femoral neck fracture
2. Which is the mechanism by which this injury most likely occurs?
   A. Axial force applied to hip in flexed, adducted, and internally rotated position
   B. External rotation to hip when femoral head is fixed in joint
   C. Axial force applied to hip in abducted and externally rotated position
   D. Posterior force applied to hip in flexed and externally rotated position

3. A common complication associated with this diagnosis is nerve injury. Which nerve is most likely to be injured in this patient?
   A. Obturator
   B. Sciatic
   C. Femoral
   D. Saphenous
4. Which of the following would be the most appropriate first step in treatment for this patient?
   A. Hip replacement
   B. Physical therapy
   C. Reduction
   D. Rest and ice hip

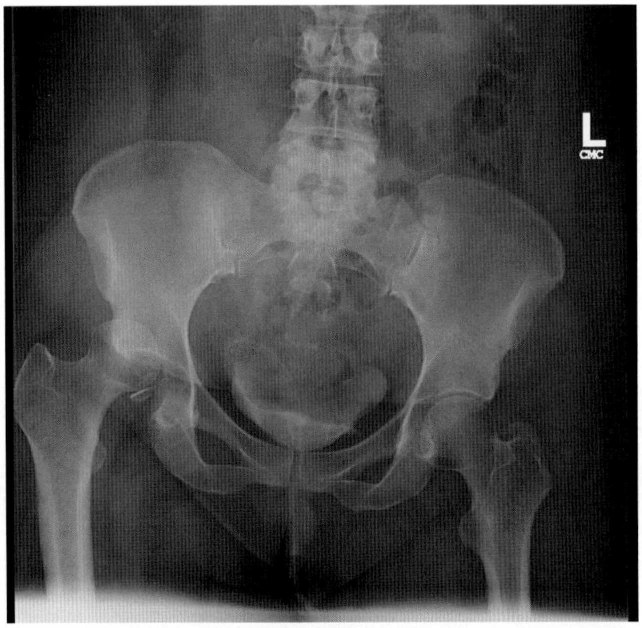

Fig. 47.1

Case 48

History: An adolescent male presents to the ED holding his left wrist. He has come directly to the ED from his intermural football league.

1. Which of the following would be included in the differential diagnosis for the imaging findings presented? (Choose all that apply.)
   A. Salter Harris fracture type II
   B. Salter Harris fracture type I
   C. Scaphoid fracture
   D. Salter Harris fracture type III
2. Which is the most common type of Salter Harris fracture?
   A. Type I
   B. Type II
   C. Type III
   D. Type IV

3. This is a common fracture in which population?
   A. Elderly
   B. Debilitated patients
   C. Children
   D. Vitamin D deficient patients
4. This type of fracture is most commonly the result of which of the following?
   A. Metabolic disease
   B. Abuse
   C. Genetics
   D. Sports-related injury
5. Which of the following type of fractures has a Tillaux pattern that is secondary to injury after the medial distal tibial growth plate has fused?
   A. Type II
   B. Type III
   C. Type IV
   D. Type V

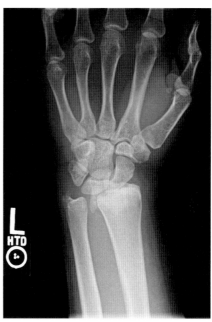

Fig. 48.2

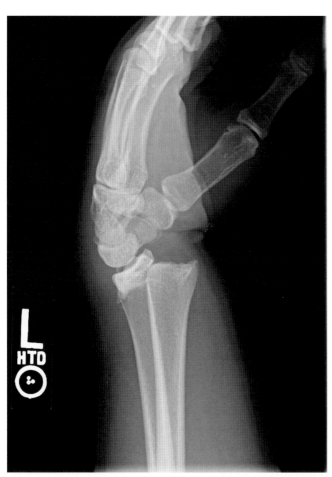

Fig. 48.1

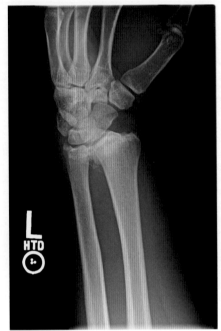

Fig. 48.3

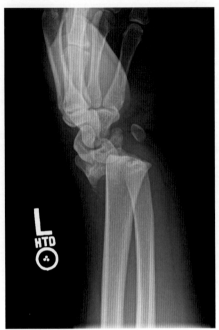

Fig. 48.4

Case 49

History: A 19-year-old female gymnast presents with pain and swelling around the knee.

1. Which of the following would be included in the differential diagnosis for the imaging findings presented? (Choose all that apply.)
   A. Patellofemoral pain syndrome
   B. Patellar dislocation
   C. Pes anserinus bursitis
   D. Femoral fracture
2. Associated nerve damage is often seen in patients suffering from this condition. Which pair of nerves is most likely to be injured?
   A. Sciatic and peroneal
   B. Obturator and saphenous
   C. Peroneal and tibial
   D. Sciatic and saphenous

3. To assess the ligaments in this area, which type of imaging would you order next for this patient?
   A. CT scan
   B. Angiogram
   C. X-ray
   D. MRI
4. The Schenck classification system is often used for knee injuries. If both cruciate ligaments were disrupted completely, but the collateral ligaments remained intact, which classification would this patient's injury receive?
   A. KDI
   B. KDII
   C. KDIII
   D. KDIV

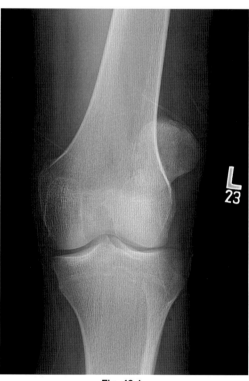

Fig. 49.1

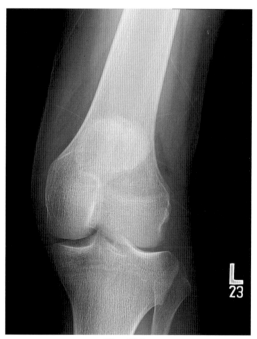

Fig. 49.2

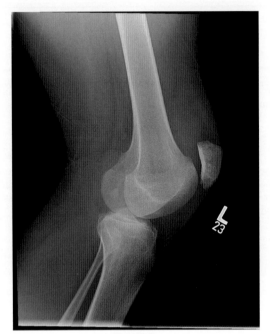

Fig. 49.3

Case 50

History: 45-year-old female who fell resulting in pain and swelling.

1. Which of the following would be included in the differential diagnosis for the imaging findings presented? (Choose all that apply.)
   A. Supination-adduction injury
   B. Supination external rotation injury
   C. Pronation-abduction injury
   D. Pronation-external rotation injury

2. Which is the Danis–Weber classification for the injury present?
   A. Type A
   B. Type B
   C. Type C
   D. None of the above

3. Which is the first stage of the ankle injury present on imaging?
   A. Anterior tibiofibular ligament rupture
   B. Lateral malleolar fracture
   C. Posterior tibiofibular ligament rupture
   D. Deltoid ligament rupture

4. Which is the last stage of the ankle injury present on imaging?
   A. Anterior tibiofibular ligament rupture
   B. Posterior malleolar fracture
   C. Deltoid ligament rupture or medial malleolar fracture
   D. None of the above

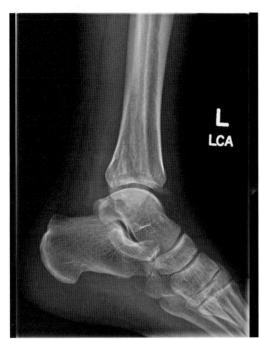

Fig. 50.1

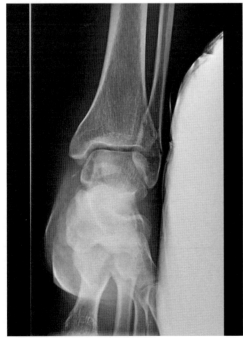

Fig. 50.3

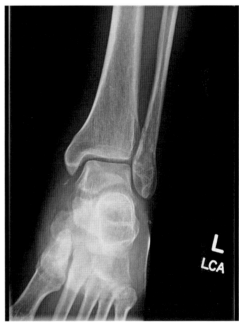

Fig. 50.2

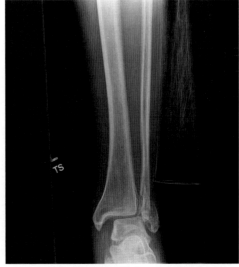

Fig. 50.4

Case 51

History: 40-year-old man with Crohn's disease presents with fever and lower pelvic pain.

1. Which of the following would be included in the differential diagnosis for the imaging findings presented? (Choose all that apply.)
   A. Anorectal abscess
   B. Anorectal cellulitis
   C. Normal examination finding
   D. None of the above
2. Which is the most common type of anorectal abscess?
   A. Perianal
   B. Ischiorectal
   C. Intersphincteric
   D. None of the above
3. Which is the most common cause of an anorectal abscess?
   A. Infected anal gland
   B. Diverticulitis
   C. Crohn's disease
   D. Trauma
4. Supralevator abscess may be caused by which of the following?
   A. Superior extension of an intersphincteric abscess
   B. Inferior extension of an infectious or inflammatory process
   C. Both A and B
   D. None of the above

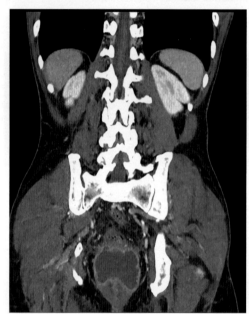

Fig. 51.3

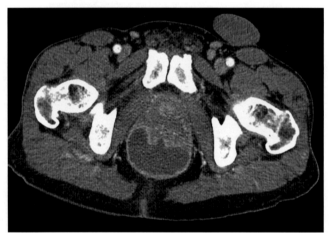

Fig. 51.1

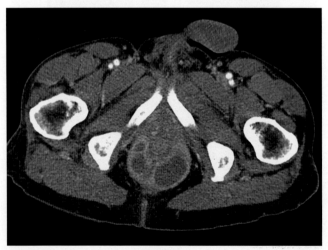

Fig. 51.2

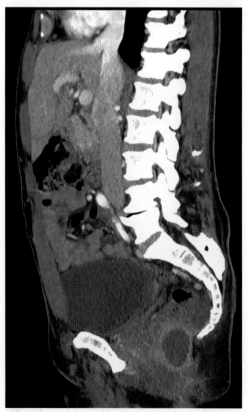

Fig. 51.4

Case 52

History: 69-year-old male presents to ED with constipation.

1. Which of the following would be included in the differential diagnosis for the imaging findings presented? (Choose all that apply.)
   A. Cecal volvulus
   B. Sigmoid volvulus
   C. Pseudoobstruction of bowel
   D. Acute small bowel obstruction

2. Which of the following is correct regarding the incidence of large bowel volvulus?
   A. Cecal > Sigmoid > Transverse colon
   B. Sigmoid > Transverse > Cecal
   C. Sigmoid > Cecal > Transverse
   D. All have nearly equal incidence of volvulus.

3. Which of the following is not described in the imaging findings of sigmoid volvulus?
   A. Coffee bean sign
   B. Bird beak sign
   C. X marks the spot sign
   D. Doughnut sign

4. Which is the most common management of suspected sigmoid volvulus in ER setting?
   A. No management required; this is a transient condition.
   B. Surgical management with resection of sigmoid colon
   C. Rectal tube insertion
   D. Follow-up kidney, ureter, bladder (KUB) radiographs every 6 hours

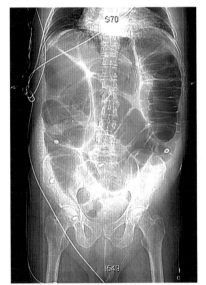

Fig. 52.1

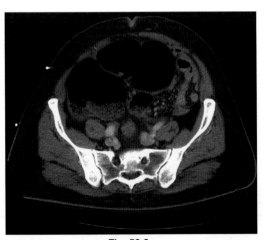

Fig. 52.2

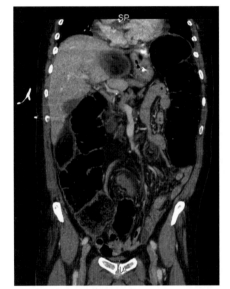

Fig. 52.3

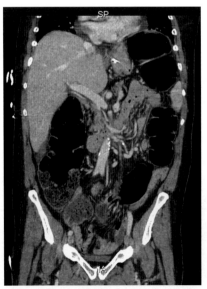

Fig. 52.4

Case 53

History: 34-year-old man involved in an unrestrained motor vehicle accident (MVA) hitting the windshield.

1. Which of the following would be included in the differential diagnosis for the imaging findings presented? (Choose all that apply.)
   A. Concussion
   B. Diffuse axonal injury
   C. Epidural hematoma
   D. Subdural hematoma
2. Which is the most accurate modality for making this diagnosis?
   A. Computed tomography (CT)
   B. Magnetic resonance imaging (MRI)
   C. Ultrasound (US)
   D. X-ray
3. Which of the following is NOT a characteristic imaging finding?
   A. Atrophy
   B. Edema
   C. Hematoma
   D. Multiple petechial hemorrhages
4. Which is the most likely prognosis?
   A. Death
   B. Focal neurologic deficits
   C. Full recovery
   D. Coma and long-term cognitive impairment

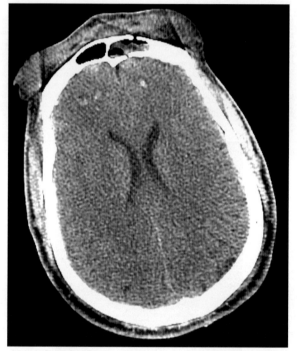

Fig. 53.2

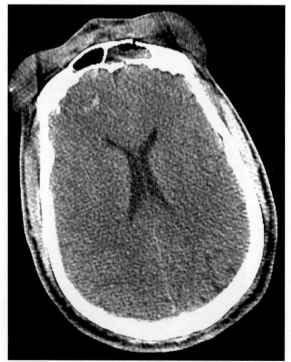

Fig. 53.1

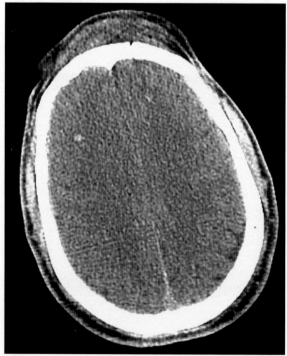

Fig. 53.3

Case 54

History: 37-year-old man, a restrained passenger, presents via emergency medical services (EMS) after a motor vehicle accident (MVA).

1. Which of the following would be included in the differential diagnosis for the imaging findings presented? (Choose all that apply.)
   A. Open book type pelvic fracture
   B. Femoral dislocation
   C. Burst fracture
   D. Intertrochanteric fracture
2. This lesion is often associated with:
   A. Loss of bladder control
   B. Leg weakness
   C. Pancreatic injuries
   D. All of the above

3. Which modality is of limited diagnostic value in evaluating these patients?
   A. Clinical examination
   B. Radiography (XR)
   C. CT
   D. MR
4. Which of the following statements is true?
   A. This location is atypical for this injury.
   B. This injury is not associated with neurologic deficits.
   C. This is high mechanism associated with intraabdominal injuries.
   D. This injury is associated with axial loading.

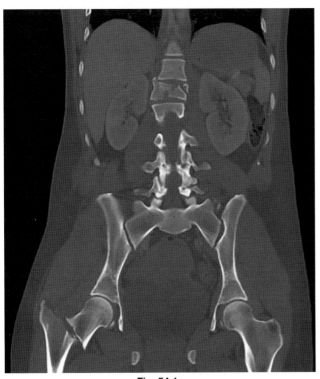

Fig. 54.1

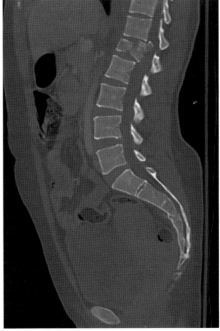

Fig. 54.2

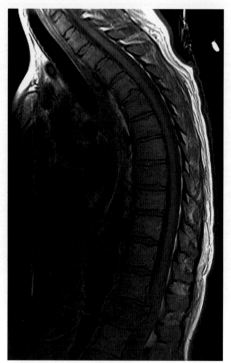

Fig. 54.3

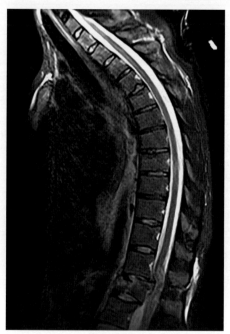

Fig. 54.4

Case 55

History: 61-year-old woman with diffuse abdominal pain.

1. Which of the following would be included in the differential diagnosis for the imaging findings presented? (Choose all that apply.)
   A. Small bowel obstruction
   B. Large bowel obstruction
   C. Ileus
   D. Pneumoperitoneum
2. Imaging findings on the CT represent:
   A. Sigmoid volvulus
   B. Small bowel volvulus
   C. Cecal volvulus
   D. Transverse colon volvulus

3. Which of the following are the types of cecal volvulus?
   A. Axial type
   B. Loop type
   C. Cecal bascule
   D. Both A and B
   E. All of the above
4. Which is the most common site of gastrointestinal volvulus in adults?
   A. Sigmoid colon
   B. Stomach
   C. Cecum
   D. Small bowel

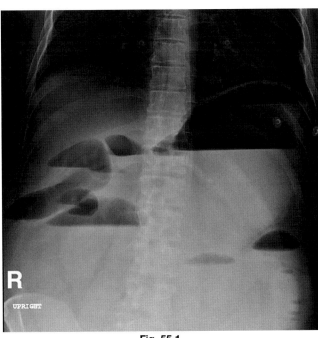

Fig. 55.1

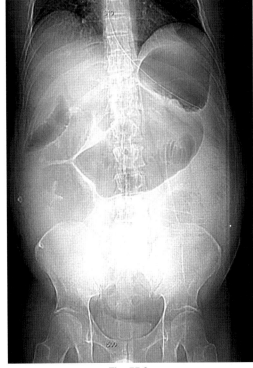

Fig. 55.2

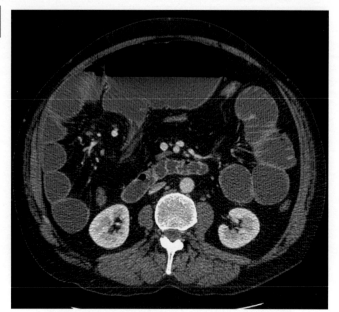

Fig. 55.3

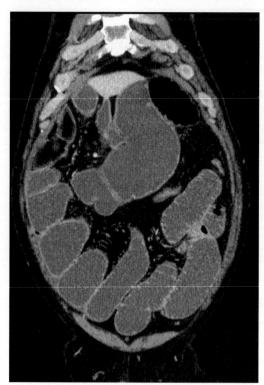

Fig. 55.4

Case 56

History: 40-year-old woman with human immunodeficiency virus (HIV), headache, and lethargy.

1. Which of the following would be included in the differential diagnosis for the imaging findings presented? (Choose all that apply.)
   A. Tumoral edema
   B. Herpes encephalitis
   C. Infarction
   D. Ischemic small vessel disease
2. These imaging findings are often associated with:
   A. History of metastatic disease
   B. Neurologic deficits
   C. Seizures
   D. All of the above

3. Which modality has the greatest diagnostic value in evaluating these patients?
   A. CT head, noncontrast
   B. CT head, contrast
   C. MR head, noncontrast
   D. MR head, contrast
4. Which of the following statements regarding MR findings is false?
   A. Localized edema is a common.
   B. Variable leptomeningeal enhancement on post-contrast sequences.
   C. Diffuse-weighted imaging (DWI) is more sensitive than T2-weighted images.
   D. Hemorrhage is more common in neonates.

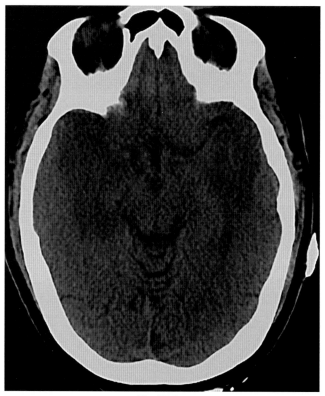

Fig. 56.1

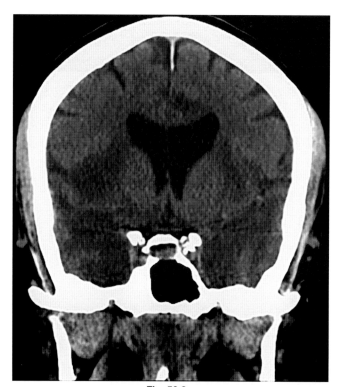

Fig. 56.2

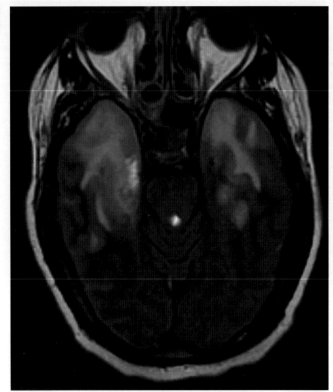

Fig. 56.3

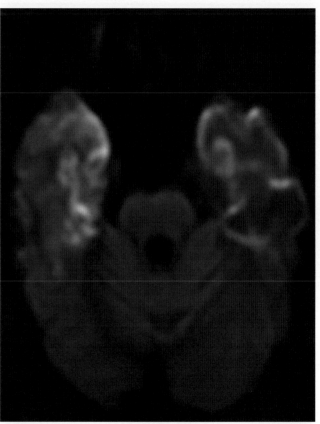

Fig. 56.4

Case 57

History: 47-year-old man with HIV, hypertension, and intravenous (IV) drug abuse complaining of headache and visual changes.

1. Which of the following would be included in the differential diagnosis for the imaging findings presented? (Choose all that apply.)
   A. Traumatic vitreal hemorrhage
   B. Endophthalmitis
   C. Orbital cellulitis
   D. Orbital pseudotumor
2. This lesion is often associated with:
   A. Diabetes
   B. Immunosuppression
   C. Fungemia
   D. All of the above
3. Diagnosis of this entity is usually made by:
   A. Clinical examination
   B. US
   C. CT
   D. MR

4. Which of the following statements is true?
   A. A presumptive diagnosis can be made only if fungus is isolated from ocular samples.
   B. Amphotericin therapy has good systemic coverage but poor vitreous penetration.
   C. Untreated cases are at little risk for sight loss.
   D. This condition has a female preponderance.

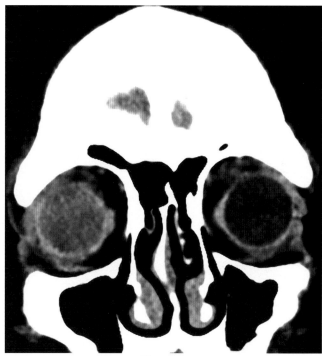

Fig. 57.2

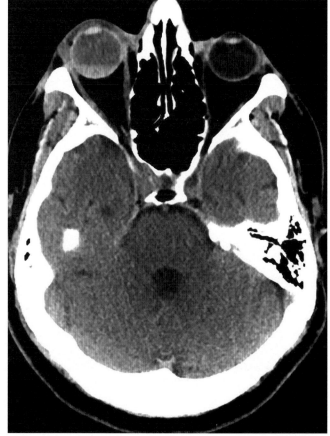

Fig. 57.1

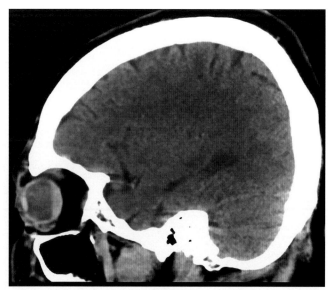

Fig. 57.3

Case 58

History: 24-year-old man with pain after injury playing football.

1. Which of the following would be included in the differential diagnosis for the imaging findings presented? (Choose all that apply.)
   A. Clavicular fracture
   B. Anterior shoulder dislocation
   C. Posterior shoulder dislocation
   D. Acromioclavicular/coracoclavicular separation

2. This type of injury is typically associated with all of the following, except:
   A. Direct blow
   B. Fall onto adducted arm
   C. Osteoarthritis
   D. None of the above

3. This type of injury can be classified using which classification system?
   A. Rockwood
   B. Tossy
   C. Allman
   D. Clinton

4. Which imaging modality is most commonly used for evaluation and diagnosis?
   A. Radiography (XR)
   B. US
   C. CT
   D. MR

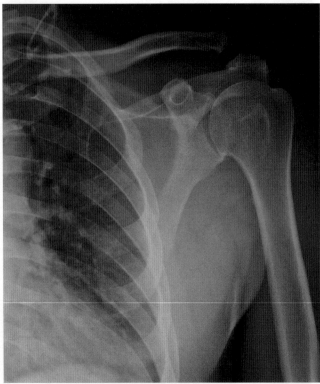

Fig. 58.1

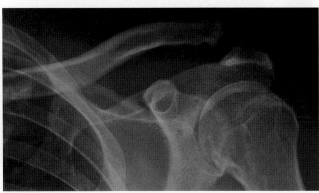

Fig. 58.2

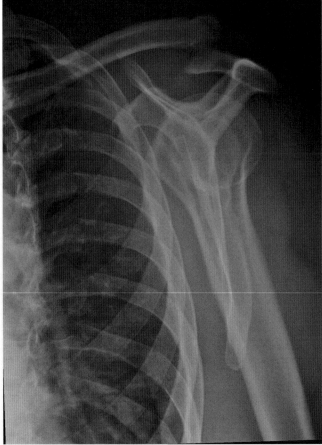

Fig. 58.3

Case 59

History: 41-year-old male with back pain, bilateral lower extremities pain, and numbness.

1. Which of the following would be included in the differential diagnosis for the imaging findings presented? (Choose all that apply.)
   A. Degeneration
   B. Infection
   C. Trauma
   D. Metastases
   E. Canal stenosis
2. MRI findings at L3-L4 are suggestive of:
   A. Pyogenic spondylitis
   B. Tuberculous spondylitis
   C. *Brucella* spondylitis
   D. *Aspergillus*-induced spondylitis

3. All of the following MR findings favor tuberculous spondylitis over pyogenic spondylitis, except:
   A. Subligamentous spread of infection to three or more vertebral bodies
   B. Early involvement of the intervertebral disk
   C. Chronicity and insidious progression
   D. Skip lesions and large paraspinal abscesses
4. Conditions that mimic spinal infection include:
   A. Modic type 1 degeneration
   B. SAPHO syndrome
   C. Acute cartilaginous node
   D. Andersson lesion

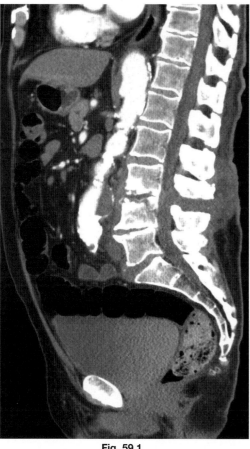

Fig. 59.1

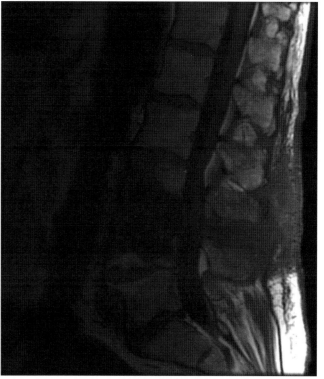

Fig. 59.2

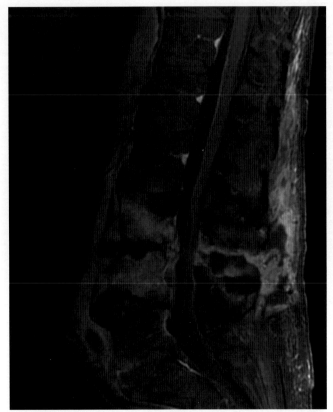

Fig. 59.3

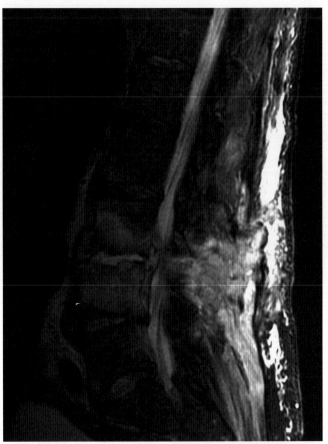

Fig. 59.4

Case 60

History: 62-year-old peanut farmer with a prior cerebrovascular accident presents to the emergency department (ED) with cough that lasted for 5 days.

1. Which of the following would be included in the differential diagnosis for the imaging findings presented? (Choose all that apply.)
   A. Right lower lobe atelectasis caused by mucus plug
   B. Right lower lobe atelectasis caused by aspirated foreign body
   C. Right lower lobe atelectasis caused by intrabronchial mass
   D. None of the above
2. Which statement is *false* in regard to tracheobronchial foreign body aspiration?
   A. Foreign bodies may be found more proximally than the right or left mainstem bronchus in younger children owing to their trachea being smaller in caliber.
   B. Foreign bodies more often lodge in the right mainstem bronchus rather than the left mainstem bronchus in adults and older children.
   C. Foreign bodies more often lodge in the left mainstem bronchus rather than the right mainstem bronchus in adults and older children.
   D. None of the above
3. Which finding is a secondary sign of tracheobronchial aspiration?
   A. Atelectasis
   B. Air trapping
   C. Postobstructive pneumonia
   D. All of the above
4. Which is the first-line imaging modality in patients with suspected foreign body aspiration?
   A. Radiography
   B. Fluoroscopy
   C. CT
   D. MRI

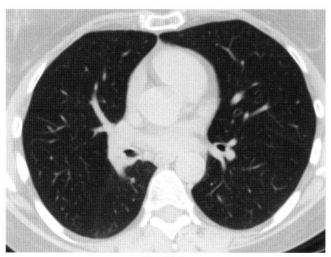

Fig. 60.1

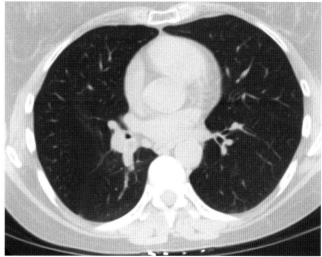

Fig. 60.2

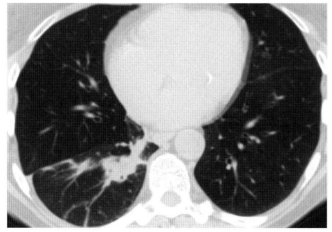

Fig. 60.3

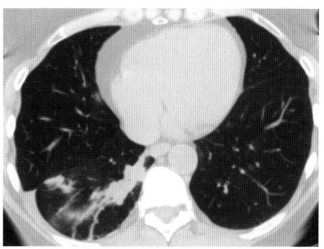

Fig. 60.4

Case 61

History: 65-year-old male status post assault.

1. Which of the following would be included in the differential diagnosis for the CT images presented? (Choose all that apply.)
   A. Normal right lens
   B. Posterior subluxation of right lens
   C. Posterior dislocation of right lens
   D. Posterior dislocation of left lens
2. Which is the most common cause of ectopia lentis?
   A. Marfan syndrome
   B. Ehlers-Danlos syndrome
   C. Homocystinuria
   D. Trauma

3. Which is the most common type of lens dislocation?
   A. Anterior
   B. Posterior
   C. Inferonasal
   D. Superotemporal
4. Which is the imaging modality of choice for orbital trauma?
   A. Ultrasound
   B. MRI
   C. CT
   D. Funduscopy

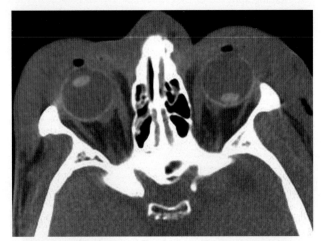

Fig. 61.1

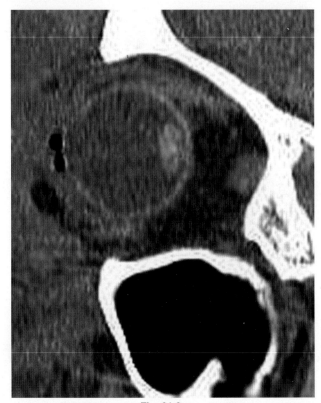

Fig. 61.2

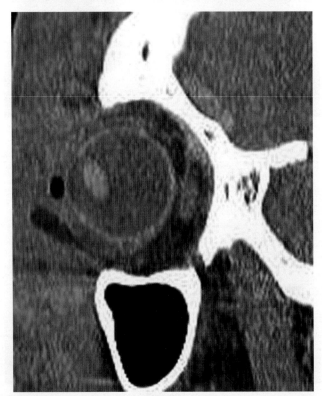

Fig. 61.3

Case 62

History: 35-year-old female status post assault.

1. Which of the following would be included in the differential diagnosis for the imaging findings presented? (Choose all that apply.)
   A. Orbital fracture
   B. Traumatic iritis
   C. Retinal detachment
   D. Globar rupture
2. Which of the following should NOT be performed during the diagnosis of globar rupture?
   A. Tonometry for intraocular pressure
   B. Evaluation for pupillary defects
   C. Visual acuity tests
   D. Full examination of eyes, including lids, cornea, and pupils

3. Which of the following can be seen in a CT scan for globar rupture?
   A. Destruction of the orbital bone
   B. Impaired visual acuity
   C. Intraocular air or a foreign body
   D. Carotid cavernous fistula
4. What is the most common cause of globar rupture?
   A. Orbital trauma
   B. Bacterial conjunctivitis
   C. Diplopia
   D. Exophthalmos

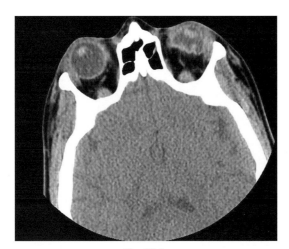

Fig. 62.1

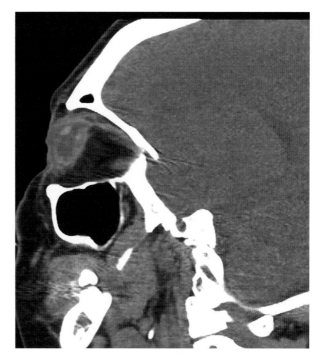

Fig. 62.2

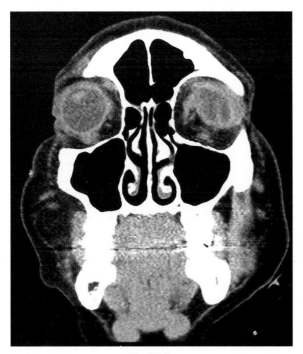

Fig. 62.3

Case 63

History: 46-year-old woman with foot swelling.

1. Which of the following would be included in the differential diagnosis for the imaging findings presented? (Choose all that apply.)
   A. Cellulitis
   B. Ulceration
   C. Laceration
   D. Osteomyelitis
2. These imaging findings are often associated with:
   A. Hypercholesterolemia
   B. Nonhealing ulcers
   C. Diabetes
   D. None of the above

3. Which modality has the greatest diagnostic value in evaluating these patients?
   A. Radiography
   B. CT
   C. Nuclear Medicine (NM) bone scan
   D. MR
4. Common organisms associated with this entity in the adult population include all of the following, except:
   A. *Staphylococcus aureus*
   B. Salmonella spp.
   C. Escherichia coli
   D. Group B streptococci

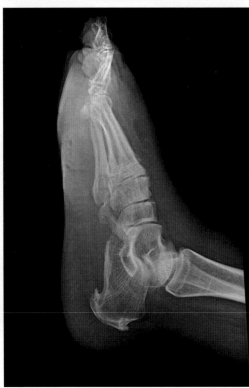

Fig. 63.1

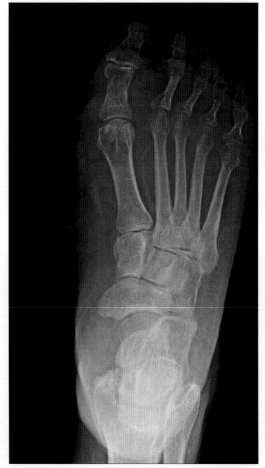

Fig. 63.2

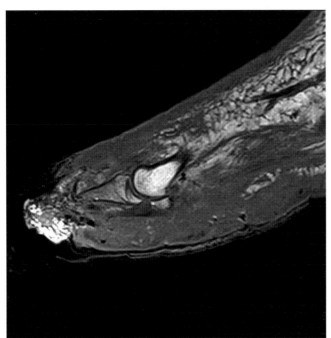

Fig. 63.3

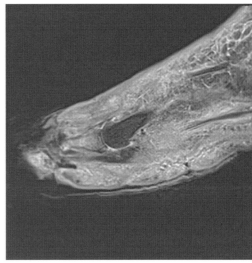

Fig. 63.4

Case 64

History: 40-year-old male presents to the ED with stomach pain radiating to his back, anorexia, nausea, and fever. He drinks often and has a family history of diabetes.

1. Which of the following would be included in the differential diagnosis for the imaging findings presented? (Choose all that apply.)
   A. Appendicitis
   B. Pancreatitis
   C. Hepatic abscess
   D. Abdominal aortic aneurysm
2. Which of the following is the most common cause of hepatic abscess in North America?
   A. Appendicitis
   B. Biliary disease
   C. Trauma
   D. Recent bowel surgery

3. Which of the following organisms are NOT commonly associated with hepatic abscess formation?
   A. *Escherichia coli*
   B. *Klebsiella* sp.
   C. *Entamoeba histolytica*
   D. *Shigella flexneri*
4. Which of the following is NOT a common risk factor for hepatic abscess formation?
   A. Smoking
   B. Diabetes
   C. Alcoholism
   D. Recent bowel surgery

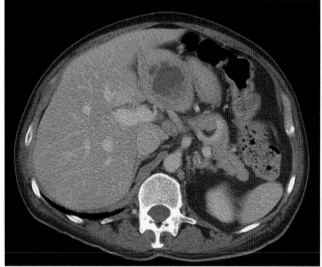

Fig. 64.1

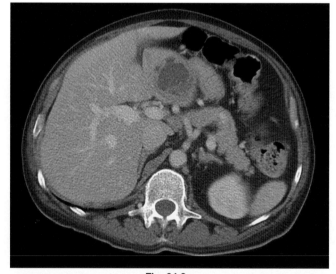

Fig. 64.2

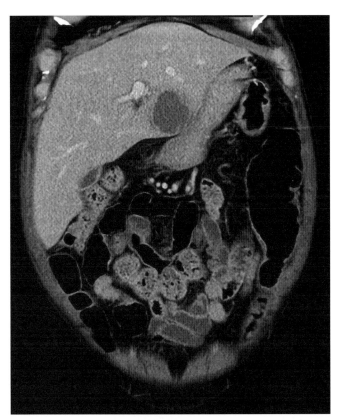

Fig. 64.3

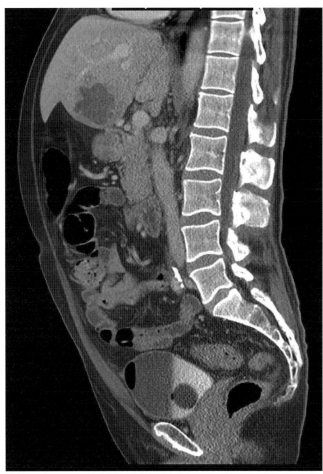

Fig. 64.4

Case 65

History: 36-year-old man with face pain.

1. Which of the following would be included in the differential diagnosis for the imaging findings presented? (Choose all that apply.)
   A. Periapical cyst
   B. Dental caries
   C. Tonsillar abscess
   D. Odontogenic abscess
2. Complications of this entity include:
   A. Osteomyelitis
   B. Meningitis
   C. Ludwig angina
   D. None of the above
3. If a diagnosis is suggested clinically, which modality is appropriate for evaluating potential complications?
   A. Radiography
   B. CT
   C. US
   D. MR
4. Management includes all of the following, except:
   A. Antibiotics
   B. Watchful waiting
   C. Drainage
   D. Surgical exploration

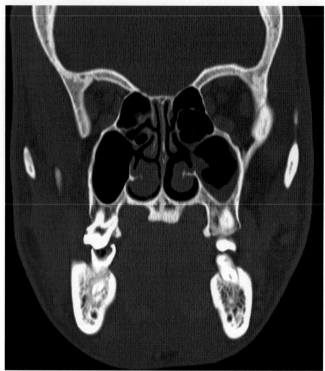

Fig. 65.2

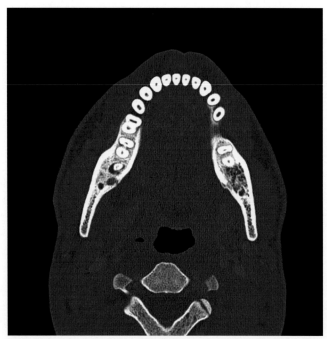

Fig. 65.1

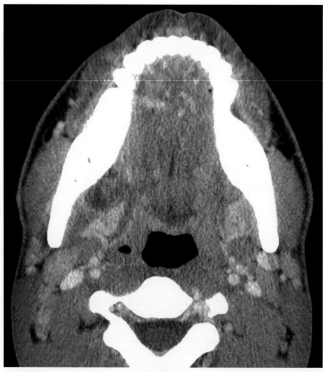

Fig. 65.3

Case 66

History: 49-year-old female presents with acute chest pain and blood pressure reading of 200/110.

1. Which of the following would be included in the differential diagnosis for the imaging findings presented? (Choose all that apply.)
   A. Acute aortic dissection
   B. Intramural hematoma
   C. Penetrating atherosclerotic ulcer
   D. Acute aortitis
2. Which of the following is the best CT protocol for the evaluation of acute aortic syndrome?
   A. CT of chest without contrast
   B. CT angiography (CTA) of chest without and with contrast
   C. CTA of chest without and CTA of chest and abdomen with IV contrast
   D. CTA of chest and abdomen without and with IV contrast

3. What is the most common cause of acute aortic syndrome (AAS)?
   A. Acute intramural hematoma (IMH)
   B. Aortic dissection (AD)
   C. Penetrating atherosclerotic ulcer (PAU)
   D. Hypertension
4. Which of the following is true regarding management of AAS?
   A. All cases require surgical or endovascular management.
   B. Can be managed medically using vasodilators and then IV beta blockade
   C. Can be managed medically using IV beta blockade and then vasodilators
   D. Surgical management only in Stanford type B aortic dissection and IMH

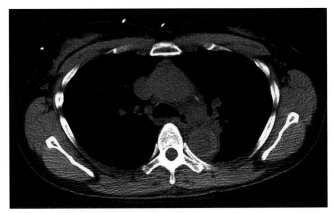

Fig. 66.1

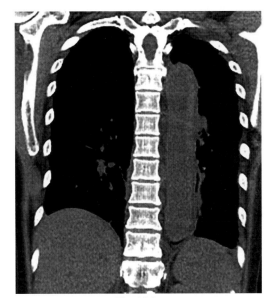

Fig. 66.2

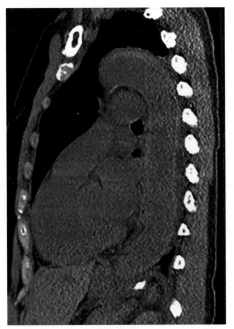

Fig. 66.3

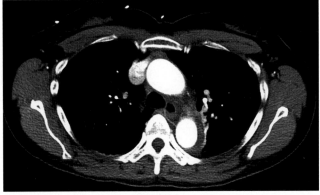

Fig. 66.4

Case 67

History: 27-year-old man in MVA.

1. Which of the following would be included in the differential diagnosis for the imaging findings presented? (Choose all that apply.)
   A. C2 instability
   B. C3 compression fracture
   C. Occipitocervical distraction
   D. Esophageal intubation with prevertebral swelling
2. These imaging findings are often associated with:
   A. Intubation in the field by EMS
   B. High-energy trauma
   C. Spondylosis
   D. None of the above

3. Which modality has diagnostic value in evaluating these patients?
   A. Radiography
   B. CT
   C. US
   D. MR
4. This injury is more common in adults than in children.
   A. True
   B. False

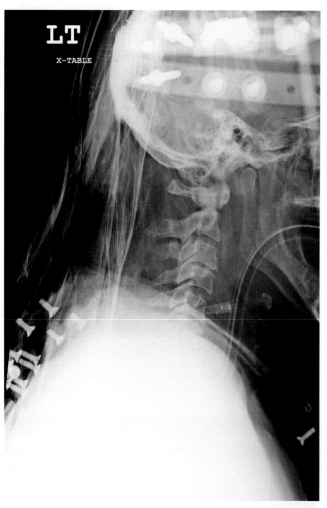

Fig. 67.1

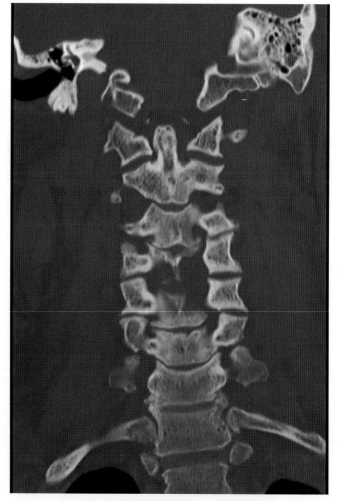

Fig. 67.2

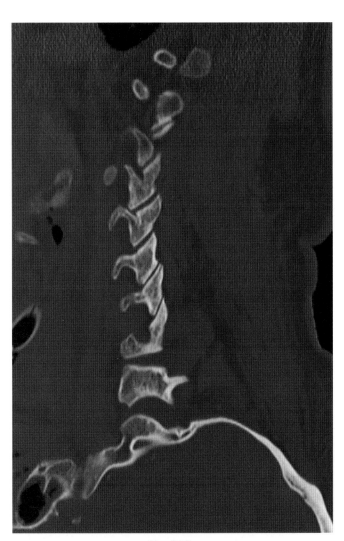

Fig. 67.3

Case 68

History: 45-year-old woman with neck pain after pharyngitis.

1. Which of the following would be included in the differential diagnosis for the imaging findings presented? (Choose all that apply.)
   A. Listhesis
   B. Odontoid fracture
   C. Grisel syndrome
   D. Mach effect
2. Which is the best imaging finding to suggest rotary fixation rather than torticollis?
   A. Reversal of the rotation of C1 on C2
   B. Shift of lateral mass and spinous process
   C. Asymmetry of the lateral masses
   D. Presence of anterolisthesis

3. An injury to the upper cervical spinal vertebrae (C1–C4) would NOT cause which of the following?
   A. Impairment or reduced ability to speak
   B. Difficulty breathing, coughing, controlling bladder, or bladder movements
   C. Paralysis in arms, legs, trunk, or hands
   D. Impairment in control of trunk muscles, but normal upper-body movement
4. Which of the following occurs in an atlanto-axial rotary fixation?
   A. C1 is not oriented in line with the head.
   B. Fracture to the C3 vertebra
   C. An excess of keratin sulphate secondary to a deficit in the degradation pathway
   D. The absence of one X chromosome (45XO)

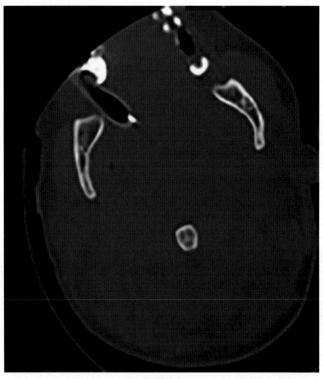

Fig. 68.1

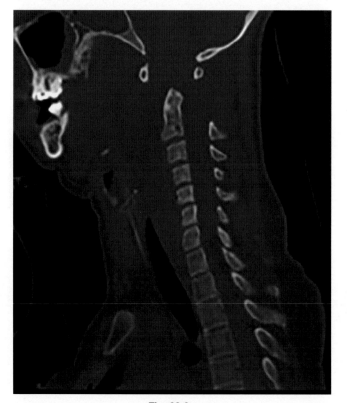

Fig. 68.2

Case 69

History: 23-year-old man with neck pain after an MVA.

1. Which of the following would be included in the differential diagnosis for the imaging findings presented? (Choose all that apply.)
   A. Muscle spasm
   B. Epiglottitis
   C. Dens fracture
   D. C2 pars interarticularis fracture
2. The mechanism of this injury is:
   A. Hyperextension
   B. Hyperflexion
   C. Axial loading
   D. Distraction

3. Which modality is commonly used as first-line imaging for this entity?
   A. Radiography
   B. CT
   C. US
   D. MR
4. Associations of this entity include?
   A. High rate of neurologic impairment
   B. Vertebral artery injury
   C. Suicidal hanging
   D. MVA

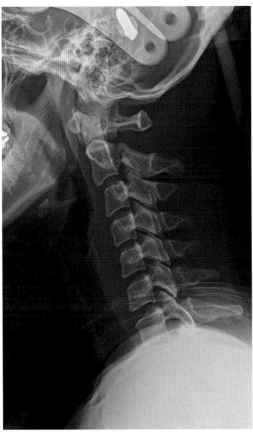

Fig. 69.1

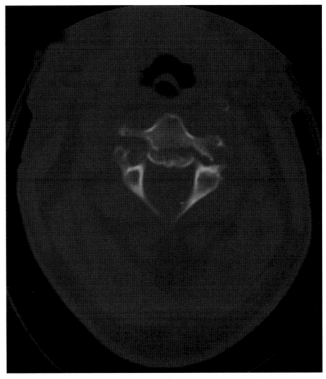

Fig. 69.2

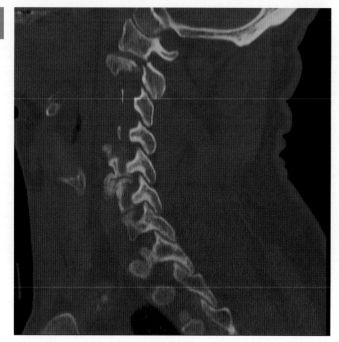

Fig. 69.3

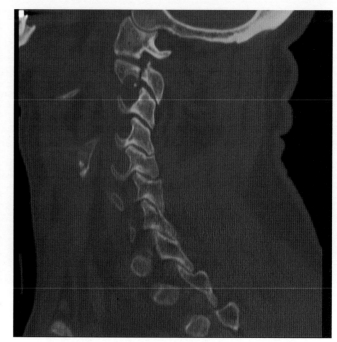

Fig. 69.4

Case 70

History: 37-year-old male with severe knee pain after falling on ice.

1. Which of the following would be included in the differential diagnosis for the imaging findings presented? (Choose all that apply.)
   A. Patellar tendon rupture
   B. Septic joint
   C. Lipohemarthrosis
   D. Synovial chondromatosis
2. Presence of a lipohemarthrosis is indicative of:
   A. Chronic degenerative joint disease
   B. Intraarticular fracture
   C. Foreign-body reaction
   D. Meniscal injury
3. Which of the following statements regarding lipohemarthrosis is most correct?
   A. May be seen on plain film, CT, and MRI
   B. Absence of a lipohemarthrosis excludes intraarticular fracture
   C. Best seen on weight-bearing views
   D. Is most frequently seen in the elbow
4. All of the following are true regarding lipohemarthrosis, except:
   A. A cross table lateral view best demonstrates a knee lipohemarthrosis.
   B. On CT and MRI, three layers may be seen.
   C. The presence of fat is related to escape of fat from the bone marrow.
   D. Size of the lipohemarthrosis correlates with severity of injury.

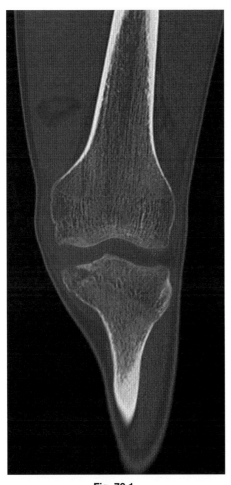

Fig. 70.1

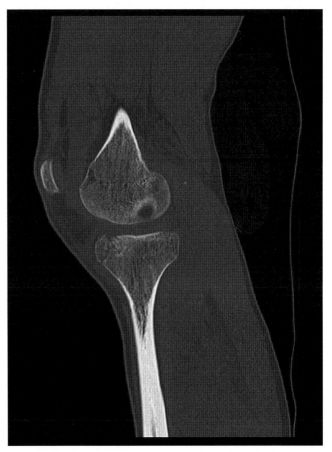

Fig. 70.2

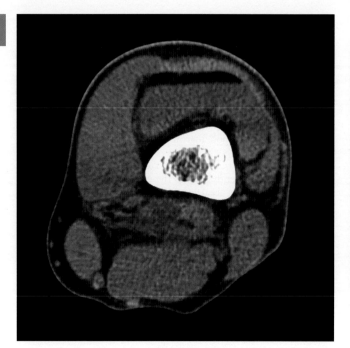

Fig. 70.3

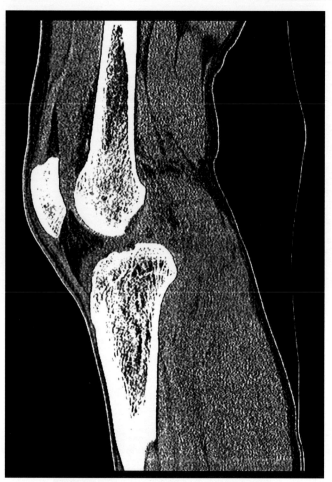

Fig. 70.4

Case 71

History: 24-year-old female status post MVA.

1. Which of the following would be included in the differential diagnosis of the imaging findings presented? (Choose all that apply.)
   A. Bilateral perched facets
   B. Unilateral facet dislocation
   C. Bilateral facet dislocation
   D. Disruption of discoligamentous complex (DLC)
2. The following is true for cervical facet dislocation, except:
   A. Unilateral facet dislocation is associated with neurologic deficits in 30% of patients.
   B. Unilateral facet dislocation results in usually greater than 25% anterior translation of the vertebral body relative to the one below.
   C. Unilateral facet dislocation results in usually less than 25% anterior translation of the vertebral body relative to the one below.
   D. Facet dislocations are associated with disruption of the DLC.
3. Morphology of this injury according to SLIC (sub-axial cervical spine injury classification system) classification is:
   A. Compression
   B. Burst
   C. Distraction
   D. Rotation-translation
4. SLIC classification includes the following parameter(s):
   A. Morphology
   B. Discoligamentous integrity
   C. Neurologic status
   D. All of the above

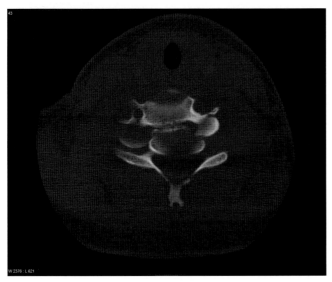

Fig. 71.1

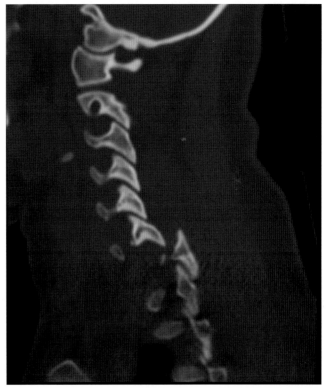

Fig. 71.2

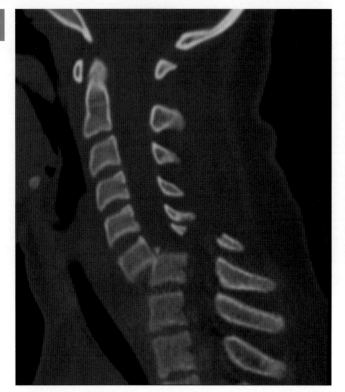

Fig. 71.3

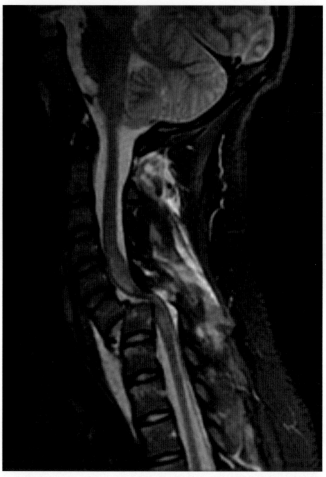

Fig. 70.4

Case 72

History: 54-year-old male with chest pain and violent coughing.

1. Which of the following would be included in the differential diagnosis of causes for the imaging findings presented? (Choose all that apply.)
   A. Pneumomediastinum
   B. Pneumothorax
   C. Pneumopericardium
   D. Subcutaneous emphysema
2. Which of the following would be included as causes for the imaging findings presented? (Choose all that apply.)
   A. Recent surgery
   B. Penetrating trauma
   C. Mechanical ventilation
   D. Vomiting

3. Which of the following are present in this case? (Choose all that apply).
   A. Tracheal foreign body with suspected perforation, pneumomediastinum, and subcutaneous emphysema
   B. Esophageal foreign body with suspected perforation, pneumomediastinum, and subcutaneous emphysema
   C. Normal esophagus
   D. Tension pneumothorax
4. Which is the most appropriate treatment plan for patients with this entity?
   A. Watchful waiting
   B. Endotracheal tube (ETT) placement
   C. Pleural catheter placement
   D. Removal of foreign body and treatment of any underlying injury

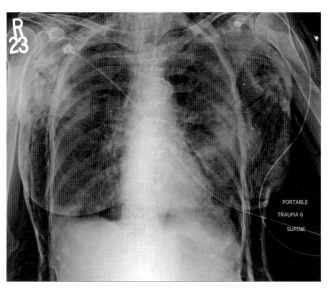

Fig. 72.1

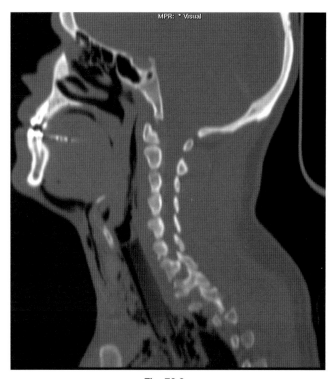

Fig. 72.2

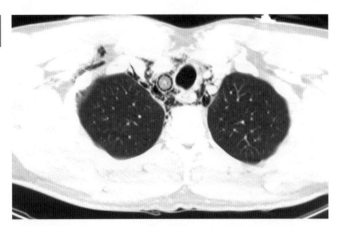

Fig. 72.3

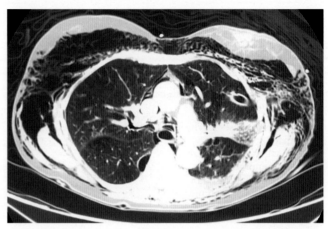

Fig. 72.4

Case 73

History: 23-year-old presents with shortness of breath (SOB) and coughing after sustaining a gunshot wound to the right upper chest.

1. Which of the following would be included in the differential diagnosis for the imaging findings presented? (Choose all that apply.)
   A. Aspiration pneumonia
   B. Atelectasis
   C. Pulmonary hemorrhage
   D. Pulmonary contusion
   E. Neoplasm
2. Which is the most appropriate imaging modality in evaluating a pulmonary contusion?
   A. Chest x-ray
   B. Ventilation-perfusion scan
   C. Chest CT
   D. US

3. Which is the most rapidly lethal untreated blunt chest injury?
   A. Pulmonary contusion
   B. Aortic injury
   C. Pneumothorax
   D. Cardiac contusion
4. Which is the ideal positioning of the ETT tube on chest radiography?
   A. 21 cm ETT tube insertion depth
   B. 23 cm ETT tube insertion depth
   C. At the carina
   D. 2 to 6 cm above the carina

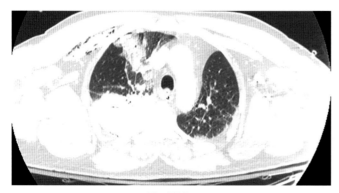

Fig. 73.1

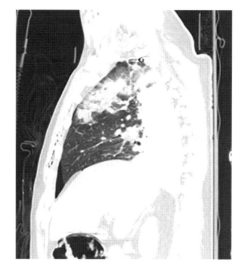

Fig. 73.3

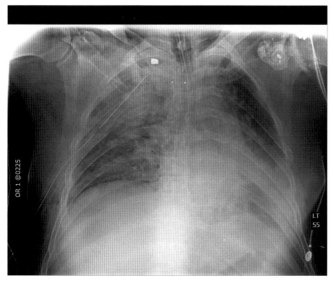

Fig. 73.2

Case 74

History: 21-year-old male with gunshot wound to the torso.

1. Which of the following would be included in the differential diagnosis for the imaging findings presented? (Choose all that apply.)
   A. Bochdalek hernia
   B. Diaphragmatic rupture
   C. Diaphragm eventration
   D. Aspiration
2. Which imaging sign of diaphragm is demonstrated?
   A. Dependent viscera sign
   B. Collar sign
   C. Hump sign
   D. Contiguous injury

3. Which imaging sign is the most sensitive direct sign for detecting diaphragmatic injury in blunt trauma?
   A. Intrathoracic herniation of viscera
   B. Collar sign
   C. Dependent viscera sign
   D. Discontinuity of the diaphragm
4. Which part of the diaphragm is most commonly injured in diaphragmatic injury?
   A. Central tendon
   B. Right hemidiaphragm
   C. Left hemidiaphragm
   D. Bilateral hemidiaphragms

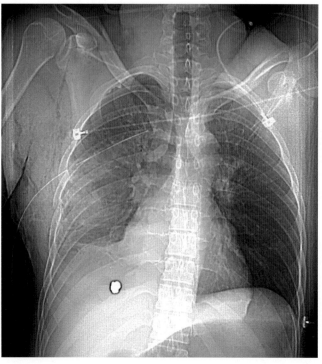

Fig. 74.1

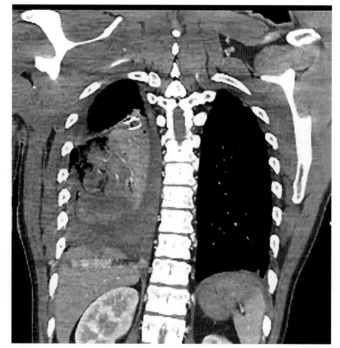

Fig. 74.2

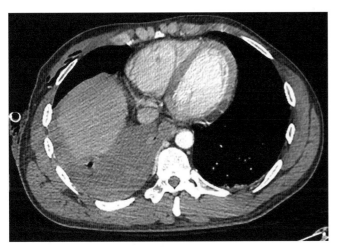

Fig. 74.2

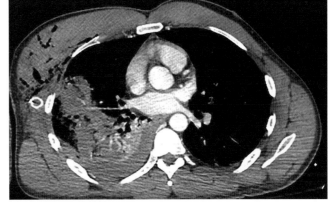

Fig. 74.4

Case 75

History: 20-year-old male presents with dysphagia.

1. Which of the following would be included in the differential diagnosis for the imaging findings presented? (Choose all that apply.)
   A. Mallory-Weiss tear
   B. Esophageal foreign body
   C. Tracheal foreign body
   D. Esophagitis
2. Which of the following presentations is an indication for emergency intervention?
   A. Chest pain
   B. Nausea and vomiting
   C. Hypersalivation and the inability to swallow saliva
   D. Dysphagia
3. At what level does esophageal foreign body impaction frequently occur?
   A. Cricopharyngeus muscle
   B. Aortic arch
   C. Left main bronchus
   D. Gastroesophageal junction
4. Which of the following is responsible for most of the esophageal impaction cases in adults?
   A. Coin
   B. Meat bolus
   C. Vinyl glove
   D. Plastic bread bag clip

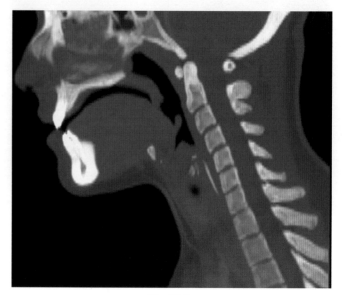

Fig. 75.2

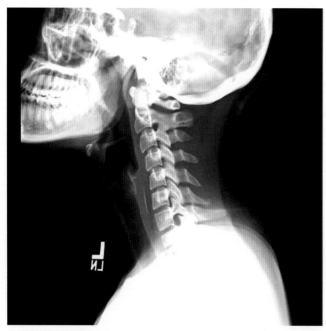

Fig. 75.1

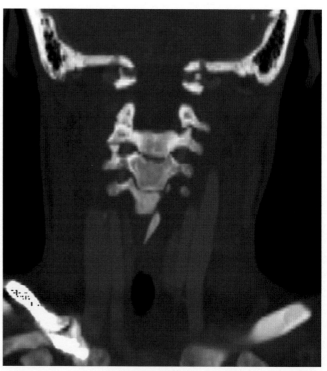

Fig. 75.3

Case 76

History: 45-year-old male presents with sudden onset of severe substernal chest pain following endoscopy.

1. Which of the following would be included in the differential diagnosis of the imaging findings presented? (Choose all that apply.)
   A. Esophageal diverticulum
   B. Esophageal perforation
   C. Tracheobronchial aspiration
   D. Boerhaave's syndrome
2. Which is the most common cause of esophageal perforation?
   A. Trauma
   B. Instrumentation
   C. Emesis
   D. Foreign body

3. Which of the following is true regarding imaging findings of esophageal perforation?
   A. Pneumomediastinum and subcutaneous gas can be seen on plain radiograph.
   B. Esophageal wall thickening can be an indirect imaging sign on CT.
   C. Fluid in mediastinum and pleural space is not uncommon.
   D. All of the above
4. What is the most common location of esophageal rupture in Boerhaave's syndrome?
   A. Cervical esophagus
   B. Mid/thoracic esophagus
   C. Right anterolateral distal esophagus
   D. Left anterolateral distal esophagus

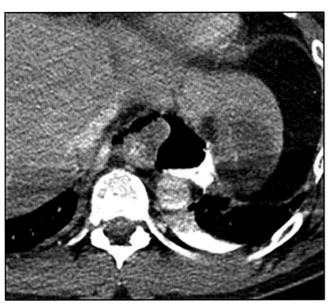

Fig. 76.1

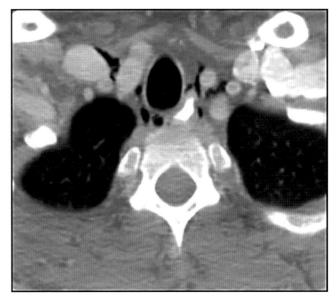

Fig. 76.2

Case 77

History: 65-year-old male who had fallen down.

1. Which of the following would be included in the differential diagnosis for the imaging findings presented? (Choose all that apply.)
   A. Pericardial effusion
   B. Pericardial rupture
   C. Cardiac tamponade
   D. Retrograde aortic dissection
2. Potential etiology of this diagnosis can include: (Choose all that apply.)
   A. Pneumopericardium
   B. Retrograde extension of aortic dissection
   C. Severe heart failure
   D. Uremic pericarditis

3. Which of the following has the greatest effect on patient presentation?
   A. Density of accumulated fluid
   B. Quantity or volume of accumulated fluid
   C. Rate of accumulated fluid
   D. Cardiac size
4. Administration of intravenous contrast in these patients during scanning may show:
   A. Increased risk of infiltration into the extremity
   B. Collateralization with flow seen through chest wall arterial vessels
   C. Reflux of contrast material into the inferior vena cava, internal jugular, or azygos vein
   D. Earlier than expected arterial opacification

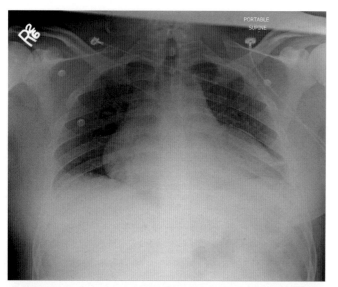

Fig. 77.1

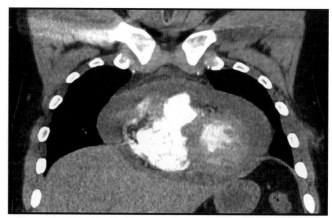

Fig. 77.3

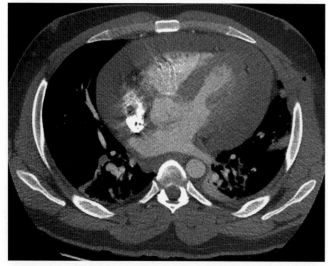

Fig. 77.2

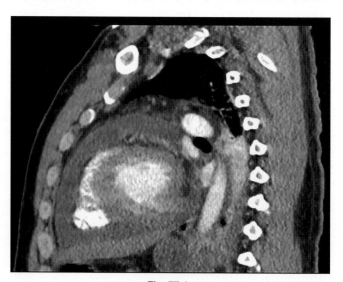

Fig. 77.4

Case 78

History: 33-year-old male who crashed car into a light pole and concrete wall.

1. Which of the following would be included in the differential diagnosis for the imaging findings presented? (Choose all that apply.)
   A. Acute traumatic aortic injury (ATAI) with aortic transection
   B. ATAI with aortic pseudoaneurysm
   C. ATAI involving the distal descending thoracic aorta with ductus diverticulum
   D. ATAI with active vascular extravasation
2. Which is the most common location for ATAI?
   A. Ascending thoracic aorta and aortic root
   B. Aortic arch
   C. Aortic isthmus
   D. Distal descending thoracic aorta at the diaphragmatic hiatus

3. The following are the direct CT signs of ATAI, except:
   A. Mediastinal hematoma
   B. Intimal flap
   C. Pseudoaneurysm
   D. Sudden change in aortic caliber—aortic pseudocoarctation
   E. Intraluminal thrombus
4. Which is the imaging modality of choice for ATAI?
   A. MRI chest with IV contrast
   B. Transesophageal echoaortography
   C. Multidetector computed tomography chest with IV contrast
   D. Conventional angiogram
   E. Intravascular ultrasound

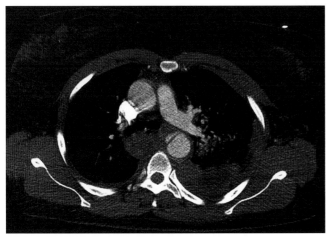

Fig. 78.1

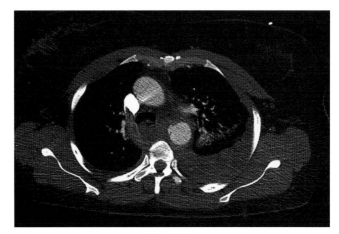

Fig. 78.2

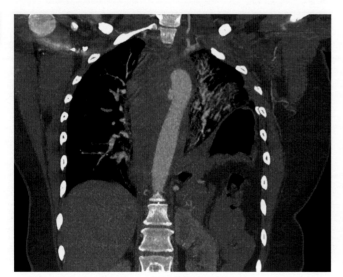

Fig. 78.3

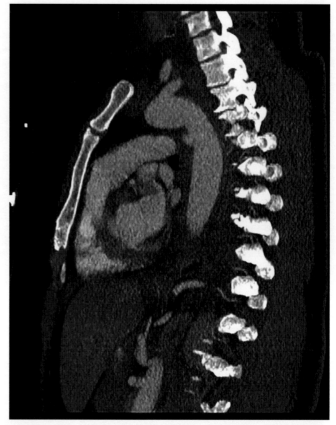

Fig. 78.4

Case 79

History: 73-year-old man with back pain.

1. Which of the following would be included in the differential diagnosis for the imaging findings presented? (Choose all that apply.)
   A. Muscle spasm
   B. Epiglottitis
   C. Dens fracture
   D. C2 pars interarticularis fracture
2. The mechanism of this injury is:
   A. Hyperextension
   B. Hyperflexion
   C. Axial loading
   D. Distraction

3. Which modality is commonly used as a first-line imaging modality for this entity?
   A. Radiography
   B. CT
   C. US
   D. MR
4. Associations of this entity include:
   A. High rate of neurologic impairment
   B. Vertebral artery injury
   C. Suicidal hanging
   D. MVA

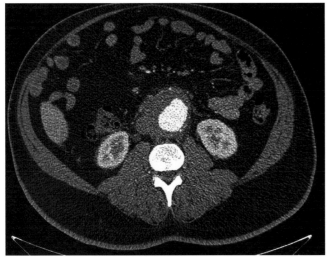

Fig. 79.1

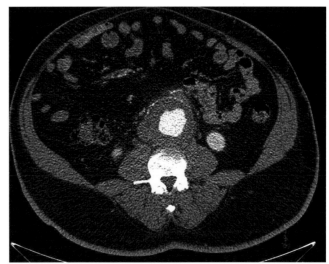

Fig. 79.2

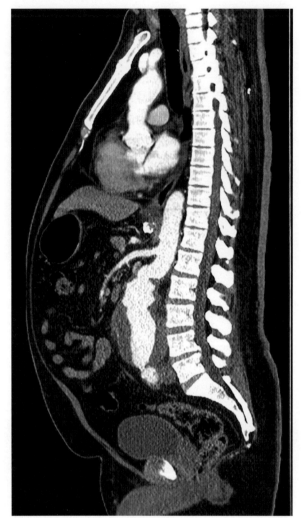

Fig. 79.3

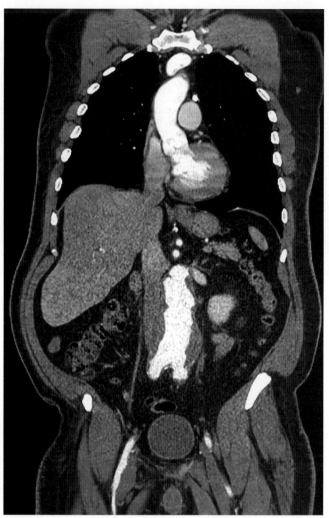

Fig. 79.4

Case 80

History: 23-year-old male with altered mental status brought to the ED by law enforcement.

1. Which of the following would be included in the differential diagnosis for the imaging findings presented? (Choose all that apply.)
   A. Complications of body packing
   B. Complications of nephrolithiasis
   C. Complications of cholecystectomy
   D. Complications of constipation
2. This finding is often associated with:
   A. Drug trafficking
   B. Poor diet
   C. Surgical error
   D. All of the above
3. Which modality is of limited diagnostic value in evaluating these patients?
   A. Clinical examination
   B. Radiography
   C. CT
   D. MR
4. Which of the following statements is true?
   A. Patients are often brought to the ED by law enforcement.
   B. Most patients are asymptomatic.
   C. Urinalysis may be positive.
   D. All of the above.

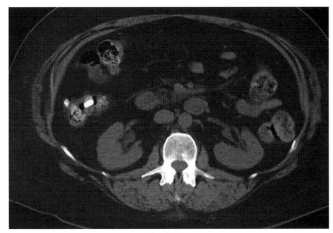

Fig. 80.1

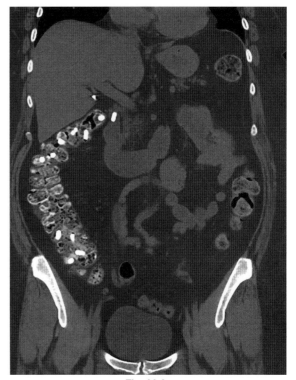

Fig. 80.2

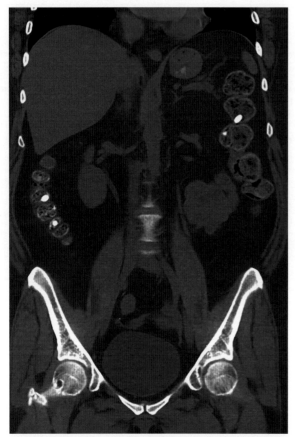

Fig. 80.3

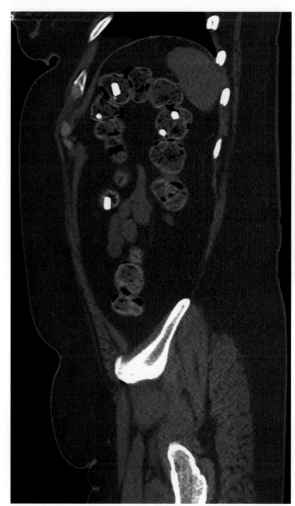

Fig. 80.4

Case 81

History: 35-year-old female presents to ED with right upper quadrant abdominal pain.

1. Which of the following findings would be included in the differential diagnosis of the imaging findings presented? (Choose all that apply.)
   A. Gallbladder sludge
   B. Acute cholecystitis
   C. Choledocholithiasis
   D. Intrahepatic biliary ductal dilatation
2. Which of the following is a known risk factor for primary choledocholithiasis?
   A. Obesity
   B. Crohn's disease
   C. Anatomic abnormalities of bile ducts
   D. Total parenteral nutrition

3. Magnetic resonance cholangiopancreatography is based on acquisition of which of the following sequences?
   A. T1-weighted images
   B. Post-contrast T1-weighted images
   C. T2 FLAIR
   D. Heavily T2-weighted images
4. Which of the following best describes Mirizzi syndrome?
   A. Fusiform dilatation of common bile duct
   B. Stone impacted within the cystic duct or Hartmann's pouch of the gallbladder causing extrinsic compression on the common hepatic duct
   C. Inflammation and obliterative fibrosis of intrahepatic and extrahepatic bile ducts
   D. Congenital dilatations of intrahepatic bile ducts with normal extrahepatic ducts

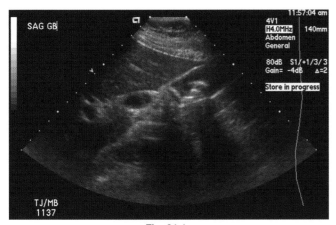

Fig. 81.1

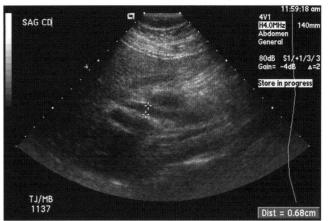

Fig. 81.3

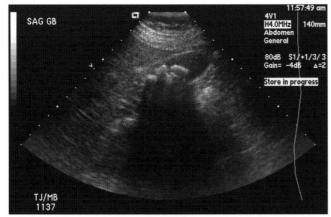

Fig. 81.2

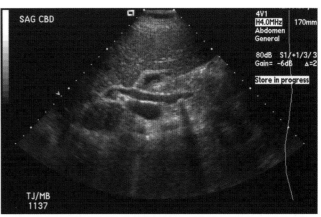

Fig. 81.4

Case 82

History: 33-year-old woman presents to ED with left flank pain and fever.

1. Which of the following findings would be included in the differential diagnosis of the imaging findings presented? (Choose all that apply.)
   A. Renal cell carcinoma
   B. Left hydronephrosis
   C. Right nephrolithiasis (staghorn stones)
   D. Renal abscess
2. Which of the following is the best possible diagnosis within the given clinical context?
   A. Renal cell carcinoma
   B. Renal abscess
   C. Multilocular cystic nephroma
   D. Oncocytoma

3. Which of the following renal lesions is usually hyperechoic on ultrasound?
   A. Renal abscess
   B. Renal cell carcinoma
   C. Angiomyolipoma
   D. Focal bacterial nephritis
4. Which of the following statements regarding urinary tract infection in adults is true?
   A. Renal parenchyma is the most common site of involvement.
   B. Routine radiologic imaging is essential for diagnosis and treatment of urinary tract infections.
   C. Patients with renal abscess can have a negative urine culture.
   D. When bacterial pyelonephritis is suspected, antibiotic therapy is started even before the collection of urine for culture and antibiotic sensitivity testing.

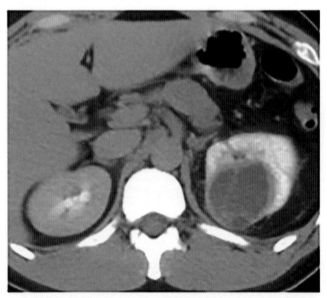

Fig. 82.1

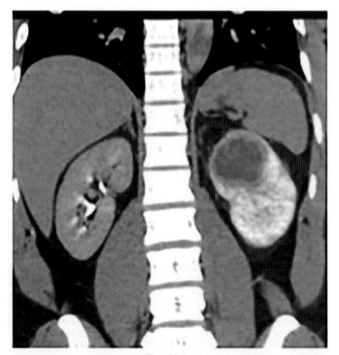

Fig. 82.2

118

Case 83

History: 59-year-old male with severe abdominal pain and history of appendectomy.

1. Which of the following would be included in the differential diagnosis for the imaging findings presented? (Choose all that apply.)
   A. Enteritis
   B. Ileus
   C. Closed loop small bowel obstruction
   D. Bowel ischemia/infarction
2. Portal venous gas may be distinguished from pneumobilia by its propensity to accumulate in the central hepatic parenchyma.
   A. True
   B. False

3. The preferred CT protocol includes use of both IV and positive oral contrast agents.
   A. True
   B. False
4. All of the following are true in the management of this entity, except:
   A. Surgical exploration and resection of necrotic bowel
   B. Anticoagulation
   C. Endoscopic decompression
   D. Possible thrombolysis

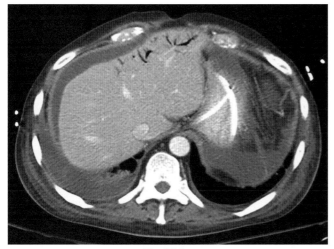

Fig. 83.1

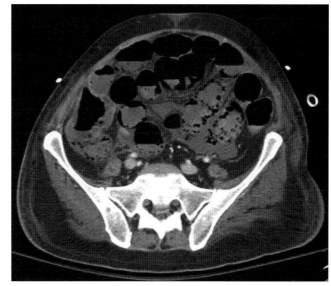

Fig. 83.3

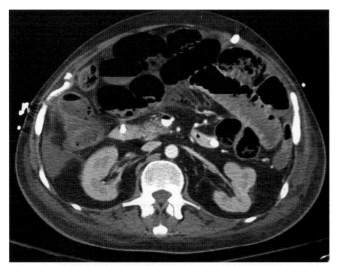

Fig. 83.2

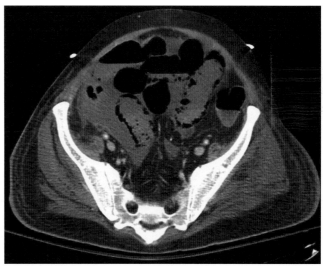

Fig. 83.4

Case 84

History: 37-year-old male presents with abdominal pain status post assault.

1. Which of the following would be included in the differential diagnosis for the imaging findings presented? (Choose all that apply.)
   A. Bowel contusion
   B. Shock bowel
   C. Colitis
   D. Penetrating bowel perforation
2. Which of the following is the least helpful CT signs in detecting bowel injury?
   A. Extraluminal contrast extravasation
   B. Extraluminal air
   C. Hemoperitoneum
   D. Bowel wall discontinuity
3. Which of the following is not true?
   A. Hematomas can occur in the intraperitoneal cavity, retroperitoneum, or both.
   B. Mesenteric stranding can occur without bowel perforation.
   C. Extraluminal contrast extravasation is not indicative of bowel perforation.
   D. The presence of ascites in intraparenchymal contusion raises suspicion of concomitant bowel injury.
4. Which is the most helpful imaging modality for the detection of bowel injury?
   A. MR
   B. CT
   C. US
   D. Radiography

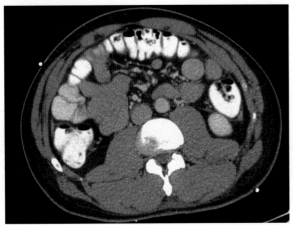

Fig. 84.1

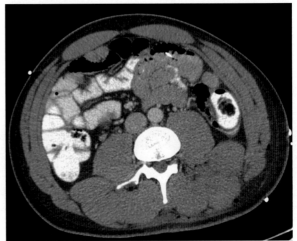

Fig. 84.3

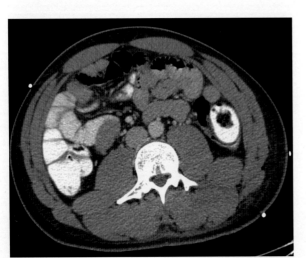

Fig. 84.2

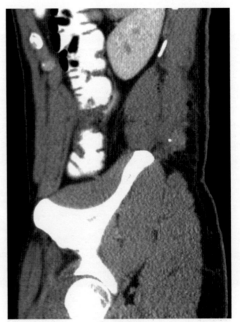

Fig. 84.4

Case 85

History: 30-year-old male treated in an outside hospital for diverticulitis, presents to ED with constant severe and sharp lower abdominal pain.

1. Which of the following would be included in the differential diagnosis for the imaging findings presented? (Choose all that apply.)
   A. Omental infarction
   B. Epiploic appendagitis
   C. Colitis
   D. Diverticulitis

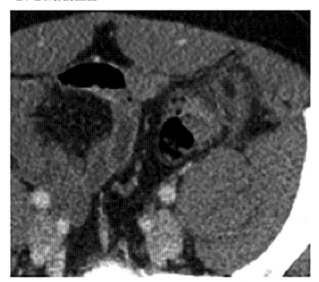

Fig. 85.1

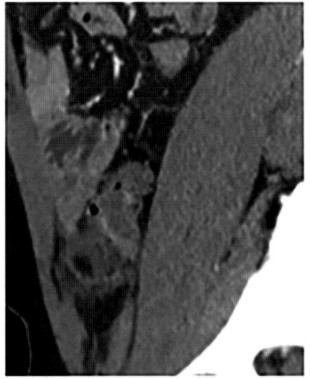

Fig. 85.2

2. Which of the following is true regarding CT finding of epiploic appendagitis?
   A. Often associated with acute diverticulitis
   B. Central hyperdense dot sign is essential for diagnosis.
   C. Colonic wall thickening is very frequent finding.
   D. Oval fat attenuation lesion that abuts the anterior colonic wall with thin enhancing rim surrounded by inflammatory changes

3. Which is most common location of epiploic appendagitis?
   A. Rectum
   B. Descending colon
   C. Ascending colon
   D. Sigmoid colon

4. Which of the following is true regarding acute epiploic appendagitis?
   A. Intestinal obstruction and abscess formation following epiploic appendagitis are common.
   B. Surgical resection is necessary in most cases.
   C. The condition is self-limited, and most patients recover with conservative management in less than 10 days.
   D. Acute epiploic appendagitis is more common in second and third decade of life and predominantly occurs in women.

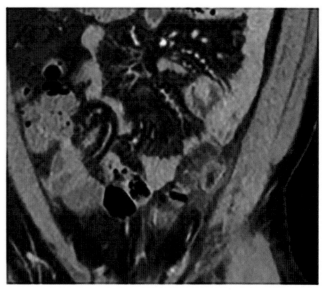

Fig. 85.3

Case 86

History: 64-year-old male with urinary retention.

1. Which of the following would be included in the differential diagnosis for the images presented? (Choose all that apply.)
   A. Bladder cancer
   B. Bladder hematoma
   C. Prostatomegaly
   D. Prostate cancer
2. Which additional finding(s) are of note?
   A. Atherosclerosis of the abdominal aortic aneurysm
   B. Misplacement of the urinary catheter
   C. Cardiac valvular calcification
   D. All of the above

3. Where is the catheter balloon inflated?
   A. Penile urethra
   B. Bulbar urethra
   C. Prostatic urethra
   D. Bladder
4. In the emergent setting, which additional imaging is warranted?
   A. Contrast CT
   B. Transrectal US
   C. Abdominal US
   D. MR pelvis
   E. None of the above

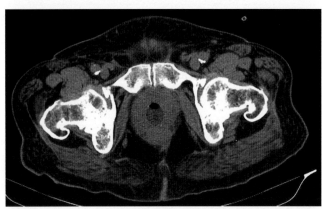

Fig. 86.1

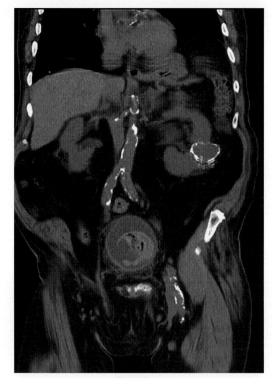

Fig. 86.2

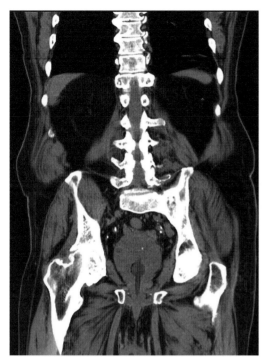

Fig. 86.3

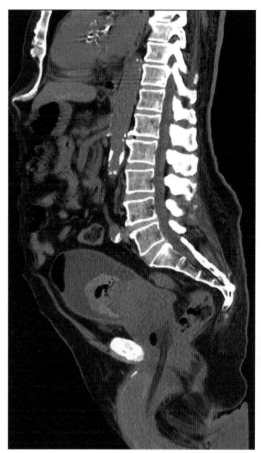

Fig. 86.4

Case 87

History: 34-year-old male presents to the ED via EMS after a fall down a flight of concrete steps.

1. Which of the following would be included in the differential diagnosis for the imaging findings presented? (Choose all that apply.)
   A. Splenic lymphoma
   B. Splenic infarction
   C. Splenic abscess
   D. Splenic laceration
2. There is a focus of high density within the splenic parenchyma. Which entities should be included in the differential for this finding?
   A. Pseudoaneurysm
   B. Active extravasation of contrast and acute hemorrhage
   C. Normally opacified splenic hilar vessel
   D. Traumatic arteriovenous fistula

3. Which of the following findings is not used for grading splenic trauma per the American Association for the Surgery of Trauma (AAST) scale?
   A. Length and number of lacerations
   B. Active extravasation of contrast
   C. Hilar vascular injury
   D. Subcapsular hematoma surface area
4. Which imaging finding predicts failure when using nonoperative management for blunt splenic trauma?
   A. Hemoperitoneum
   B. Splenic laceration (2 cm, grade II)
   C. Pseudoaneurysm
   D. Devascularized spleen

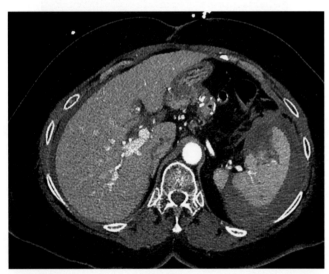

Fig. 87.1

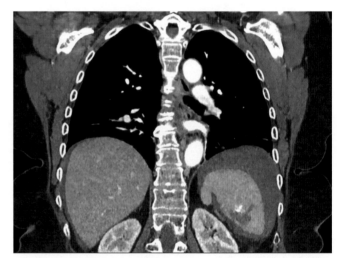

Fig. 87.3

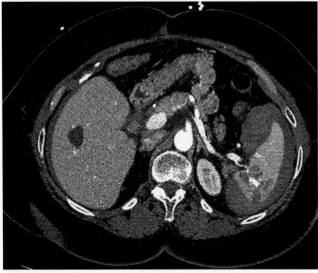

Fig. 87.2

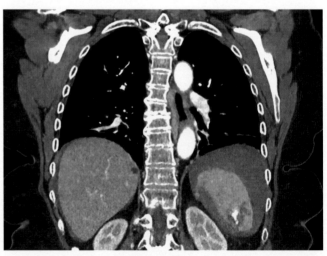

Fig. 87.4

Case 88

History: Unidentified, unrestrained passenger status post MVA.

1. Which of the following would be included in the differential diagnosis for the imaging findings presented? (Choose all that apply.)
   A. Renal laceration
   B. Liver laceration
   C. Traumatic renal artery dissection
   D. Urinoma
2. What is the next step in imaging this patient?
   A. Delayed imaging through the abdomen and pelvis
   B. Delayed imaging through the kidneys only
   C. Renal US
   D. No further imaging required

3. Based on the images provided, which is the correct AAST grade for the renal laceration?
   A. Grade 1
   B. Grade 2
   C. Grade 3
   D. Grade 4
4. What is the most common cause of renal injury?
   A. Penetrating trauma
   B. Iatrogenic injury
   C. Blunt abdominal trauma
   D. None of the above

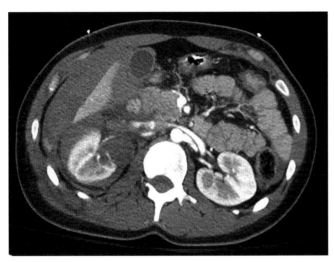

Fig. 88.1

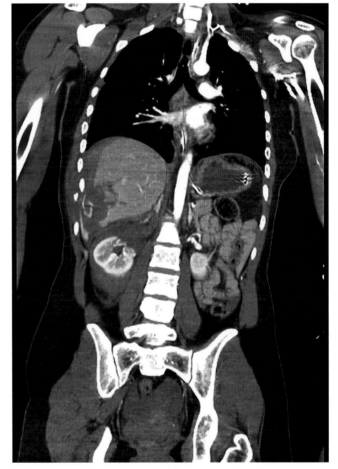

Fig. 88.2

Case 89

History: 12-year-old boy with upper abdominal pain after a bicycle accident.

1. Which of the following should be included in the differential diagnosis for the imaging findings presented? (Choose all that apply.)
   A. Pancreatitis
   B. Portal venous thrombosis
   C. Left renal vein thrombosis
   D. Pancreatic transection
2. Injury to this organ is one of the two most commonly injured organs in the setting of abdominal trauma.
   A. True
   B. False

3. This injury is associated with all of the following, except:
   A. Penetrating trauma
   B. Child abuse
   C. Endoscopy
   D. Bicycle handlebar injury
4. Delay in diagnosis may result in all of the following, except:
   A. Fistula
   B. Pancreatitis
   C. Abscess
   D. Pseudocyst
   E. All of the above may present as delayed complications of pancreatic injury.

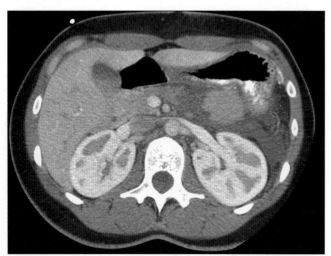

Fig. 89.1

Case 90

History: 42-year-old male on therapy for deep vein thrombosis presents to the ED with abdominal pain.

1. Which of the following would be included in the differential diagnosis for the imaging findings presented? (Choose all that apply.)
   A. Portal vein thrombosis
   B. Bilateral renal masses
   C. Bilateral adrenal hemorrhage
   D. Adrenal cortical carcinoma
2. Which is the most common cause of bilateral adrenal hemorrhage in adults?
   A. Trauma
   B. Primary adrenal lesions
   C. Anticoagulation therapy
   D. Stress
3. Which of the following conditions/lesions predispose to spontaneous adrenal hemorrhage?
   A. Waterhouse-Frederickson syndrome
   B. Pheochromocytoma
   C. Adrenocortical carcinoma
   D. All of the above

4. Which of the following statement is true regarding adrenal hemorrhage?
   A. Hypodense lesion in non enhanced CT (NECT) is diagnostic.
   B. More common in adults than in children or neonates
   C. Traumatic adrenal hemorrhage is often bilateral.
   D. Most cases of spontaneous adrenal hemorrhage are treated conservatively.

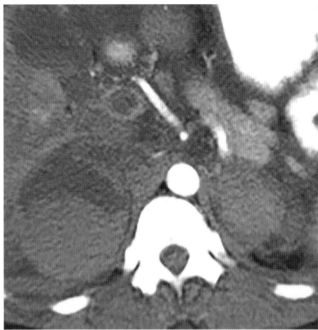

Fig. 90.2

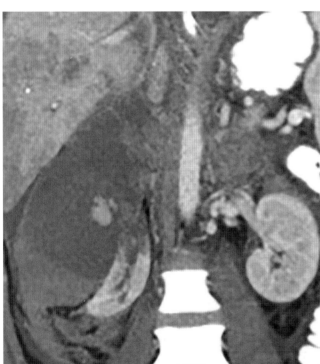

Fig. 90.1

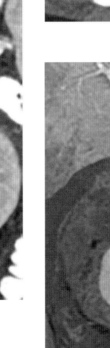

Fig. 90.3

Case 91

History: 21-year-old male in MVA.

1. Which of the following would be included in the differential diagnosis for the imaging findings presented? (Choose all that apply.)
   A. Bowel perforation
   B. Bladder rupture
   C. Aortic injury
   D. Renal collecting system injury
2. Which is the most common cause of urinary bladder rupture?
   A. MVAs
   B. Pelvic crush injuries
   C. Penetrating injury with knife or gunshot
   D. Fall from height

3. Which percentage of bladder rupture is associated with pelvic fracture?
   A. 20%
   B. 50%
   C. 80%
   D. 100%
4. Which injury is properly matched with its mechanism of injury?
   A. Intraperitoneal rupture: perforation by bone shards from pelvic fracture
   B. Intraperitoneal rupture: shear injury owing to distortion of pelvic ring
   C. Extraperitoneal rupture: shear injury owing to distortion of pelvic ring
   D. Extraperitoneal rupture: sudden rise in intravesical pressure

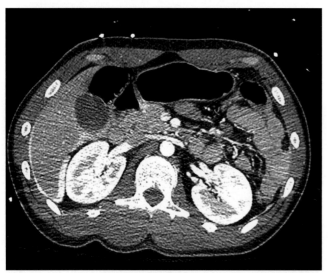

Fig. 91.1

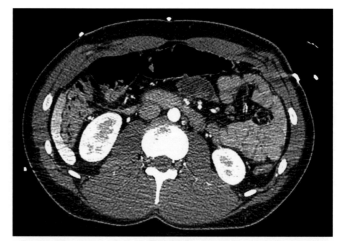

Fig. 91.2

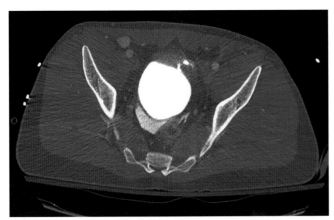

Fig. 91.3

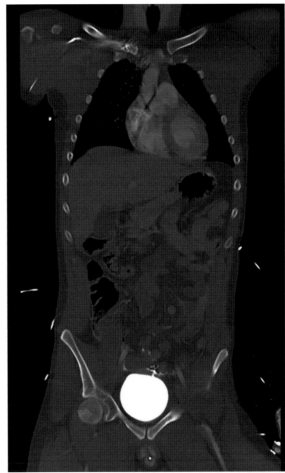

Fig. 91.4

Case 92

History: 42-year-old male pedestrian hit by an automobile.

1. Which of the following would be included in the differential diagnosis for the imaging findings presented? (Choose all that apply.)
   A. Intraperitoneal hemorrhage
   B. Retroperitoneal hemorrhage
   C. inferior vena cava (IVC) injury
   D. Abdominal aortic injury
2. According to the zonal anatomy from the surgical perspective, the presented images represent retroperitoneal hemorrhage predominantly involving which zone?
   A. Zone I
   B. Zone II
   C. Zone III
   D. All of the above
3. The most common location of IVC injury in blunt trauma is?
   A. Infrarenal IVC
   B. Retrohepatic IVC
   C. Junction of IVC and right atrium
   D. IVC bifurcation
4. According to the zonal anatomy from the surgical perspective, the most common location for retroperitoneal hemorrhage is:
   A. Zone I
   B. Zone II
   C. Zone III
   D. Zones I and II

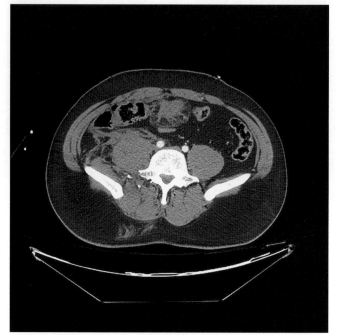

Fig. 92.2

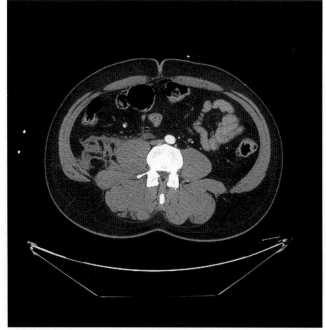

Fig. 92.1

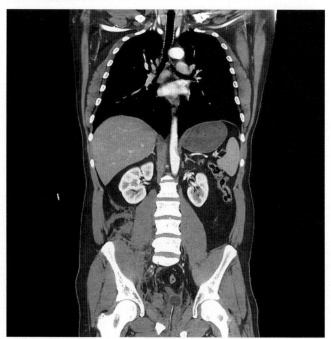

Fig. 92.3

Case 93

History: 68-year-old presents to the ED after a motor vehicle collision.

1. Which of the following would be included in the differential diagnosis for the imaging findings presented? (Choose all that apply.)
   A. Hyperflexion injury
   B. Compression fracture
   C. Hyperextension injury
   D. Burst fracture
2. What is the name of the sign demonstrated by the injury in this case, when viewed on axial CT images?
   A. Overriding facet sign
   B. Holdsworth sign
   C. Incomplete ring sign
   D. Naked facet sign

3. Which of the following is NOT a component of SLIC?
   A. Morphologic findings
   B. Posterior element integrity
   C. Neurologic status
   D. Discoligamentous integrity
4. Which injury has, by definition, greater than 50% of anterior translation of the cranial vertebral body with respect to the caudal vertebral body?
   A. Burst fracture
   B. Bilateral interfacetal dislocation
   C. Atlanto-axial rotatory fixation
   D. Unilateral interfacetal dislocation

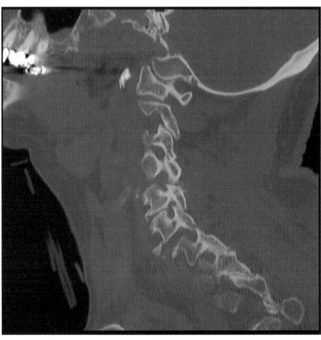

Fig. 93.1

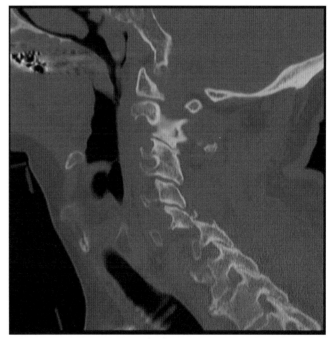

Fig. 93.2

Case 94

History: 58-year-old man with hypertension, headaches, and visual changes.

1. Which of the following would be included in the differential diagnosis for the imaging findings presented? (Choose all that apply.)
   A. Adrenal pheochromocytoma
   B. Adrenal carcinoma
   C. Adrenal metastasis
   D. Renal cell carcinoma
2. This lesion is always associated with hypertension.
   A. True
   B. False

3. The majority of cases of this entity are:
   A. Associated with multiple endocrine neoplasia type 2 (MEN II)
   B. Associated with known malignancy
   C. Sporadic
   D. Associated with hematuria
4. Which imaging modality is least likely to yield an accurate diagnosis?
   A. Radiography
   B. NM
   C. CT
   D. MR

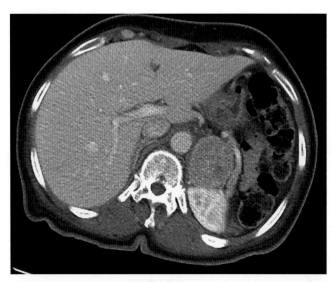

Fig. 94.1

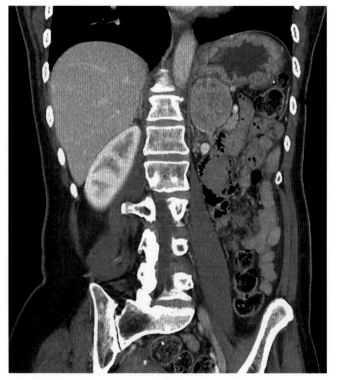

Fig. 94.2

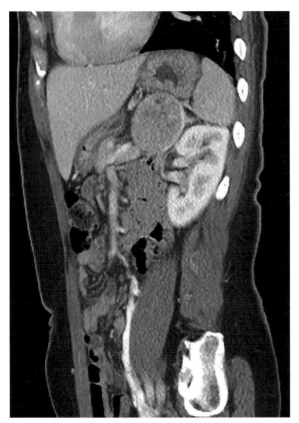

Fig. 94.3

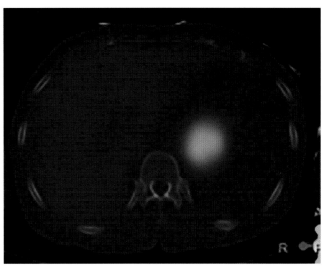

Fig. 94.4

Case 95

History: 53-year-old female with intermittent abdominal pain.

1. Which of the following would be included in the differential diagnosis for the imaging findings presented? (Choose all that apply.)
   A. Endometriosis
   B. Intestinal lipomatosis
   C. Adenocarcinoma
   D. Foreign body ingestion
2. This finding is often associated with:
   A. Intussusception
   B. Anemia
   C. No signs or symptoms
   D. All of the above

3. Which is the most common location for this entity?
   A. Esophagus
   B. Stomach
   C. Small intestine
   D. Colon
4. Which of the following statements is true?
   A. Gastrointestinal tract (GIT) lipomas are common.
   B. GIT lipomas most commonly occur in the young (age 20 to 40 years).
   C. The vast majority of GIT are submucosal.
   D. Local excision is warranted.

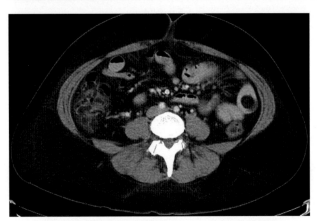

Fig. 95.1

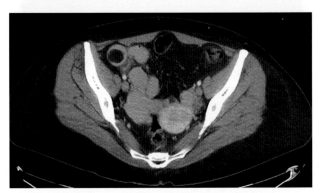

Fig. 95.2

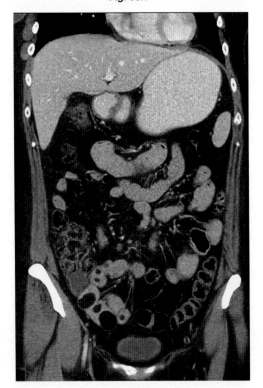

Fig. 95.3

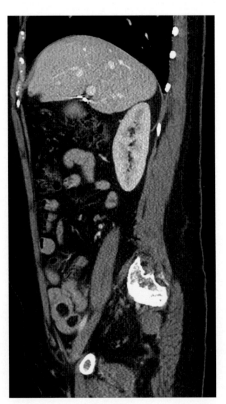

Fig. 95.4

Case 96

History: 19-year-old female presents with lower abdominal and pelvic pain.

1. Which of the following would be included in the differential diagnosis for the imaging findings presented? (Choose all that apply.)
   A. Ectopic pregnancy
   B. Pelvic inflammatory disease (PID)
   C. Urinary tract infection
   D. Interstitial cystitis
2. A pregnant woman is diagnosed with PID. Which clinical treatment course is most appropriate?
   A. Hospitalization with 1 to 2 days of oral antibiotic therapy
   B. A 14-day course of oral antibiotics with no need for hospitalization
   C. Hospitalization with oral antibiotic therapy for 14 days
   D. Hospitalization and IV therapy. Parental antibiotics should be used for 24 to 48 hours after clinical improvement. The patient can then be transitioned to oral antibiotics therapy for 14 days.

3. *Neisseria gonorrhoeae* antibiotic monotherapy is widely recommended.
   A. True
   B. False
4. A patient with longstanding PID has an acute onset of nausea and vomiting with accompanying severe, sharp pain in the right upper quadrant, especially over the area of the gallbladder. She describes her pain as pleuritic and extending into the right shoulder. Ultrasound shows "violin string" adhesions of the parietal peritoneum to the liver. From which complication is this patient suffering?
   A. Viral hepatitis
   B. Cholecystitis
   C. Fitz-Hugh-Curtis syndrome
   D. Pleurisy

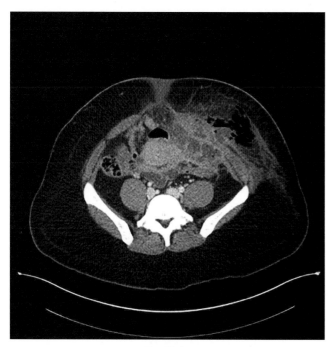

Fig. 96.1

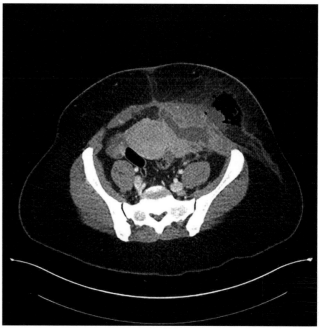

Fig. 96.2

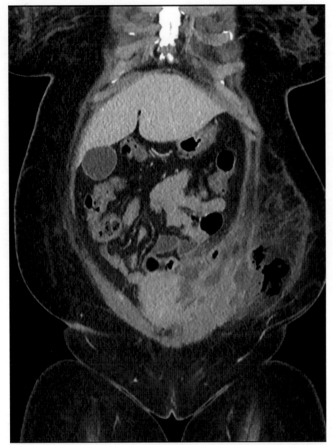

Fig. 96.3

Fig. 96.4

Case 97

History: 28-year-old female with mental status changes.

1. Which of the following would be included in the differential diagnosis for the imaging findings presented? (Choose all that apply.)
   A. Parafalcine hemorrhage
   B. Acute infarction
   C. Osteogenic tumor of the frontal bone
   D. Frontal lobe encephalomalacia
2. This finding is often associated with:
   A. Prior trauma
   B. Cerebrovascular incident
   C. Acute trauma
   D. Metastatic disease
3. The imaging findings are most likely:
   A. Acute
   B. Subacute
   C. Chronic
4. Which of the following statements is true?
   A. 20% to 30% of severe closed head injuries are associated with contusion.
   B. Cognitive decline may be seen in the long term.
   C. Brain herniation may be seen in the acute setting.
   D. All of the above

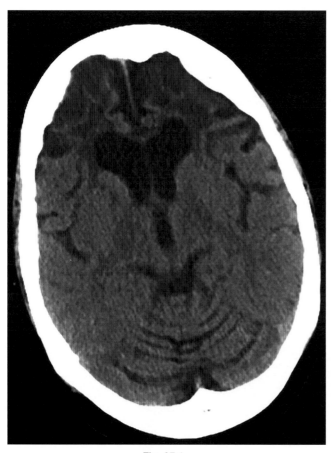

Fig. 97.1

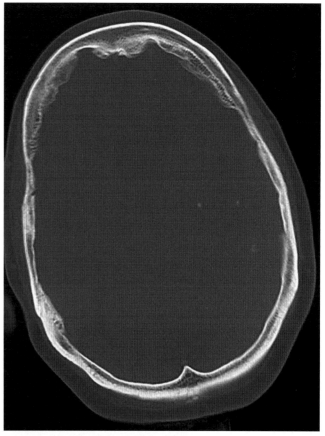

Fig. 97.2

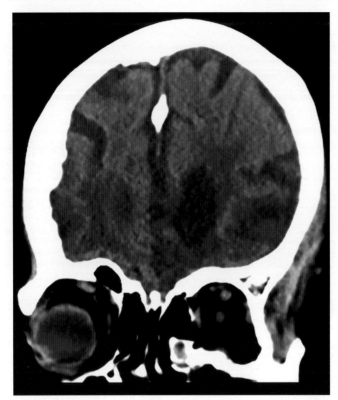

Fig. 97.3

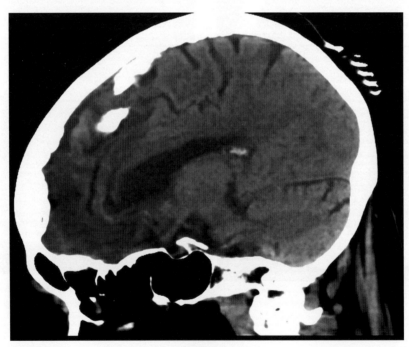

Fig. 97.4

Case 98

History: 58-year-old male smoker with difficult and painful swallowing. Rule out foreign body.

1. Which of the following would be included in the differential diagnosis for the imaging findings presented? (Choose all that apply.)
   A. Pharyngitis
   B. Uvulitis
   C. Tonsillitis
   D. Foreign body
2. This finding is often associated with:
   A. Bacterial infection
   B. Viral infection
   C. Fungal infection
   D. Allergic reaction
3. Primary diagnosis is made by:
   A. Clinical examination
   B. Radiography
   C. US
   D. CT
4. Which of the following statements is true?
   A. Critical findings of airway compromise should be relayed immediately to the clinical team.
   B. The abscess is easily drainable.
   C. Retropharyngeal extension is present.
   D. The epiglottis is involved.

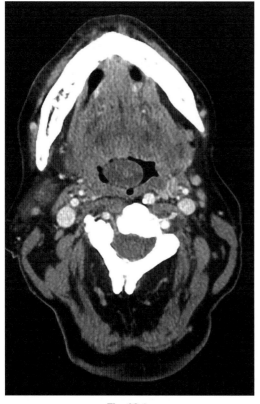

Fig. 98.1

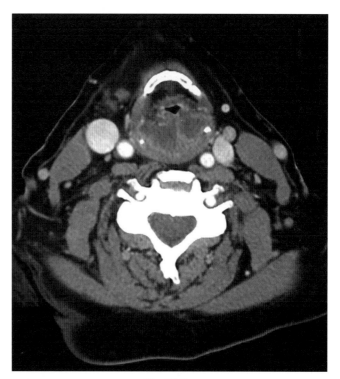

Fig. 98.2

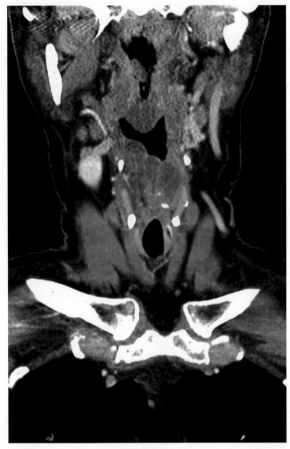

Fig. 98.3

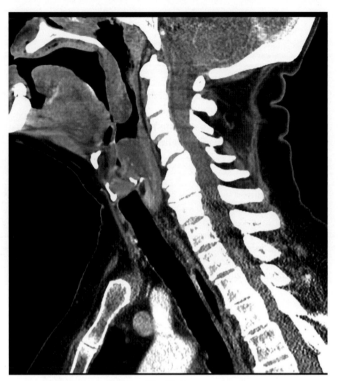

Fig. 98.4

Case 99

History: 32-year-old woman presents to the ED via EMS after a high-speed motor vehicle collision.

1. Which of the following would be included in the differential diagnosis for the imaging findings presented? (Choose all that apply.)
   A. Pregnancy
   B. Trauma
   C. Bladder extrophy
   D. Hyperthyroidism
2. If the patient is hemodynamically unstable, what is the next step in treating this patient?
   A. Retrograde urethrogram
   B. Catheter angiography and embolization
   C. CT
   D. Application of a pelvic binder

3. When classifying pelvic ring disruption based on the force to the pelvis, which force would best describe the resultant injuries seen?
   A. Lateral compression
   B. Combined mechanism
   C. Anteroposterior compression
   D. Vertical shear injury
4. In patients with pelvic ring disruption and macroscopic hematuria, which further imaging tests can be performed in immediate setting to evaluate for injury to the urinary tract? (Choose all that apply.)
   A. CT
   B. CT cystogram
   C. Urethrography
   D. All of the above

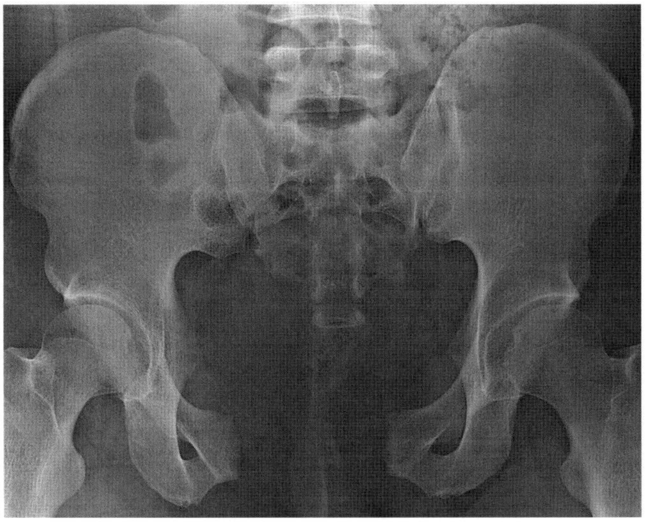

Fig. 99.1

Case 100

History: 32-year-old female who had severe chest pain during exercise.

1. Which of the following would be included in the differential diagnosis for the imaging findings presented? (Choose all that apply.)
   A. Anomalous origin of the right coronary artery
   B. High origin of the left coronary artery
   C. Anomalous origin of the left coronary artery
   D. Anomalous origin of the circumflex coronary artery
2. Which of the following course of this artery is considered to carry the highest risk of myocardial ischemia and sudden cardiac death?
   A. Septal
   B. Subpulmonic
   C. Interarterial
   D. Retroaortic

3. The most commonly seen anomalous course of the coronary arteries is:
   A. Right coronary artery arising from left coronary cusp
   B. Left coronary artery arising from right coronary cusp
   C. Left coronary artery arising from the main pulmonary trunk
   D. Left coronary artery arising from the noncoronary cusp
4. Which would be the recommended action for this diagnosis?
   A. Balloon angioplasty and stenting
   B. Beta-blockers and vasodilator therapy
   C. Bypass grafting or reimplantation
   D. Unroofing of the vessel

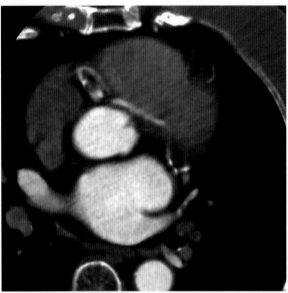

Fig. 100.1

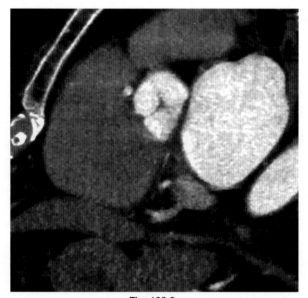

Fig. 100.2

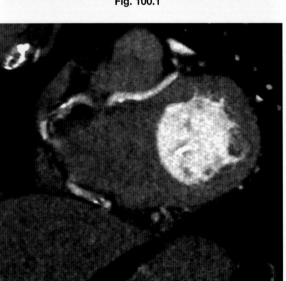

Fig. 100.3

Case 101

History: 35-year-old male presents with heel pain.

1. Which of the following would be included in the differential diagnosis for the imaging findings presented? (Choose all that apply.)
   A. Calcaneal spur
   B. Haglund deformity
   C. Calcaneal fracture
   D. Os calcaneus secundarius
2. Which of the following causes of heel pain has been associated with calcaneal spurs?
   A. Achilles tendinopathy
   B. Plantar fasciitis
   C. Tarsal tunnel syndrome
   D. Sever disease

3. On the lateral radiograph, what is the name of the angle formed by the intersection of the tangent to the superior edge of the calcaneal tuberosity and a line drawn between the highest points of the anterior process of the calcaneus and the posterior facet?
   A. Calcaneal inclination angle
   B. Lateral talocalcaneal angle
   C. Gissane angle
   D. Bohler angle
4. In the setting of a fall from a height, a calcaneal fracture should raise suspicion for which of the following injuries?
   A. Tibial fracture
   B. Lumbar spine fracture
   C. Pelvic fracture
   D. Femoral fracture

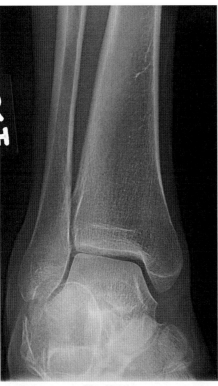

Fig. 101.1

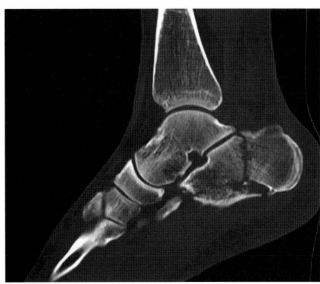

Fig. 101.3

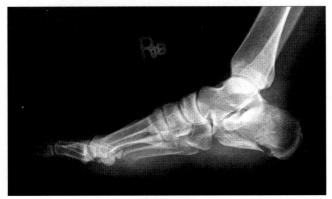

Fig. 101.2

Case 102

History: 34-year-old female with history of dilation and curettage (D&C) 3 weeks ago now presents with new heavy bleeding and the passage of four lemon-sized clots with accompanying cramping back and abdominal pain.

1. Which of the following would be included in the differential diagnosis for the imaging findings presented? (Choose all that apply.)
   A. Blood clot within the endometrial cavity
   B. Endometritis
   C. Retained products of conception (RPOC)
   D. Ectopic pregnancy
2. Which is the first-line imaging modality for suspected RPOC?
   A. Gray-scale/Doppler US
   B. MRI: T1, T2, T1 C+ (Gd)
   C. CT
   D. Positron emission tomography

3. The reported incidence of retained products of conception seems to depend on the gestational age of pregnancy. RPOC most frequently occur in:
   A. Second-trimester delivery
   B. First-trimester delivery
   C. Second-trimester termination of pregnancy
   D. Both A and C
4. The most sensitive finding of RPOC at gray-scale US is a thickened endometrial echo complex.
   A. True
   B. False

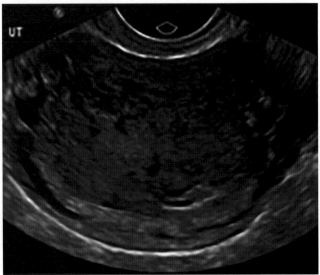

Fig. 102.1

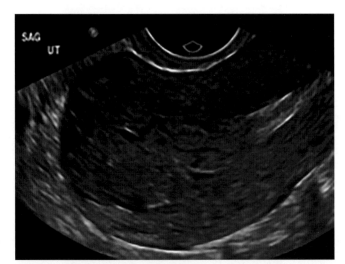

Fig. 102.2

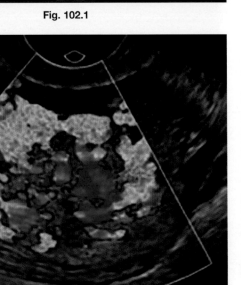

Fig. 102.3

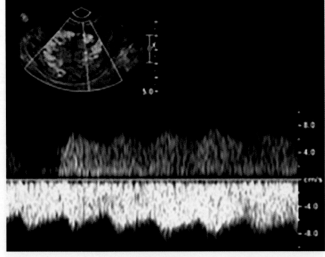

Fig. 102.4

Case 103

History: 55-year-old male, unrestrained, ejected passenger in MVA with facial instability on examination.

1. Which of the following would be included in the differential diagnosis for the imaging findings presented? (Choose all that apply.)
   A. intracranial hemorrhage (ICH)
   B. Le Fort I fracture
   C. Le Fort II fracture
   D. Le Fort III fracture
   E. Isolated zygomatic fracture
2. Which is the most common fracture of the mid-facial skeleton?
   A. Nasal bones
   B. Zygomatic arch
   C. Mandible
   D. Orbits

3. Tripod fractures of the zygoma most commonly involve:
   A. Orbital floor, body of zygoma, and lateral wall of maxilla
   B. Orbital floor, zygomaticofrontal suture, and medial wall of maxilla
   C. Orbital floor, zygomaticofrontal suture, posterior portion of the zygomatic arch, and lateral wall of maxilla
   D. Zygomatic arch, lateral wall of the maxilla, and greater wing of the sphenoid
4. Mandible fractures generally occur after a blow to the mandibular body. Which is the most common location of a mandible fracture?
   A. Through the parasymphyseal area or mental foramen area on the side of the blow and angle or subcondylar fracture on opposite side
   B. Parasymphyseal fracture
   C. Bilateral condylar fractures
   D. Dental socket

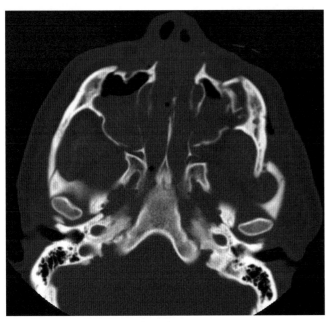

Fig. 103.1

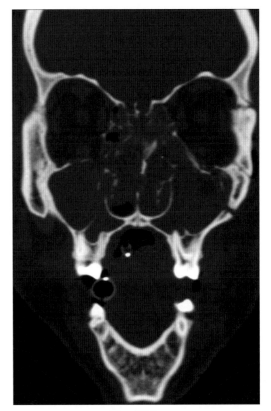

Fig. 103.2

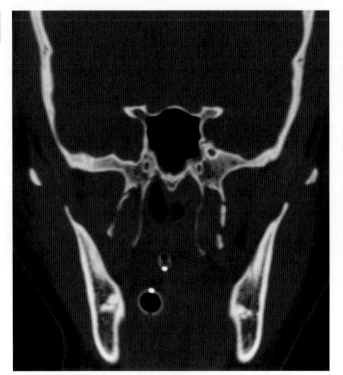

Fig. 103.3

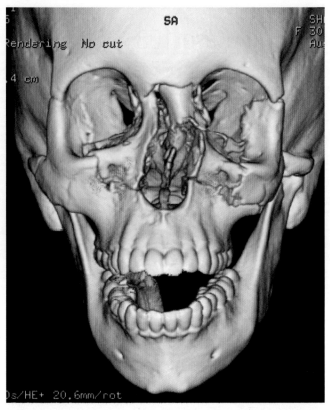

Fig. 103.4

Case 104

History: 50-year-old female with altered mental status.

1. Which of the following would be included in the differential diagnosis for the imaging findings presented? (Choose all that apply.)
   A. Elevated hematocrit
   B. Hyperdense middle cerebral artery (MCA) with acute stroke
   C. Contrast administration
   D. Calcified atherosclerotic plaques

2. Which is the earliest CT finding in acute ischemic stroke?
   A. Loss of gray-white differentiation
   B. Insular ribbon sign
   C. Hyperdense MCA sign
   D. Gyral swelling

3. Assuming that prerequisite criteria are met, which is the recommended definitive treatment for acute proximal MCA (M1) thrombus when there are no contraindications?
   A. Aspirin
   B. Heparin administration
   C. Intravenous tissue plasminogen activator
   D. Endovascular clot retrieval

4. To what does the "dot sign" refer?
   A. Thrombus of an M2 branch in the Sylvian fissure
   B. Hyperenhancing focus on CTA in intracranial hemorrhage
   C. Dense material near a presumed site of hemorrhage
   D. A typical appearance of neurocysticercosis

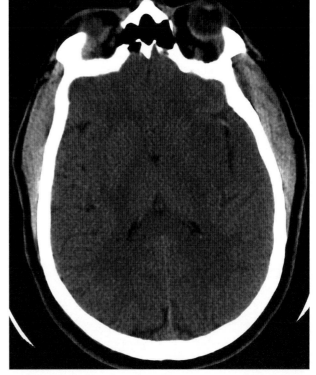

Fig. 104.2

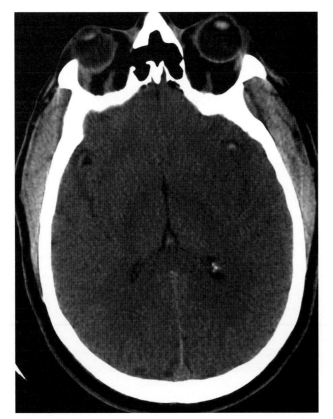

Fig. 104.1

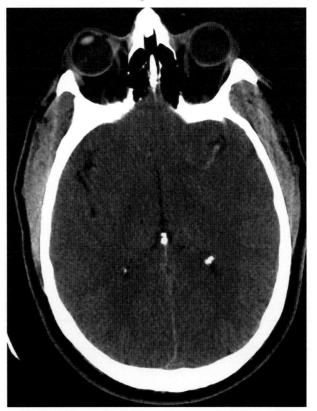

Fig. 104.3

Case 105

History: 19-year-old male status post MVA.

1. Which of the following would be included in the differential diagnosis for the images presented? (Choose all that apply.)
   A. Extraperitoneal urinary contrast extravasation
   B. Intraperitoneal urinary contrast extravasation
   C. Abnormal position of the Foley bulb
   D. Urethral injury
   E. Bladder neck injury
2. The retrograde urethrogram (RUG) image demonstrates urethral injury to:
   A. Penile urethra
   B. Bulbar urethra
   C. Posterior urethra with contrast extravasation above the urogenital diaphragm
   D. Posterior urethra with contrast extravasation below the urogenital diaphragm

3. The following statements are true regarding urethral injuries except:
   A. Posterior urethral injuries are commonly associated with pelvic fractures.
   B. Most common cause of anterior urethral injury is straddle injury.
   C. Posterior urethral injuries are more common than anterior urethral injuries.
   D. Anterior urethral injuries are more common than posterior urethral injuries.
4. According to the unified classification proposed by Goldman et al., the RUG findings are consistent with what type of urethral injury?
   A. Type I
   B. Type II
   C. Type III
   D. Type IV
   E. Type V

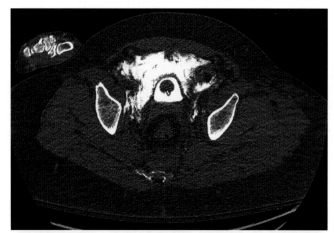

Fig. 105.1

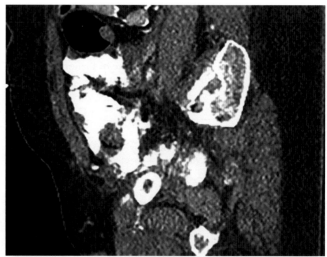

Fig. 105.3

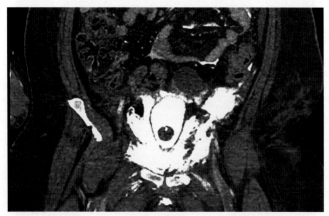

Fig. 105.2

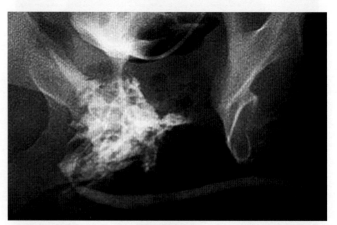

Fig. 105.4

Case 106

History: 32-year-old with palpable neck mass.

1. Which of the following would be included in the differential diagnosis given the imaging findings presented? (Choose all that apply.)
   A. Necrotic lymph node
   B. Ranula
   C. Abscess
   D. Thyroglossal duct cyst
2. The plunging types of this entity extend into which space?
   A. Sublingual space
   B. Retropharyngeal space
   C. Submandibular space
   D. Oral cavity

3. Which of the following statements is true?
   A. Uncomplicated ranulas appear as thick-walled cystic lesions with central low attenuating fluid.
   B. Infected ranulas may contain hyperattenuating central fluid and may occasionally resemble a nonenhancing soft-tissue mass.
   C. Ranulas result from obstruction of the submandibular gland.
   D. Incision and drainage is a commonly accepted treatment.
4. Evaluation with magnetic resonance (MR) should include gadolinium administration.
   A. True
   B. False

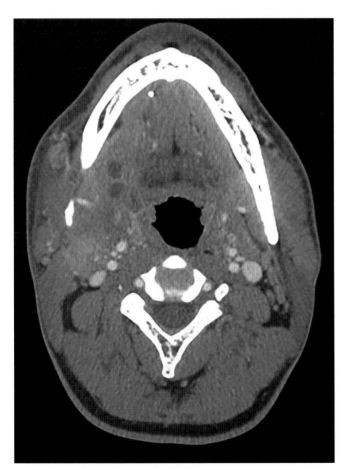

Fig. 106.1

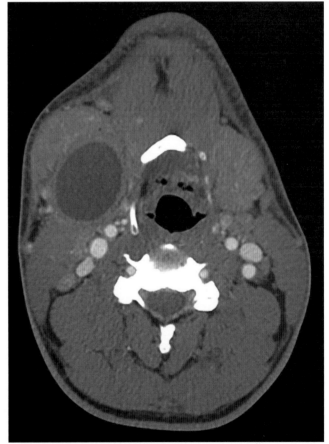

Fig. 106.2

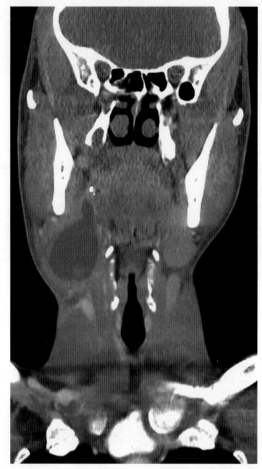

Fig. 106.3

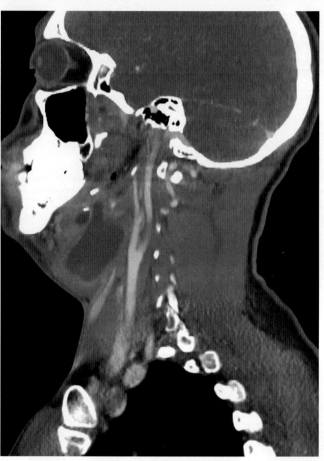

Fig. 106.4

Case 107

History: 34-year-old woman with facial pain and mild swelling. Symptoms began after dinner.

1. Which of the following would be included in the differential diagnosis for the images presented? (Choose all that apply.)
   A. Sjogren's syndrome
   B. Sarcoidosis
   C. Sialadenosis
   D. Sialadenitis
2. Bacterial sialadenitis is commonly caused by:
   A. *Escherichia coli*
   B. *Staphylococcus aureus*
   C. *Streptococcus viridans*
   D. *Streptococcus salivarius*

3. Which location is the most common location of obstructive sialadenitis?
   A. Accessory salivary ducts
   B. Parotid ducts
   C. Submandibular ducts
   D. Sublingual ducts
4. Epidemic parotitis is associated with which disease?
   A. Measles
   B. Rubella
   C. Diphtheria
   D. Mumps

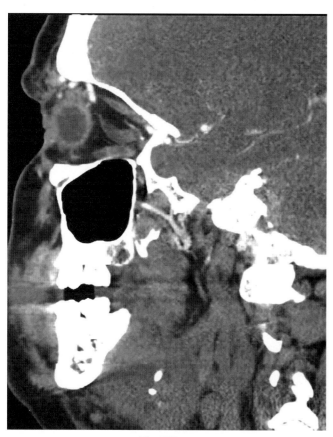

Fig. 107.1

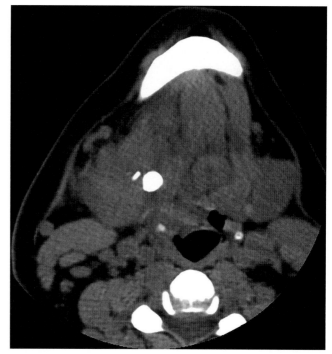

Fig. 107.2

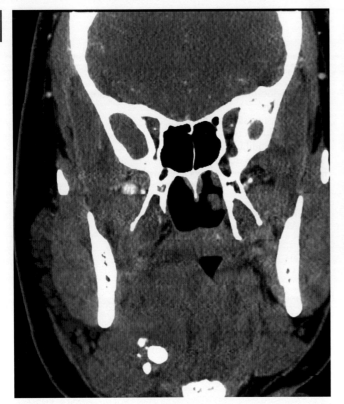

Fig. 107.3

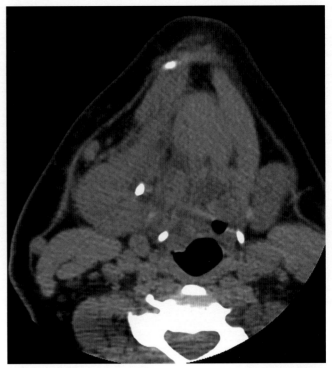

Fig. 107.4

Case 108

History: 42-year-old man with fever, facial pain, and mild swelling.

1. Which of the following would be included in the differential diagnosis for the images presented? (Choose all that apply.)
   A. Necrotic lymph node
   B. Ludwig angina
   C. Sialadenosis
   D. Sialadenitis
2. Ludwig angina is commonly caused by:
   A. *E. coli*
   B. *Staphylococcus* sp.
   C. *Streptococcus* sp.
   D. *Bacteroides* sp.

3. Which locations can be involved?
   A. Submandibular space
   B. Sublingual space
   C. Submental space
   D. Retropharyngeal space
4. Most cases of Ludwig angina are associated with:
   A. Sialadenitis
   B. Epiglottitis
   C. Odontogenic infection
   D. Penetrating trauma

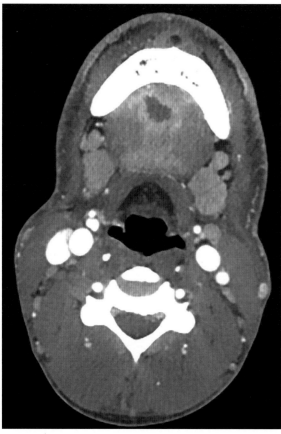

Fig. 108.1

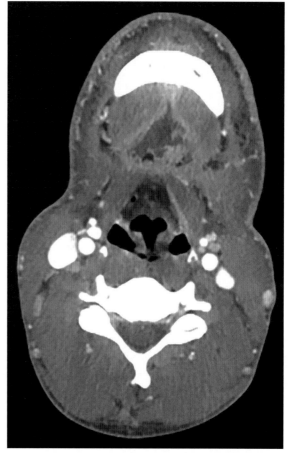

Fig. 108.2

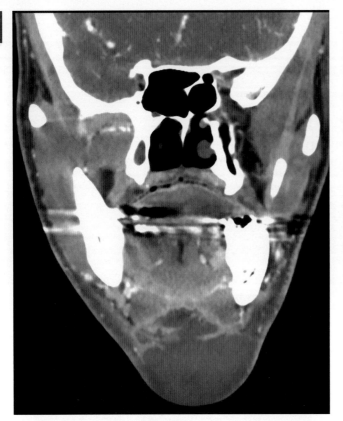

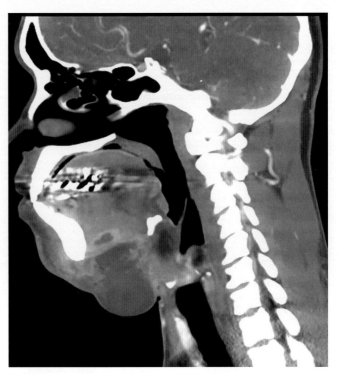

Fig. 108.4

Fig. 108.3

Case 109

History: 19-year-old man with fever, facial pain, neck swelling.

1. Which of the following would be included in the differential diagnosis for the images presented? (Choose all that apply.)
   A. Necrotic lymph node
   B. Ludwig angina
   C. Lemierre syndrome
   D. Sialadenitis
2. Distant septic emboli are most commonly noted in the:
   A. Lungs
   B. Liver
   C. Hips
   D. Brain

3. Which bacteria are commonly associated with this entity?
   A. *S. aureus*
   B. *Fusobacterium necrophorum*
   C. *Streptococcus* sp.
   D. *E. coli*
4. This entity is associated with tonsillitis with or without abscess.
   A. True
   B. False

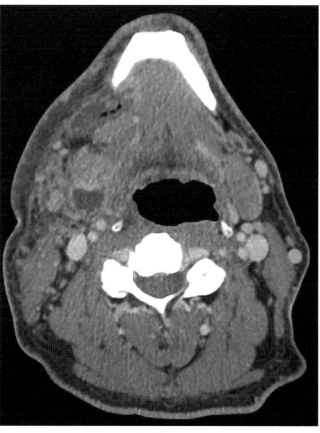

Fig. 109.1

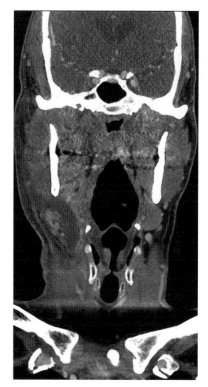

Fig. 109.2

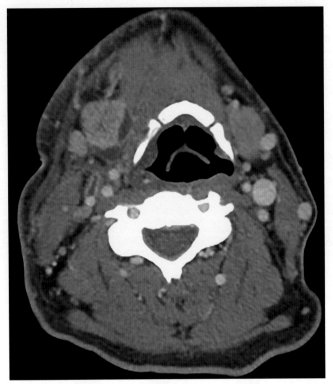

Fig. 109.3

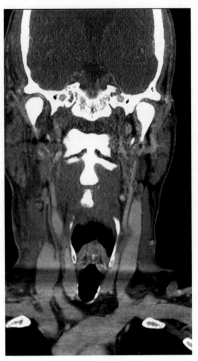

Fig. 109.4

Case 110

History: 53-year-old female with eye pain.

1. Which of the following would be included in the differential diagnosis for the imaging findings presented? (Choose all that apply.)
   A. Lymphoproliferative lesions
   B. Sarcoidosis
   C. Orbital cellulitis
   D. Glaucoma
2. Which of the following finding best indicates an orbital pseudotumor?
   A. Uveal involvement
   B. Bone damage and intracranial extension
   C. Poorly marginated, mass-like enhancing soft tissue involving any area of the orbit
   D. A focal intraorbital mass

3. Which of the following is a typical presentation for individuals affected with orbital pseudotumor?
   A. Sudden, painful proptosis, redness, and edema
   B. Inflammation, fibrosis, and blindness
   C. Nausea, headaches, and difficulty breathing
   D. Macular edema, arteritis, and headaches
4. Which of the following is NOT indicative of exophthalmos?
   A. Optic nerve dysfunction
   B. Proptosis
   C. Inflammation, redness, or irritation
   D. Refractive errors

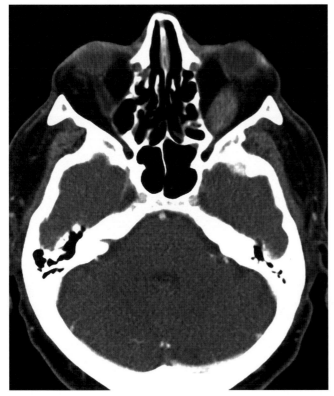

Fig. 110.1

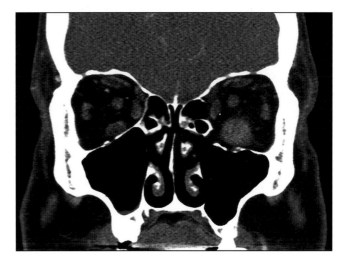

Fig. 110.2

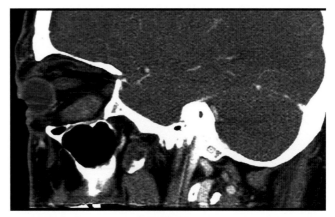

Fig. 110.3

Case 111

History: 67-year-old male with claudication.

1. Which of the following would be included in the differential diagnosis for the imaging findings presented? (Choose all that apply.)
   A. Atherosclerosis
   B. High-grade stenosis of the popliteal artery
   C. Duplicated femoral arteries
   D. Thrombosis of the fem-fem bypass graft

2. Which of the following is the age-adjusted prevalence of peripheral arterial disease (PAD)?
   A. 5%
   B. 8%
   C. 10%
   D. 12%

3. Which of the following is a risk factor for PAD?
   A. Diabetes
   B. Smoking
   C. Hypertension
   D. Obesity
   E. All of the above
   F. None of the above

4. Which modality would not be indicated in the evaluation of PAD in the emergent setting?
   A. XR
   B. CT
   C. MR
   D. Angiography

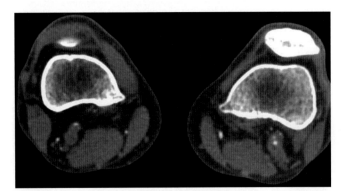

Fig. 111.1

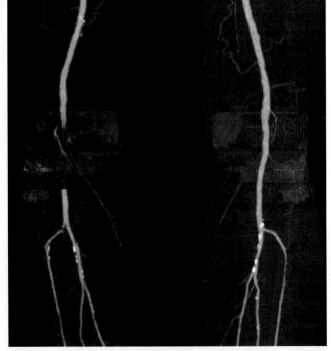

Fig. 111.2

Case 112

History: 45-year-old female with abdominal pain.

1. Which of the following would be included in the differential diagnosis for the imaging findings presented? (Choose all that apply.)
   A. Lymphoma
   B. Graft vs. host disease
   C. Crohn's disease
   D. Intestinal angioedema
2. This entity may be associated with:
   A. Hereditary deficiency of C1 inhibitor enzyme
   B. Dietary deficiency of B_{12}
   C. Medications such as beta blockers
   D. Environmental toxins such as parabens

3. In addition to abdominal pain, other common symptoms include:
   A. Cough
   B. Hematemesis
   C. Vomiting
   D. Syncope
4. This entity excludes the large bowel.
   A. True
   B. False

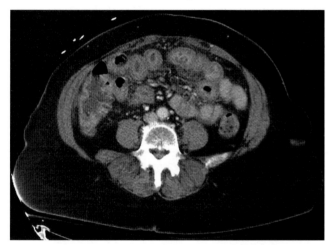

Fig. 112.1

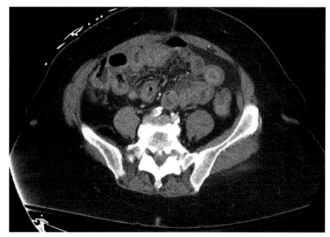

Fig. 112.2

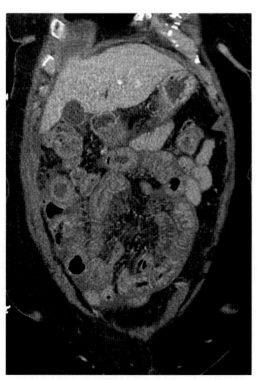

Fig. 112.3

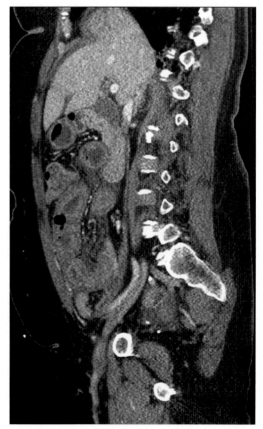

Fig. 112.4

Case 113

History: 19-year-old man status post after a motor vehicle accident (MVA).

1. Which of the following would be included in the differential diagnosis for the images presented? (Choose all that apply.)
   A. Tracheal diverticulum
   B. Tracheobronchial injury
   C. Foreign body ingestion
   D. Achalasia
2. Expected findings of an endotracheal tube balloon in this setting include:
   A. Herniation into airway defect
   B. Overinflation
   C. Abnormal shape
   D. All of the above
3. Late complications of this entity, if not treated, include all of the following, except:
   A. Bronchiectasis
   B. Recurrent spontaneous pneumothoraces
   C. Bronchial or tracheal stenosis
   D. Recurrent infections
4. Expected findings on radiography include all of the following, except:
   A. Pneumothorax
   B. Pneumomediastinum
   C. Subcutaneous emphysema
   D. Multiple rib fractures

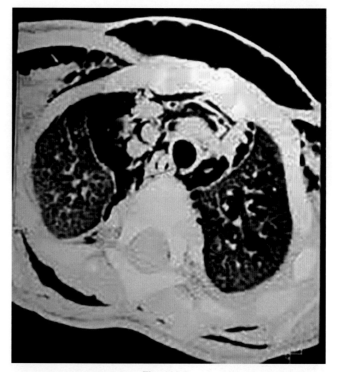

Fig. 113.2

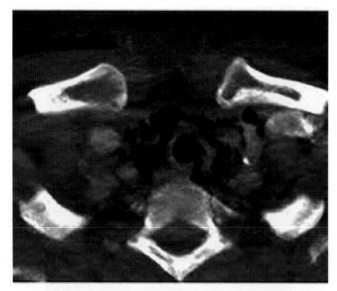

Fig. 113.1

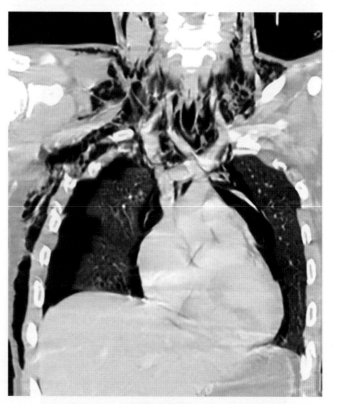

Fig. 113.3

Case 114

History: 64-year-old man with tearing chest pain.

1. Which of the following would be included in the differential diagnosis for the images presented? (Choose all that apply.)
   A. Achalasia
   B. Esophageal perforation
   C. Foreign body ingestion
   D. Tracheobronchial injury
2. Causes for this entity include all of the following, except:
   A. Iatrogenic
   B. Trauma
   C. Vomiting
   D. Gastroesophageal reflux disease

3. Fluoroscopic evaluation is most sensitive after 24 hours.
   A. True
   B. False
4. The most common cause of this entity is:
   A. Ingestion
   B. Vomiting
   C. Iatrogenic
   D. Malignancy

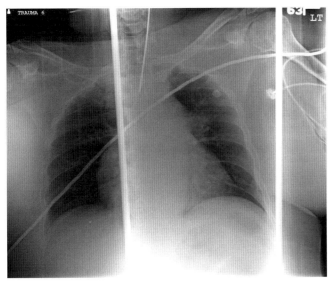

Fig. 114.1

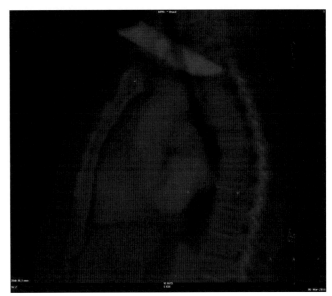

Fig. 114.2

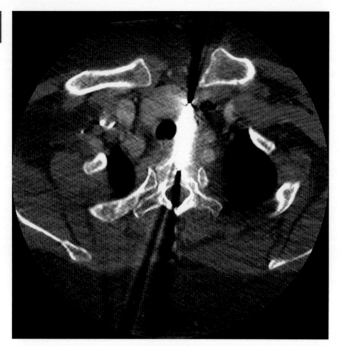

Fig. 114.3

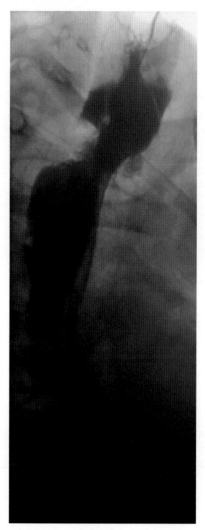

Fig. 114.4

Case 115

History: 54-year-old man with chest pain; rule out pulmonary embolism.

1. Which of the following would be included in the differential diagnosis for the images presented? (Choose all that apply.)
   A. Myocardial infarction
   B. Pulmonary embolism
   C. Aortic dissection
   D. Pericardial effusion
2. Causes for this entity include all of the following, except:
   A. Anemia
   B. Hypertension
   C. Hypercholesterolemia
   D. Hypercoagulopathy

3. CT is the first-line modality for the evaluation of this entity.
   A. True
   B. False
4. Silent ischemia may occur in patients with:
   A. Malignancy
   B. Prior infarcts
   C. Diabetes
   D. Anemia

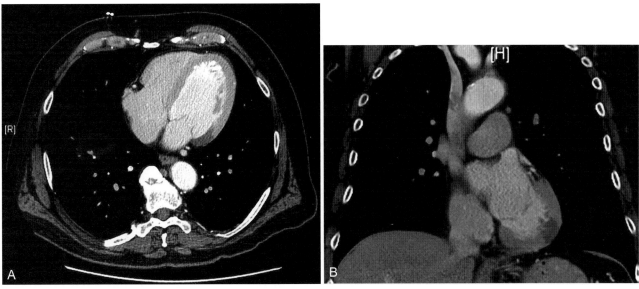

Fig. 115.1A and B

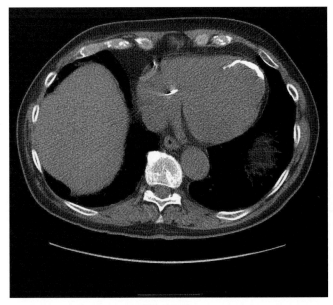

Fig. 115.2

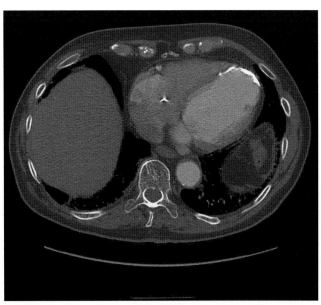

Fig. 115.3

Case 116

History: 33-year-old male with gunshot wound to the chest.

1. Which of the following would be included in the diagnosis for the imaging findings presented? (Choose all that apply.)
   A. Pericardial hemorrhage
   B. Myocardial laceration
   C. Sternal fracture
   D. Cardiac tamponade
2. Potential etiologies of myocardial injury related to trauma can include:
   A. Penetrating trauma
   B. Blunt trauma
   C. Iatrogenic injury
   D. Ischemic

3. Myocardial injury can be detected with which of the following:
   A. Electrocardiogram
   B. Laboratory markers
   C. MR imaging
   D. Nuclear scintigraphy
   E. CT imaging
4. Which is the most common procedures or treatment for myocardial injuries in trauma?
   A. CT angiography
   B. Conventional angiography
   C. Surgical revascularization
   D. None

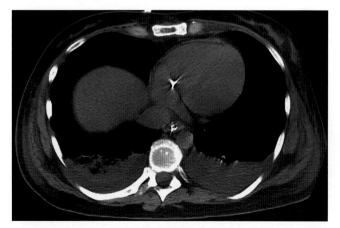

Fig. 116.1

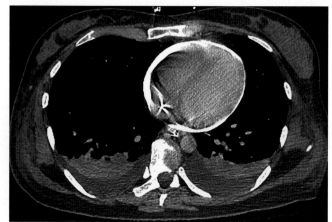

Fig. 116.2

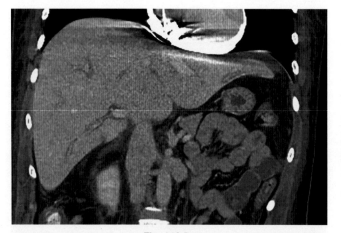

Fig. 116.3

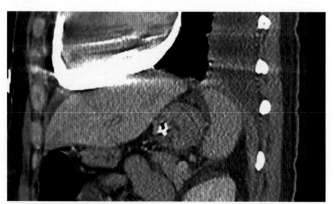

Fig. 116.4

Case 117

History: 60-year-old man with difficulty swallowing.

1. Which of the following would be included in the differential diagnosis for the imaging findings presented? (Choose all that apply.)
   A. Foreign body ingestion
   B. Ludwig angina
   C. Sialolith obstruction
   D. Tonsillitis
2. The most common location for this entity is a finding often associated with:
   A. Pharynx
   B. Submandibular
   C. Parotid
   D. Epiglottis

3. Which statement is false?
   A. Sialolithiasis is the most common disease of the salivary glands.
   B. 80% to 90% of sialoliths are noted in the submandibular glands and ducts.
   C. 80% to 90% of sialoliths are noted in the parotid glands and ducts.
   D. The salivary secretions in the parotid glands are more viscous than in the mandibular gland and predisposes to sialolithiasis.
4. This condition can be associated with which of the following?
   A. Pain associated with eating
   B. Airway compromise
   C. Abscess formation
   D. Fatty atrophy

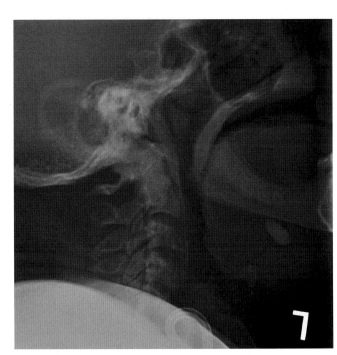

Fig. 117.1

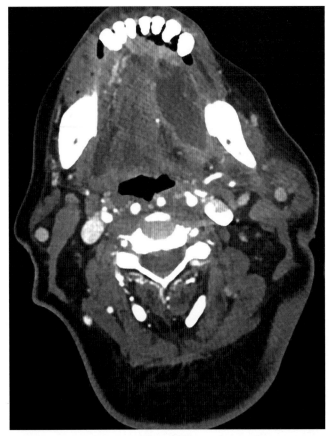

Fig. 117.2

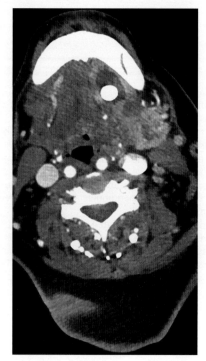

Fig. 117.3

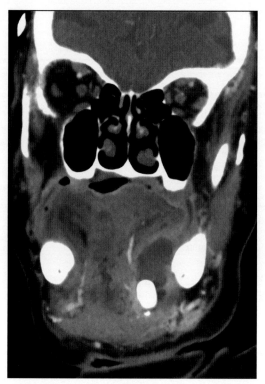

Fig. 117.4

Case 118

History: 59-year-old man with blood in stool.

1. Which of the following would be included in the diagnosis for the imaging findings presented? (Choose all that apply.)
   A. Ingested foreign body
   B. Enteric contrast
   C. Gastrointestinal (GI) bleed
   D. Luminal calcification
2. Potential etiologies of lower GI bleeding (LGIB) can include:
   A. Inflammatory bowel disease
   B. Angiodysplasia
   C. Malignancy
   D. Steroids

3. Which is the correct estimated detection rate of bleeding by modality?
   A. Nuclear medicine: >0.5 mL/min
   B. CTA: >0.35 mL/min
   C. Angiography: <0.1 mL/min
4. Contraindications for CTA in patients with LGIB include?
   A. Rapid LGIB bleeding
   B. Suspected malignancy
   C. Claustrophobia
   D. Impaired renal function

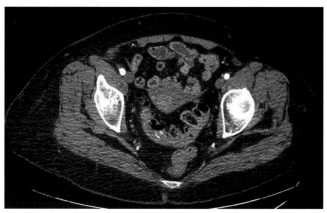

Fig. 118.1

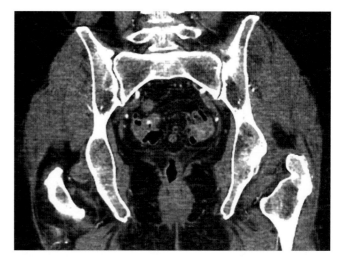

Fig. 118.2

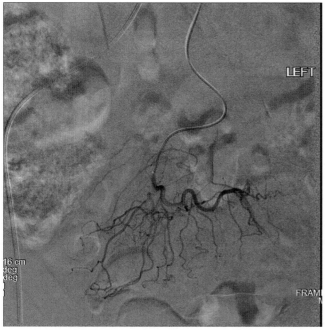

Fig. 118.3

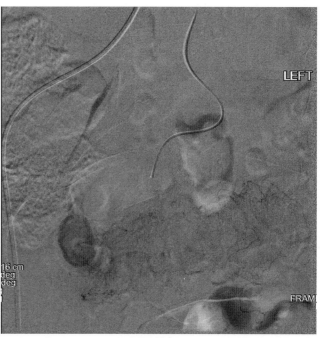

Fig. 118.4

Case 119

History: 23-year-old male status post MVA.

1. Which of the following would be included in the diagnosis for the imaging findings presented? (Choose all that apply.)
   A. Ischemic bowel
   B. Hypotension complex
   C. Radiation enteritis
   D. Submucosa hemorrhage
2. Which is the most common etiology for this diagnosis?
   A. Cardiac arrest
   B. Septic shock
   C. Spinal injury
   D. Posttraumatic hypovolemic shock

3. Which location is the most common site of involvement in this entity?
   A. Small bowel
   B. Pancreas
   C. Adrenal glands
   D. Spleen
4. Which of the following statements is false regarding inferior vena cava (IVC) and aortic involvement in this condition?
   A. Small caliber aorta: <13 mm
   B. Small caliber IVC: <9 mm
   C. High-density fluid surrounding the IVC
   D. Small-caliber aorta is seen in approximately 30% of patients.

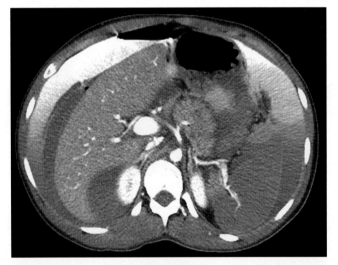

Fig. 119.1

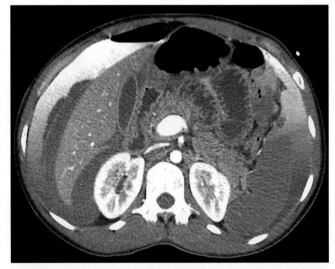

Fig. 119.2

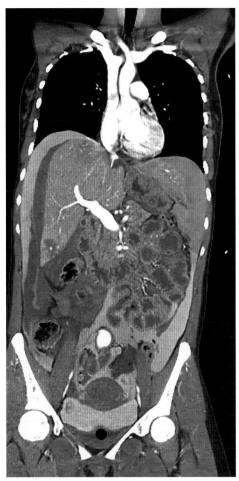

Fig. 119.3

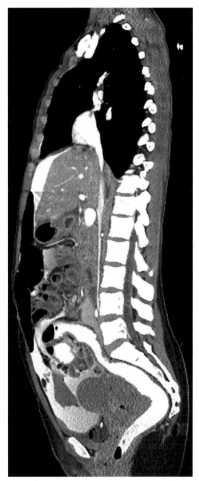

Fig. 119.4

Case 120

History: 23-year-old woman with fever and pelvic pain status post 5 days after spontaneous vaginal delivery.

1. Which of the following would be included in the diagnosis for the imaging findings presented? (Choose all that apply.)
   A. Endometritis
   B. Retained products of conception
   C. Endometrial carcinoma
   D. Intrauterine gestation
2. Which are common ultrasound (US) findings with this diagnosis?
   A. Increased vascularity on Doppler US
   B. Intracavitary and cul-de-sac fluid
   C. Thickened/heterogeneous endometrium
   D. Echogenic foci with posterior acoustic shadowing

3. Obstetric risk factors include:
   A. Retained products of conception
   B. Prolonged labor
   C. Premature rupture of membranes
   D. Misoprostol administration
4. Which of the following statements is false regarding this entity?
   A. Can occur in the acute or chronic settings
   B. Can occur in the obstetric or gynecologic settings
   C. Can complicate 3% of vaginal deliveries
   D. Can complicate 20% of Cesarean sections

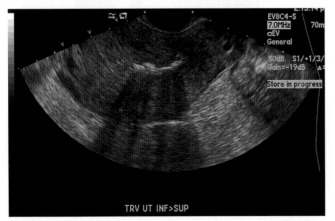

Fig. 120.1

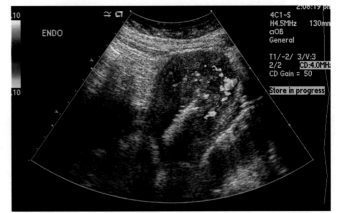

Fig. 120.3

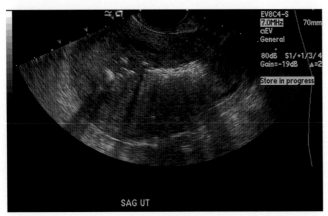

Fig. 120.2

Case 121

History: 28-year-old woman with spotting and cramping; history of pregnancy, but no prenatal care.

1. Which of the following would be included in the diagnosis for the imaging findings presented? (Choose all that apply.)
   A. Retained products of conception
   B. Placentomegaly
   C. Placental abruption
   D. Fibroids
2. During which time frame is this entity encountered?
   A. 4th week of gestation
   B. 8th week of gestation
   C. 12th week of gestation
   D. 20th week of gestation

3. Which is an associated risk factor?
   A. Advanced maternal age
   B. Smoking tobacco or cocaine use
   C. Preeclampsia
   D. Maternal trauma
4. Conservative therapy for this entity includes:
   A. Serial sonographic examinations
   B. Assessment of antepartum heart rate
   C. Monitoring maternal symptoms
   D. Strict bedrest

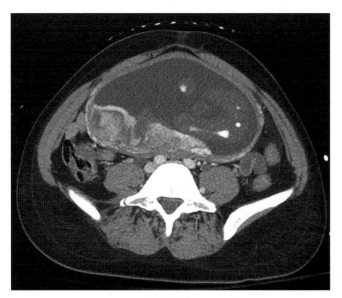

Fig. 121.1

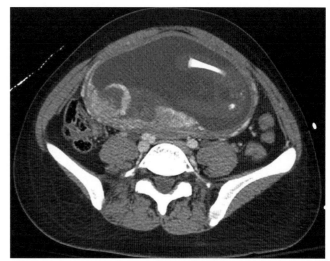

Fig. 121.2

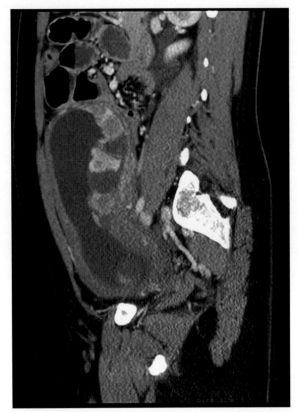

Fig. 121.3

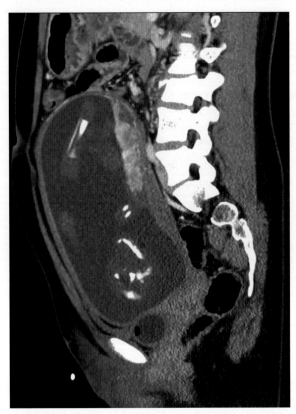

Fig. 121.4

Case 122

History: 28-year-old woman with spotting and cramping; history of pregnancy but no prenatal care.

1. Which of the following would be included in the diagnosis for the imaging findings presented? (Choose all that apply.)
   A. Submucosa fibroid
   B. Placenta previa
   C. Endometrial polyp
   D. Myometrial contraction
2. Which is the earliest gestational age before which this entity is unlikely to be detected on US?
   A. 4th week of gestation
   B. 8th week of gestation
   C. 12th week of gestation
   D. 20th week of gestation
3. Which is the best modality for assessing the placenta and its relationship to the cervix?
   A. X-ray
   B. US
   C. CT
   D. MR
4. Risk factors for this condition include:
   A. Prior C-section
   B. Increased maternal age
   C. Advanced maternal age
   D. Large placentas

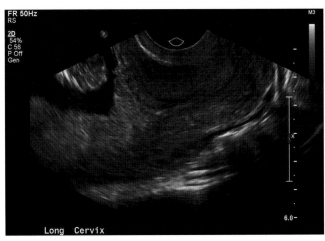

Fig. 122.1

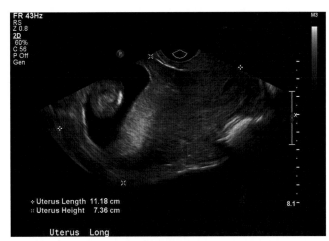

Fig. 122.2

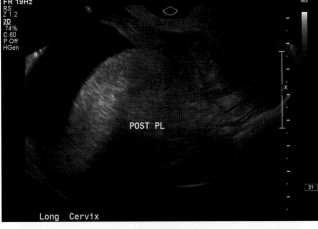

Fig. 122.3

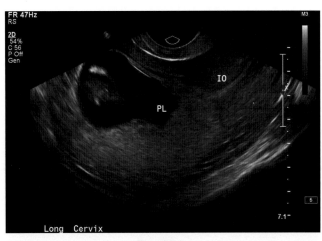

Fig. 122.4

Case 123

History: 62-year-old man with scrotal swelling.

1. Which of the following would be included in the diagnosis for the imaging findings presented? (Choose all that apply.)
   A. Abscess
   B. Perforated viscus
   C. Cellulitis
   D. Fournier gangrene
2. Which is not a risk factor for developing this condition?
   A. Smoking
   B. Alcoholism
   C. Immunosuppression
   D. Diabetes

3. Which bacteria are often involved in this condition?
   A. *Proteus*
   B. *Staphylococcus*
   C. *E. coli*
   D. *Klebsiella*
4. Management includes all, except:
   A. Radical surgical debridement
   B. Hyperbaric therapy
   C. Outpatient oral antibiotics
   D. Intravenous antibiotics

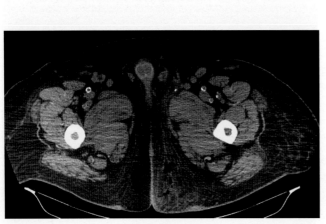

Fig. 123.1

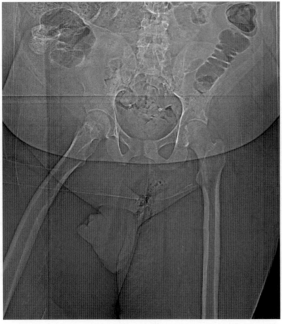

Fig. 123.2

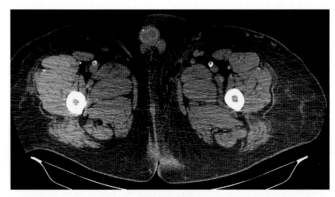

Fig. 123.3

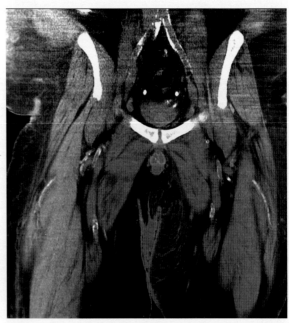

Fig. 123.4

Case 124

History: 37-year-old man with pain.

1. Which of the following would be included in the diagnosis for the imaging findings presented? (Choose all that apply.)
   A. External foreign body
   B. Rectal foreign body
   C. Urethral foreign body
   D. Buttock foreign body
2. Which are factors usually associated with this case?
   A. Psychiatric illness
   B. Autoerotic stimulation
   C. Intoxication
   D. Cigarette smoking

3. Which is the next imaging step?
   A. Retrograde urethrography
   B. US
   C. CT
   D. MRI
4. Complications include:
   A. Stricture
   B. False lumen development
   C. Mucosal tears
   D. Foreign body migration

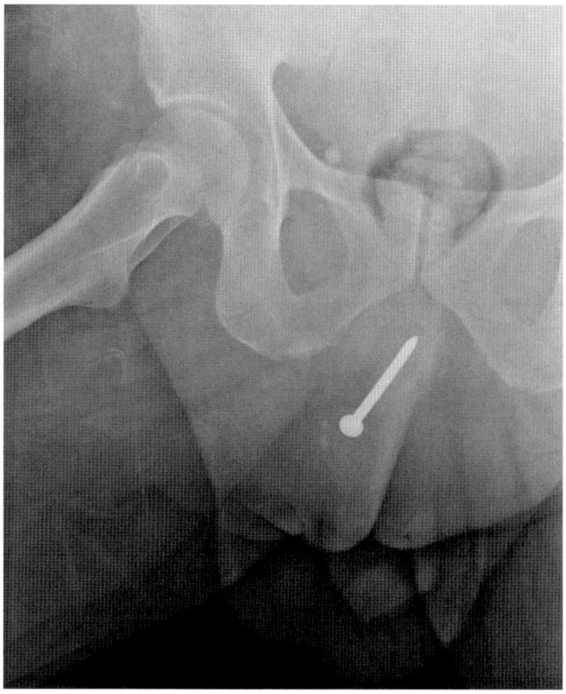

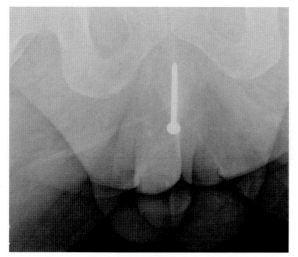

Fig. 124.1

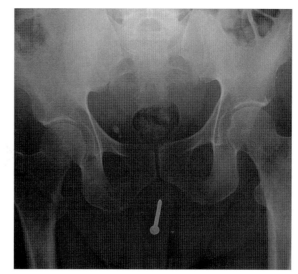

Fig. 124.3

Fig. 124.2

Case 125

History: 22-year-old man thrown from a horse and trampled.

1. Which of the following would be included in the differential diagnosis for the images presented? (Choose all that apply.)
   A. Testicular cancer
   B. Testicular hematoma
   C. Testicular fracture
   D. Late testicular torsion
2. Which finding helps distinguish the correct diagnosis from the other above options?
   A. Disruption of the tunica albuginea
   B. Hematocele
   C. Heterogeneity of the testicle
   D. All of the above

3. Late complications of this entity include:
   A. Infertility
   B. Posttraumatic ischemia
   C. Recurrent infections
   D. All of the above
4. Expected findings on sonography include all of the following, except:
   A. Hematocele
   B. Heterogeneity of the testicle
   C. Disrupted testicular contour
   D. Scrotal swelling
   E. All of the above

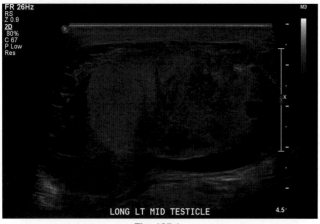

Fig. 125.1

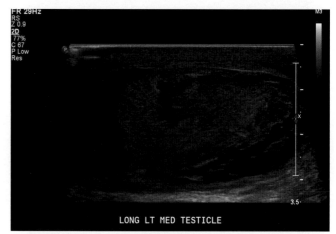

Fig. 125.3

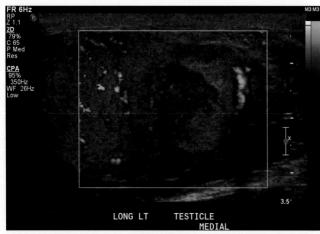

Fig. 125.2

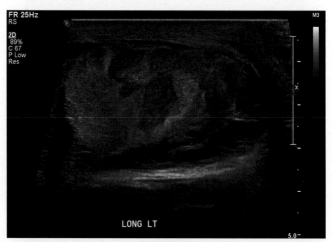

Fig. 125.4

Opening Round

CASE 1

Acute Appendicitis

1. **A, C.** Acute appendicitis and pelvic inflammatory disease (PID) may have similar symptoms, and both should be listed in the differential diagnosis.
2. **B.** Inability to pass gas is sometimes seen in patients with acute appendicitis, indicating an obstruction.
3. **A.** Computed tomography (CT) has a sensitivity of 97% to 100% and specificity of 95%. Answer B, Ultrasonography has a 75% to 90% sensitivity with 86% to 100% specificity.
4. **B.** Lumen obstruction is not always the cause of acute appendicitis even though it is the most commonly accepted etiology.

Comments

CT Scan
Acute appendicitis on CT (Figure 1-1 axial and Figure 1-2 sagittal) includes a thickened appendix with or without surrounding fluid and inflammatory changes in the right lower quadrant of the abdomen.

Acute Appendicitis in the Young. CT Versus Ultrasonography
Appendicitis is the most frequent cause of abdominal pain in children and young adults requiring surgery. It is important to note that the thickened appendix and the fluid that may be present may be difficult to detect in young children, thereby decreasing the usefulness of CT in this population. Ultrasonography should be considered. It has the added benefit of no ionizing radiation.

Accuracy of CT in Acute Appendicitis
Computed tomography has a 97% to 100% sensitivity and 95% specificity for detecting acute appendicitis.

CASE 2

Acute Stroke/Cerebrovascular Accident (CVA)

1. **C.** Although a transient ischemic attack (TIA) and a cerebrovascular accident (CVA) would be included in the differential diagnosis for acute right hemiparesis, the imaging findings are consistent with a nonhemorrhagic, left middle cerebral artery (MCA) territory CVA.
2. **B.** All four answers are conceivable reasons for increased density within an intracranial blood vessel; however, the hyperdense MCA sign represents proximal MCA/M1 thrombosis. Contrast material would be more dense and present throughout all the visualized intracranial vascular structures. Generally, hemoconcentration manifests as symmetrically increased density within the bilateral middle cerebral and basilar arteries.
3. **D.** The penumbra represents hypoperfused, at-risk tissue at the periphery of the acute infarction and has increased mean transit time (MTT). However, the penumbra can have either moderately decreased cerebral blood flow (CBF) with normal or increased cerebral blood volume (CBV). Similarly, it can also have markedly reduced CBF and moderately reduced CBV.

4. **A.** In order to receive intravenous tissue plasma activator (tPA), it is generally accepted that treatment should start within 4.5 hours in patients who have less than one-third involvement of the MCA territory.

Comments

Background
Signs and symptoms of acute CVA are common indications for imaging in the emergency department and, much as in myocardial infarction, early intervention can improve outcomes. In the United States, approximately 800,000 people/year suffer CVAs resulting in more than 130,000 deaths, making it the fifth most common cause of death.

Diagnosis
Imaging's primary goal acutely is to differentiate ischemic or hemorrhagic CVA. Imaging can identify the involved vascular territory, the presence of intravascular thrombus, and possibly the extent of the penumbra. The noncontrast head CT remains the first-line examination owing to its widespread availability, rapid image acquisition, and high sensitivity for hemorrhagic changes, which will guide tPA administration.

When windowed and leveled appropriately, a noncontrast head CT has a sensitivity and specificity as high as 71% and 100%. The hyperdense MCA sign represents an acute intravascular thrombus within the proximal MCA M1 segment, which may be seen on CT angiography (CTA) imaging as an arterial cut-off or absence of the distal vascular opacification owing to proximal intravascular thrombosis. Two additional findings on the noncontrast head CT involve the loss of the gray-white differentiation in the insular cortex, known as the insular ribbon sign, and obscuration of the lentiform nucleus. Once intracranial hemorrhage has been excluded via the noncontrast head CT, tPA can be administered. Strong evidence exists that tPA infusion within 4.5 hours improves outcomes; however, if the infarcted tissue involves more than one-third of the MCA territory, treatment is contraindicated owing to increased rates of intracranial hemorrhage.

Computed tomography angiography of the head and neck allows for rapid evaluation of both the extracranial and intracranial blood supply. CT perfusion imaging is useful for evaluating the penumbra by measuring specific perfusion parameters, including CBV, CBF, and MTT. In the penumbra, this tissue will demonstrate increased MTT with moderately decreased CBF (>60%) or severely decreased CBF (>30%). Cerebral blood volume can be either normal or increased owing to physiologic autoregulation, or moderately reduced. Infarcted tissue demonstrates severely decreased CBF (<30%), decreased CBV (<40%), and increased MTT. MTT and CBV maps are the most sensitive and specific indicators of an acute stroke. If a discrete penumbra is present, tPA therapy may be considered.

Although CT imaging is very important to the management algorithms for acute CVA, magnetic resonance (MR) imaging is both more sensitive and more specific for the detection of acute cerebral ischemia, and most MR protocols include both diffuse-weighted imaging (DWI) with associated apparent diffusion coefficient (ADC) maps. These sequences demonstrate increased intensity on DWI with decreased intensity on the ADC map in the setting of acute ischemia.

CASE 3

Deep Vein Thrombosis (DVT)

1. **E.** Superficial thrombosis is rarely associated with DVT.
2. **D.** Pain in the middle of the calf is a sign of DVT, whereas pain on the right of the calf is more commonly associated with muscular injury.
3. **C.** IVC filter placement requires (1) absolute or relative contraindication to anticoagulation; (2) complication of anticoagulation, and (3) failure of anticoagulation leading to recurrent pulmonary embolism (PE) despite adequate therapy.
4. **D.** This patient failed warfarin anticoagulation and developing a DVT.

Comments

DVT Epidemiology
In the United States the incidence of first-time venous thromboembolism (VTE) is in about 100 in 100,000/year and increases with advancing age. PE is associated with one-third of patients with VTE. Mortality at 1 month for patients with DVT is 6%. Estimates suggest that 60,000 to 100,000 Americans die each year of DVT or PE.

DVT Evaluation
The most common diagnostic tool to evaluate for DVT is ultrasonography (Figure 3-1). Compressibility of the venous lumen; gray-scale evaluation of the lumen for echogenic luminal filling defects; Doppler interrogation demonstrating normal venous waveforms and luminal color flow; and respiratory variation are evaluated.

Clinical Presentation of DVT and PE
The classic clinical presentation of DVT includes extremity swelling, pain, warmth, and redness.

CASE 4

Pulmonary Embolism

1. **A.** Filling defects within the pulmonary arterial tree are compatible with PE.
2. **A.** Cyanosis is owing to low oxygen saturation and decreased pulmonary perfusion.
3. **A.** Lung scintigraphy generally delivers less radiation to the mother than conventional angiography and CT pulmonary angiography (CTPA).
4. **A.** Evidence of right-sided heart strain should prompt immediate, intensive monitoring.

Comments

Risk Factors
The risk of PE doubles every 10 years after age 60. Risk factors include immobilization or decreased mobility, active malignancy, and hypercoagulopathies. Remember the pneumonic, THROMBOSIS Trauma/Travel, Hypercoagulable state/HRT, Recreational drugs, Older, Malignancy, Birth Control, Obesity/Obstetrical, Surgery, Immobilization, and Sickness.

Symptoms
Clinical symptoms include dyspnea, chest pain, tachycardia, and/or syncope. Syncope is caused by a severely reduced hemodynamic reserve. In a more central PE, isolated dyspnea with a rapid onset will be seen. In patients with preexisting heart failure or pulmonary disease, worsening dyspnea over time may be the only symptom indicative of PE.

Treatment
The initial treatment is aimed at keeping the blood clot from getting bigger and preventing new clots from forming. Prompt treatment is essential to prevent serious complications or death. In general, anticoagulation with intravenous heparin is the initial drug of choice for PE overlapped with warfarin until the anticoagulant is effective. If the patient shows significant right ventricular stress and hypoxemia, then thrombolytic therapy (intravenous [IV] tPA 100 mg) should be given. An echocardiogram should be done in the following days to check for resolution from the right ventricle strain and pulmonary hypertension.

CASE 5

Acute Diverticulitis

1. **A, C.** Acute diverticulitis and colon adenocarcinoma both may have wall thickening and fat stranding, and both should be included in the differential diagnosis. Epiploic appendagitis will appear beside the colon as a fatty mass surrounded by a thin, hyperdense rim. Appendicitis will be seen with a distended, inflamed appendix.
2. **A.** Age is a risk factor for developing diverticulitis. Other risk factors include nonsteroidal antiinflammatory drugs (NSAIDs), obesity, and sedentary lifestyle. Avoidance of nuts, corn, or popcorn does not lower the risk of developing diverticulitis.
3. **C.** Adenocarcinoma is associated with lymphadenopathy and focal segmental bowel involvement. Adenocarcinoma classically demonstrates bowel wall shouldering rather than a gradual transition of colon wall thickness. It is not generally associated with accumulation of fluid.
4. **D.** Complications of diverticulitis include bleeding, abscesses, phlegmon, fistula, obstruction, and perforation.

Comments

Background
Diverticula develop as outpouchings of mucosa and submucosa through the muscular layer of the colon wall. Although they can form anywhere within the small bowel or colon, diverticula are most frequently found in the sigmoid or descending colon. Approximately 5% occur in the right colon. Diverticulitis of the small bowel and the transverse colon is rare. A Meckel's diverticulum is a congenital diverticulum developing from the fetal yolk stalk and appears solely in the distal ileum. Acute diverticulitis develops secondary to blockage of the neck of a diverticulum.

Signs and Symptoms
Patients commonly present with left lower quadrant pain, tenderness, fever, and abdominal distention. Other common symptoms include nausea, constipation, and diarrhea. Complicated diverticulitis can present with tachycardia and hypotension. Rebound tenderness and abdominal rigidity suggest peritonitis.

Diagnosis
Computed tomography is the most commonly employed modality. Imaging findings include diverticula, bowel wall thickening, and local inflammation. Abscess formation, perforation, fistula formation, extravasation of IV contrast (bleeding), and free peritoneal gas may be present in complicated cases.

CASE 6

Subdural Hemorrhage

1. **A, C.** Subdural and epidural hemorrhage should be considered in the setting of head trauma. On CT, subdural hemorrhage appears crescent distribution, whereas epidural hemorrhage appears lentiform. Cerebral atrophy will demonstrate vessel delineation. Subdural empyema will present with additional symptoms, such as fever, leucocytosis, and associated infarct/abscess.
2. **D.** Typically, patients with epidural hemorrhage experience a "lucid interval" where they regain normal consciousness for a period of time before gradually losing consciousness. Patients with subdural hemorrhage will gradually lose consciousness but usually do not experience a "lucid interval."
3. **C.** Small epidural hemorrhage may be difficult to differentiate from subdural hemorrhage. Larger epidural hemorrhage will appear in the typical "lentiform" (biconcave) distribution on head CT. Epidural hemorrhages do not cross sutures because they do not occur in the subdural space. Subdural hemorrhage can cross sutures.
4. **C.** Subdural empyema may present in a crescentic shape on CT, similar to subdural hemorrhage. However, subdural empyema is associated with additional symptoms, such as fever, leucocytosis, and a source of infection/abscess. Most commonly, subdural empyema is a consequence of a frontal sinusitis.

Comments

Causes

Subdural hemorrhage accumulates between the arachnoid and dural meninges. Head injury results in the tearing of the bridging veins that cross the subdural space. In young adults, subdural hemorrhages are most typically a result of motor vehicle accidents (MVAs), and make up between 10% and 20% of all head trauma cases. In the elderly, a subdural hemorrhage is typically a result of a fall. Epidural hemorrhage, in contrast, is typically caused by an arterial tear with accumulation of blood between the dura mater and the skull.

Symptoms of Subdural Hemorrhage Versus Epidural Hemorrhage

Subdural hemorrhage often presents in the setting of head trauma. Most patients will present with gradual depressed consciousness. Depression of consciousness will continue as the mass effect increases. Confusion is more common among elderly patients with subdural hemorrhage. In contrast, patients with epidural hemorrhage typically present with an immediate loss of consciousness, followed by a "lucid interval," where they regain consciousness for a short period of time. Typically, after a few hours of lucidity, these patient will gradually lose consciousness.

Imaging

In the emergent setting, CT is the most appropriate imaging modality. Follow-up CT may help assess evolution or progression of hemorrhage.

CASE 7

Epidural Hemorrhage

1. **A, B.** In the setting of head trauma, epidural and subdural hemorrhage should be considered. Typically, infections will present with additional symptoms, such as fever, leucocytosis, and an abscess/source of infection. Meningioma is not likely to present after head injury and is typically asymptomatic/present incidentally.
2. **A.** Epidural hematomas tend to be biconvex/lentiform in shape and sharply demarcated.

3. **D.** Trauma is the most common cause of an epidural hemorrhage in young adults. Typically, the patient will present with diminishing conscious with an interval of lucidity.
4. **A.** Any serious or symptomatic epidural hemorrhage needs to be treated with emergent craniotomy and clot evacuation. If the epidural hemorrhage is very small or asymptomatic, it can be managed conservatively.

Comments

Causes

Epidural hemorrhages are a result of traumatic injury. Anatomically, epidural hemorrhages result after damage to arteries, most commonly the middle meningeal artery.

Symptoms

Patients will typically present with loss of consciousness after head trauma. Headache is a common symptom. Patients experience a "lucid interval" followed by decreased consciousness. It is essential to monitor patients closely during this period of lucidity and not consider it a normal finding.

Imaging

Computed tomography is the first-line imaging modality. Epidural hemorrhage appears biconcave and hyperdense. Epidural hematomas are bound by cranial sutures and will not cross intact sutures. Magnetic resonance imaging (MRI) and angiography can assist in differentiating between trauma-induced epidural hemorrhages and other causes.

CASE 8

Community-Acquired Pneumonia, Right Middle Lobe

1. **A.** Based on radiograph, lobar consolidations should be considered.
2. **C.** Patients with human immunodeficiency virus (HIV) are at risk for a number of pulmonary infections. *Pneumocystis jiroveci* remains the most common opportunistic infection in this group, but the most common bacterial pathogen causing illness in patients with HIV is *Streptococcus pneumoniae*.
3. **C.** Assessing oxygenation and utilizing clinical judgment is sufficient for treating uncomplicated community-acquired pneumonia.
4. **D.** Type I allergic patients should avoid cephalosporins and other beta-lactam antibiotics.

Comments

Background

Pneumonia is an infection of the lung parenchyma that can be caused by bacteria, viruses, protozoa, parasites, and fungi. The most common causative agent is *Streptococcus pneumoniae*, which is usually present in 30% of the cases. However, 40% of cases show no identifiable pathogen. Damage to the lung is uncommon, and recovery is associated with complete resolution. In the pre-antibiotic era, empyema was the most common complication.

Risk Factors

Risk factors include smoking, chronic bronchitis, asthma, immune compromise, alcoholism, chronic lung diseases such as chronic obstructive pulmonary disease (COPD), cystic fibrosis, and bronchiectasis. Pneumonia is usually either community-acquired pneumonia or nosocomial/hospital-acquired pneumonia. Other types of pneumonia, such as pneumocystic pneumonia, may be seen in immune-compromised patients.

Treatment

Penicillin and its derivatives effectively treat pneumococcal pneumonia. In penicillin allergic patients, erythromycin and clarithromycin are alternatives. Generally, a 7- to 10- day course of therapy is sufficient treatment.

CASE 9

Acute Calculus Cholecystitis

1. **C.** In a middle-aged woman with acute right upper quadrant (RUQ) abdominal pain, fever, and vomiting, acute cholecystitis should be considered. The presence of gallstones, gallbladder inflammation, and pericholecystic fluid are often present on CT. Polyps may appear as echogenic foci in the gallbladder wall with vascularity. No stones are noted in the bile ducts. Adenomyomatosis is a benign condition characterized by hyperplastic changes of unknown etiology involving the gallbladder wall and causing overgrowth of the mucosa, thickening of the muscular wall, and formation of intramural diverticula or sinus tracts termed Rokitansky-Aschoff sinuses.
2. **D.** Gallstones are associated with 90% to 95% of cases of acute cholecystitis.
3. **A, B, C.** Major findings of acute cholecystitis on CT include gallstone, pericholecystic fluid, and gallbladder inflammation/thickening. Sludge may or may not be present.
4. **A, B, D.** Radiography is not routinely used to evaluate or diagnose patients with suspected acute cholecystitis.

Comment

Background

Acute cholecystitis is the inflammation of the gallbladder and a common cause of acute pain in the right upper quadrant. Persistent pain may radiate to the right shoulder. Nausea, vomiting, and fever may be noted. The majority, 90% to 95%, of cases are associated with gallstones. Less than 10% are secondary to acalculous cholecystitis. Gallstones obstruct the gallbladder neck or cystic duct. Reactive inflammation leads to increased intraluminal pressure, distention, and restricted blood flow. Secondary bacterial infection is noted in two-thirds of patients.

Diagnosis

Sonography is the preferred initial modality and is more sensitive than CT or hepatobiliary iminodiacetic acid (HIDA) scintigraphy. Cholelithiasis in combination with a sonographic Murphy's sign is the most sensitive sonographic combination for acute cholecystitis. Wall thickening greater than 3 mm and pericholecystic fluid are secondary findings. Gallbladder distention and sludge are less specific findings. HIDA scan will demonstrate nonvisualization of the gallbladder. Major CT findings include gallstones, thickening, wall hyperemia, and pericholecystic fluid. Minor CT findings include sludge and distention. MR findings may be similar to ultrasound (US) or CT. Magnetic resonance cholangiopancreatography (MRCP) may identify an obstructing stone.

Management

Urgent cholecystectomy. Complications include gangrenous cholecystitis (20%), perforation (5%), and, less often, cholecystenteric fistula, emphysematous cholecystitis, and pericholecystic abscess.

CASE 10

Scaphoid Fracture

1. **B.** The scaphoid is the most commonly fractured carpal bone. This patient suffered a scaphoid waist fracture, which is in the most common location. Scapholunate ligament injury can occur in isolation or with scaphoid fractures and can be diagnosed with scapholunate widening (>3 mm). Kienbock's disease is avascular necrosis (AVN) of the lunate and would present as lunate sclerosis. In advanced cases, lunate sclerosis and flattening or fragmentation may occur. Hook of hamate fractures are difficult to diagnose by plain radiographs.
2. **D.** Distal scaphoid fractures are associated with lower rates of nonunion owing to distribution of blood supply. Scaphoid vascular supply enters distally.
3. **C.** As scaphoid blood supply enters distally, supply to the proximal pole can be disrupted in scaphoid waist fractures. This can lead to proximal pole AVN.
4. **D.** If not properly imaged, up to 65% of scaphoid fractures remain radiographically occult. Scaphoid views can aid in the diagnosis. With clinical concern for scaphoid fracture with negative radiographs, it is a common practice to immobilize the wrist and reimage the patient in 10 to 14 days.

Comments

Background

Scaphoid fractures account for approximately 70% of all carpal fractures. The majority (80%) of scaphoid fractures occur in the scaphoid waist, followed by the proximal pole (20%) and the distal pole (10%). Because of ligamentous attachments and because the blood supply of the scaphoid enters distally, the more proximal fractures have a higher likelihood of nonunion. Chance of nonunion: distal pole virtually 0%; waist 10% to 20%; and proximal pole 30% to 40%. Owing to scaphoid blood supply, the proximal pole in scaphoid waist fractures is at risk for AVN.

Signs and Symptoms

Patients often present following hyperextension injury, such as a fall on an outstretched hand, with snuff box tenderness and swelling.

Diagnosis and Management

Anatomic snuff box tenderness has an approximate 90% sensitivity and 40% specificity for presence of a scaphoid fracture. Patients are usually treated with cast immobilization. In cases of nonunion, internal fixation is usually performed. Nondisplaced scaphoid fractures may be missed on initial radiographs. Follow-up radiographs in 7 to 10 may be helpful for further evaluation in clinical settings where concerns remain.

CASE 11

Posterior Shoulder Dislocation

1. **B.** When the humerus dislocates posteriorly, there is an internal rotation such that the humeral head appears as a light bulb (light bulb sign). There is also a loss of halfmoon overlap sign and a prominent coracoid process.
2. **D.** The most common causes of posterior shoulder dislocation are seizures and electrocution. Falling on an outstretched hand is also a cause.
3. **B.** Posterior shoulder accounts for 2% to 5% of shoulder dislocations. Anterior shoulder dislocation accounts for 95% to 97%, and inferior shoulder dislocation accounts for 0.5%.
4. **A.** Posterior dislocation presents with a shoulder flexed, internally rotated, and adducted. Anterior dislocation: externally rotated and slightly abducted. Inferior dislocation: hyperabducted.
5. **C.** Reverse Hill-Sachs lesion is an impaction fracture of the anteromedial humeral head.

Comments

Background

Posterior shoulder dislocation accounts for approximately 2% to 5% of all shoulder injuries. Of posterior shoulder dislocations,

60% to 79% are missed on initial examination. Classically, a patient will present after a seizure or electrocution. This injury can also be seen with high-energy trauma anteriorly or indirect trauma to the flexed, adducted, and internally rotated shoulder.

Presentation and Diagnosis
On examination, the shoulder will be abnormal in appearance: it will appear internally rotated with limited rotation. An axillary radiograph can confirm the diagnosis and detect other fractures and complications of the humeral head. CT and MRI can give further insight into the injury.

Associated Injuries
The most common types of injuries associated with posterior shoulder dislocation are humeral neck fracture and the lesser tuberosity fractures. A Reverse Hill-Sachs lesion, an impaction fracture of the anteromedial aspect of the humeral head, is a characteristic associated injury.

CASE 12

Pseudomembranous (*Clostridium difficile*) Colitis

1. **A.** Differential for colitis is broad. Pseudomembranous colitis, ulcerative colitis, ischemic colitis, and cytomegalovirus colitis are common. In the clinical context of prior antibiotic use, C. *difficile* causing pseudomembranous colitis is the most likely diagnosis.
2. **A.** Enteric contrast seen trapped between thickened/inflamed mucosal folds is termed accordion sign. Finding can be seen in several conditions: pseudomembranous colitis, ischemic colitis, portal hypertensive colopathy, and infectious types of colitis caused by cytomegalovirus, cryptosporidium, and salmonella.
3. **C.** Toxic megacolon is most often caused by C. *difficile*.
4. **D.** Vancomycin is recommended as first-line therapy.

Comments

Background
Pseudomembranous colitis, a common cause of antibiotic-associated diarrhea, is caused by C. *difficile*. The incidence of C. *difficile*-associated colitis has increased in the last few years because of indiscriminate use of antibiotics, higher numbers of elderly and immunocompromised patients, and high rate of hospital occupation. Untreated pseudomembranous colitis may progress to fulminant colitis, toxic megacolon, and perforation.

Imaging Findings
Computed tomography features of infectious colitides: bowel wall thickening, pericolonic stranding, and various amounts of ascites. C. *difficile* colitis produces one of the most severe degrees of colonic wall thickening among all types of colitis. The accordion sign is associated with C. *difficile* colitis but can also be seen in patients with bowel ischemia, portal hypertensive colopathy, cytomegalovirus infection, and salmonellosis. Differential for pancolitis includes pseudomembranous colitis, ulcerative colitis, cytomegalovirus, and *Escherichia coli*.

CASE 13

Avascular Necrosis

1. **D.** This is an advanced case of AVN of the femoral head, which has resulted in left femoral head collapse. Notice the flattening of the left femoral head in comparison with the right. You can see the mixed sclerosis and lucency in both femoral heads. Conversely, notice how normal the acetabula look; in cases of septic arthritis, inflammatory arthritis, or even conventional

osteoarthritis—both sides of the joint space should demonstrate changes. Transient osteoporosis of the femoral head is an uncommon disorder that presents with femoral head marrow edema and localized radiographic osteopenia; this is a painful condition, but self-limited, and does not lead to osseous destruction. Subchondral fractures, which are isolated fractures of the bone underlying the cartilage, can occur during trauma, but are rarely bilateral and would not result in the sclerosis and lucency seen in this case.
2. **E.** All of these can result in femoral head AVN.
3. **B.** Early AVN is characterized by marrow edema on MRI, but often presents with normal radiographs. If anything is detectable by radiography, it will be localized osteopenia. High-risk patients (e.g., those with sickle cell or chronic steroid users) presenting with acute only atraumatic hip pain, with negative radiographs, may warrant an MRI if there is high clinical concern for early AVN.
4. **D.** All of these statements are accurate.

Comment

Pathophysiology
As the name implies, AVN is an interruption of blood supply to the osseous cellular matrix of the femoral head, which leads to cell death. AVN can occur in virtually any bone but is most common in the epiphysis of long bones: clinically it is most frequently encountered in the femoral head. There are numerous risk factors for AVN, including trauma; hematologic disorders, such as sickle cell anemia; chronic diseases, such as lupus or Gaucher's; medications, such as corticosteroids; and alcohol usage. Ultimately, some cases of AVN are idiopathic.

Imaging Progression and Ficat Staging
The Ficat classification is the most commonly used staging system for AVN. An understanding of the Ficat stages provides a useful illustration of the imaging progression of AVN. Ficat stage 1 is normal plain radiographs or minimal femoral head osteopenia; at this stage, the patient is often symptomatic with pain, and MRI demonstrates marrow edema. Stage 2 demonstrates mixed lucency and sclerosis of the femoral head, which can be subtle, and is often the initial radiographic presentation of AVN. At stage 3, a subchondral lucent crescent may be present, which weakens the subchondral bone and leads to eventual collapse. Stage 4 is a collapsed femoral head, often with changes of secondary osteoarthritis.

Treatment
Unfortunately, most cases of AVN of the femoral head present late, with femoral head collapse and secondary osteoarthritis. At this stage, the treatment is a total hip replacement. For cases that present earlier, a core decompression can be performed. In this procedure, a single large or multiple smaller holes are drilled through the femoral neck (from a trochanteric approach), up to the femoral head. These channels relieve local pressure and encourage the formation of new blood vessels. Some surgeons combine core decompression with bone grafting in order to help rebuild bone in the femoral head and try to prevent collapse.

CASE 14

Aortic Dissection

1. **C.** A long-segment dissection flap is seen within the contrast-enhanced aorta, creating both a true and false lumen, indicative of an aortic dissection. There is no dilation of the aorta to suggest aortic aneurysm. Aortitis typically presents with fever, pain, and weight loss; classically, the imaging findings of aortitis include circumferential aortic wall thickening or calcification. No filling defects in the pulmonary arteries suggest PE.

2. **D.** Medical management may be an option for treating a descending aortic dissection. If the dissection involves the aortic arch, the ascending aorta, or includes any complications, such as organ involvement or rupture, surgery (open or minimally invasive) is necessary.

3. **B.** DeBakey category II involves a dissection in the ascending aorta. Category I includes the arch and descending aorta, and category III involves descending aorta. There is no category IV.

4. **D.** Diabetes has no known association with an increased risk of aortic dissection. Marfan's syndrome weakens the structure of the aortic wall, and chronic hypertension increases the force on the aortic wall. Smoking increases the risk of aortic dissection.

Comments

Associations With Aortic Dissection

The prevalence aortic dissection in the United States is 3/100,000/ year, with a mean age of 63 years and a 65% male dominance. Hypertension is the strongest predisposition for acute aortic dissection in these patients, followed by smoking, trauma (especially MVAs), and drugs. Genetic traits also impart an increased risk in some patients, including those with connective tissue disorders such as Marfan's or Ehlers-Danlos syndromes. Additionally, patients with inflammatory disorders such as Takayasu's disease or polyarteritis nodosa may also have an increased risk of aortic rupture.

Presentation

Patients most commonly present with severe, acute onset of chest pain or back pain, often accompanied by a recent history of strenuous activity, drugs, or blunt-force trauma. Patients may experience syncope, paraparesis, or paraplegia. New-onset aortic regurgitation, pericardial effusion, or myocardial ischemia suggest an ascending thoracic aortic dissection involving the aortic root.

Categorizations

Aortic dissection categorizations may include classification by acute versus chronic, the DeBakey system, or the Stanford system. Acute dissection occurs within 2 weeks of symptom onset, whereas chronic dissection is considered greater than 2 weeks. The DeBakey system has three main categories, as follows:

I: Tear in the ascending aorta, propagating to the arch and descending aorta
II: Tear involving only the ascending aorta
III: Tear in the descending aorta, with propagation above the diaphragm (IIIa) or below the diaphragm (IIIb)

The Stanford system is divided into type A and type B aortic dissections.

Type A: Tear involving the ascending aorta.
Type B: Tear involving any area of the aorta, including the arch, excluding the ascending aorta.

CASE 15

Triquetral Fracture

1. **D.** A small crescentic osseous fragment at the dorsal aspect of the carpus with overlying soft-tissue swelling is compatible with a (dorsal ridge) triquetral fracture. Synovial osteochondromatosis is a disorder characterized by synovial metaplasia with multiple chondral loose bodies that slowly ossify; it can occur in the wrist, but this presentation and imaging findings are not supportive of that diagnosis. The capitate and scaphoid are intact.

2. **C.** Triquetral fractures most commonly involve the dorsal ridge of the triquetrum and can occur from ligamentous avulsion or direct impaction by the ulnar styloid process. Triquetral body fractures can occur in the setting of high-energy wrist injuries, such as perilunate dislocations.

3. **E.** Dorsal triquetral fractures are not often seen on anteroposterior (AP) radiographs owing to the overlying pisiform and dorsal location of the osseous fracture fragment. In the standard 3-view radiographic series, oblique and lateral views are often diagnostic. The reverse oblique view is a nonstandard view of the wrist that can help in further evaluation of the dorsal triquetral fractures when standard views are not definitive.

4. **E.** Dorsal ridge can occur secondary to direct impingement or ligamentous avulsion. Direct impingement occurs during forced hyperextension and ulnar deviation, when the ulnar styloid impacts on the dorsal triquetral and chips it. Ligamentous avulsion occurs during hyperflexion.

Comment

Background

After scaphoid fractures, triquetral fractures are the second most common carpal fractures, with a prevalence of approximately 20%. The majority of triquetral fractures are fractures of the dorsal ridge, which can occur secondary to direct impingement or ligamentous avulsion. Impingement or chip fractures of the dorsal triquetral ridge usually result from impaction of the ulnar styloid process during hyperextension and ulnar deviation. Dorsal avulsion fractures are often caused by avulsion of the dorsal radiotriquetral and/or scaphotriquetral ligaments.

Diagnosis and Pitfalls

A small bony fragment at the dorsal aspect of the wrist, at the distal level of the first carpal row is suggestive of a triquetral fracture. Sharp osseous margins, local pain or swelling, and a visible donor site are findings that support acuity. An *os triquetrum* is a triangular ossicle that may occur on the dorsal ridge of the triquetrum. If the osseous fragment in question is closely opposed to the triquetral body, there is lack of overlying soft-tissue swelling, and the bony margins appear corticated or serrated, consider this diagnosis. In discussion with the clinician, this will be an incidental finding without local tenderness to palpation.

Management

Dorsal triquetral fractures can be treated with plaster cast immobilization (followed by physiotherapy) or splint/bandage, depending on the patient's level of discomfort and the provider's preference. There is no strong evidence comparing outcomes from these various treatment methods.

CASE 16

Ectopic Pregnancy

1. **D.** In a patient with a positive β-hCG, without a visualized gestational sac present within the uterus, an ectopic pregnancy should be considered. Although the ovarian images are not Doppler images, the presence of a fetal pole confirms the diagnosis of an ectopic pregnancy. A failed intrauterine pregnancy (IUP) would be in the differential, but the presence of an ovarian gestational sac excludes that as a likely option. In the case of a bicornuate uterus, a normal IUP is possible but unlikely and would require showing both horns of the uterus with an intrauterine gestational sac.

2. **A.** Tubal ectopic pregnancies are the most common, with 70% being found in the ampullary portion of the fallopian tube. Ovarian and cornual/interstitial ectopic pregnancies are both

quite rare, accounting for only 3% and 2% of all ectopic pregnancies, respectively.
3. **C.** At a value of 2000 mIU/mL, an IUP should be visualized by transvaginal ultrasound; however, if using transabdominal ultrasound, the discriminatory value would be 6500 mIU/mL.
4. **D.** In a stable patient, either methotrexate or expectant management can be considered. Generally, conservative management would be considered in a patient who may have an early IUP with an unproved ectopic pregnancy. A patient in that position would require close clinical and sonographic follow up. But, in the case of a patient with a proven ectopic pregnancy without findings of hemoperitoneum, treatment would be required, and intramuscular methotrexate is the treatment of choice.

Comment

Background
Although the incidence of ectopic pregnancy increased over the last half of the 20th century, it remained fairly uncommon, being found in only 2% of all pregnancies. However, the risk of death from ruptured ectopic pregnancy remains high, with approximately 10% to 15% during the first trimester. Although there is a classic clinical triad of abdominal or pelvic pain, vaginal bleeding, and a tender adnexal mass after approximately 6 to 8 weeks of amenorrhea, as many as 50% of ectopic pregnancies are actually asymptomatic. If a first-trimester pregnant female presents with abdominal pain, vaginal bleeding, or abnormal β-hCG trends, an ultrasound should be performed.

Diagnosis
On sonographic imaging, the first goal should be to locate an intrauterine gestational sac using transvaginal ultrasound. When the β-hCG level has reached the discriminatory value of 2000 mIU/mL, a transvaginal ultrasound should locate an intrauterine gestational sac. Outside of imaging, following the β-hCG trend is important. Early in a viable pregnancy, the β-hCG value will have a doubling time that occurs every 48 hours. At around 10 weeks, it will plateau and start declining significantly around 20 weeks. If the β-hCG reaches a plateau early in pregnancy or does not double every 48 hours, this is highly suggestive of either a nonviable or ectopic pregnancy.

Management
Size and location of the ectopic pregnancy can guide treatment options, which makes ultrasound valuable. Most commonly, ectopic pregnancies are tubal in location. Because they are being diagnosed earlier, it is possible to take a more conservative approach to management. In a stable patient lacking free pelvic fluid, a more conservative, nonsurgical approach can be considered. Methotrexate has become the standard of care in stable patients, especially in patients who wish to preserve future fertility. If the patient is unstable or the ectopic pregnancy demonstrates cardiac activity, suggesting a later pregnancy, then surgical intervention is often required.

CASE 17

Epididymoorchitis

1. **A, B, D.** Causes of acute scrotal pain include ischemia, trauma, infection, inflammatory conditions, and inguinal hernia (incarcerated/strangulated).
2. **D.** Gray-scale and color Doppler with high-frequency linear transducer (>10 MHz) is ideal when evaluating the scrotum.
3. **C.** Enlarged testis and epididymis; decreased echogenicity or heterogeneous echogenicity; increased vascular flow; associated hydrocele and scrotal wall edema/thickening

4. **C.** Usually medical treatment is sufficient. Surgical treatment is warranted in complications related to epididymoorchitis, such as testicular abscess, infarction, or Fournier gangrene.

Comments

Background
Epididymitis or epididymoorchitis, an infection of the epididymis and/or testis, is a common cause of acute-onset scrotal pain. The differential diagnosis for acute scrotal pain is broad and includes ischemia (testicular torsion, appendiceal torsion, testicular infarction), trauma (testicular rupture, hematoma, hematocele), infections (acute epididymitis, epididymoorchitis, abscess, Fournier gangrene), and inflammatory conditions (Henoch-Schonlein purpura vasculitis of scrotal wall, fat necrosis). An accurate clinical history and physical examination can frequently precisely define the condition. Typically, scrotal pain associated with epididymitis or epididymoorchitis is relieved when the testes are elevated over the symphysis pubis, a maneuver called the Prehn sign. In contradistinction, the pain associated with testicular torsion is not relived by this maneuver.

Acute epididymoorchitis can present with fever. Although the causative agent in epididymitis is usually not identified in the pediatric population, the infection usually originates in the prostate gland or bladder and spreads to the epididymis and testes via the vas deferens and spermatic cord lymphatics. A congenital anomaly of the urinary tract may be present. In adolescents the cause is most often a sexually transmitted infections (STI). In men younger than 35 years of age with a history of venereal infectious exposure, epididymitis is often caused by chlamydia or gonococcal infection. In older men and those with problems, such as significant benign prostatic hyperplasia, a history of urinary tract infection (UTIs), or urethral strictures disease, enteric, gram-negative bacteria related to ascending urinary infection are much more likely causes. Orchitis, secondary to infection with mumps, occurs in approximately 25% of patients who contract the disease.

Diagnosis
Doppler US and high-frequency linear transducers (>10 MHz) are ideal for evaluation of testis/scrotum. The US findings of infection and torsion are usually quite distinct. Typical sonographic features of epididymitis include an enlarged epididymis with increased blood flow on color Doppler. Enlargement of the epididymis primarily involves the head. In epididymoorchitis, there is also increased blood flow to the testis, which is often enlarged and hypoechoic owing to edema. Although the testis and epididymis are typically enlarged and hypoechoic with torsion as well, blood flow is decreased or absent in torsion. A reactive hydrocele may be an associated finding in both conditions. On gray-scale imaging findings alone, the appearance of testis may mimic a diffusely infiltrative disease, such as leukemia or lymphoma, although the clinical presentation should suggest the correct diagnosis. Scrotal wall edema is an additional finding.

Management
Initial treatment is with broad-spectrum antibiotics used with therapy further directed based on culture results. Untreated epididymoorchitis may progress to scrotal abscess or testicular infarction, which can lead to testicular atrophy. Severe scrotal infection may result in a rare condition called Fournier gangrene Follow-up scrotal US is recommended in 4 to 6 weeks after the initial episode of epididymoorchitis in all cases to ensure complete resolution of the imaging findings following appropriate interval therapy. This follow-up approach also helps to exclude an underlying testicular tumor; however, it is very uncommon for a testicular tumor to present with pain.

CASE 18

Pyelonephritis

1. **A, D.** Although many of the choices could manifest in right-sided abdominal pain, the right kidney is asymmetrically enlarged with perinephric stranding and heterogeneous enhancement. The right ureter is also hyperemic. The colon is distended with stool, and constipation could be a consideration. No diverticular disease or diverticulitis is noted. The urinary bladder appears within normal limits.
2. **B.** The constellation of symptoms can help provide insight into the diagnosis. For example: dysuria, white blood cells present in the urine, suprapubic tenderness, ± fever = high clinical suspicion for cystitis. Dysuria, ± fever, blood cells present in the urine, flank pain/tenderness = high suspicion for pyelonephritis.
3. **B.** CT scan can help determine the etiology of pyelonephritis. Pyelonephritis is commonly perpetuated by disruption of urine flow within the urinary tract, allowing for easier colonization of bacteria. Cysts, stones, strictures, tumors, or other anatomic defects are associated with pyelonephritis. A CT scan is a highly sensitive method for evaluating the complications of UTIs, in addition to providing a global assessment of involvement within the abdomen and pelvis. The use of intravenous contrast provides some functional information about the kidney. CT is able to detect parenchymal abnormalities in patients with pyelonephritis that are generally missed by US.
4. **A.** DMSA (99m-technetium-dimercaptosuccinic acid) is particularly helpful in the pediatric population; it uses a radioactive tracer that is given via IV infusion and readily absorbed by the kidneys. A series of images acquired immediately following the infusion as well as 2 to 4 hours after the infusion to allows time for the kidneys to absorb the tracer. Functionality of the kidneys can be assessed and can be helpful in assessing cortical damage caused by recurrent infections. Its limitations include the inability to differentiate renal parenchymal disease from perinephric processes.

Comment

Background

Inflammation and infection of the renal parenchyma and renal pelvis are generally a result of an ascending lower UTI. If the infection is confined to an obstructed collecting system, the infection is referred to as pyelonephritis. Gram-negative enteric pathogens are the most commonly colonized bacterial agent causing pyelonephritis. Among them, *E. coli* is the most frequent cause. This is attributed to its virulence factors, which allow adherence to urothelium, paralysis of ureter peristalsis, and colonization within the urinary tract.

Diagnosis

Noncontrasted CT or unenhanced CT imaging is helpful in identifying urinary tract gas, calculi, renal enlargement, and obstruction.

Intravenous contrasted CT imaging during the corticomedullary phase can also detect renal enlargement, obstruction, calculi, gas, and parenchymal masses. This phase also allows for the visualization of disrupted contrast flow through infected renal tubules highlighting by wedge-shaped areas or streaky zones of lesser enhancement that extend from the papilla to the renal cortex (striated nephrogram). Complications, such as abscess, can be detected. If there is a concern about a ureteral stricture/lesion, ureteric anatomic anomaly, or bladder lesion, delayed images may be helpful.

Management

Empiric antibiotics generally result in resolution of symptoms within 72 hours. If pyelonephritis is not treated promptly, the microabscesses that form during the acute phase of pyelonephritis may coalesce to form a larger renal abscess. These renal abscesses are susceptible to rupture within the perinephric space and can lead to perirenal abscess or peritonitis.

CASE 19

Crohn's Disease

1. **B, C.** Although shigellosis presents with diarrhea, it is typically not chronic in nature. The same argument can be applied to traveler's diarrhea. Celiac and Crohn's disease are distinguished by the appearance of diarrhea, with celiac presenting more as greasy stools (steatorrhea) and Crohn's disease presenting with either normal-appearing stool or bloody stool. The appendix is normal.
2. **D.** See below.
3. **A.** The submucosal fat halo sign is pathognomonic for inflammatory bowel disease. This sign represents submucosal infiltration of fat. Comb sign is also seen in other acute inflammatory diseases of the bowel and in lupus mesenteric vasculitis.
4. **E.** All of the listed choices are potential complications of Crohn's disease.

Comment

Background

Crohn's disease is an idiopathic gastrointestinal (GI) disorder characterized by transmural inflammation of the GI tract. It may involve any portion of the GI tract from mouth to the perianal area. However, 80% of patients have small bowel involvement, usually in the distal ileum. One-third of patients have ileitis exclusively. Approximately 50% of patients will have ileocolitis. Isolated colonic involvement occurs in 20% of patients. A third of the patients suffer from perianal involvement.

Diagnosis

Endoscopic evaluation of the upper or lower GI tract may be helpful based on symptomatology. Air-contrast barium examinations may be useful in detecting aphthous ulcers or sacculations seen in chronic Crohn's disease. Small bowel findings in Crohn's disease often seen on barium studies include luminal narrowing with nodularity and ulceration, which can lead to the "string" sign when narrowing becomes severe. Cobblestoning, fistulas, and abscesses may also be seen. Wireless capsule endoscopy has become more common place.

In the emergency setting, many patients undergo CT for evaluation of abdominal pain or complications of Crohn's disease. Bowel wall thickening fatty infiltration and inflammation, strictures, and fistulas may be present. Predilection for the terminal ileum is common.

Common CT Signs

Fat halo sign: As mentioned above, the fat halo sign is seen on CT of the abdomen and represents submucosal infiltration of fat between the mucosa and muscularis layers of the bowel wall.

Comb sign: Hypervascularity of the mesentery seen in active Crohn's disease, which is outlined by fibrofatty proliferation and perivascular inflammation. These form linear markings in the mesentery of the affected bowel segment, giving it the appearance of the teeth of a comb (Figure 19-3).

Given the frequency and severity of Crohn's flares, it is not unusual for patients to have frequent visits to the Emergency Department (ED). Consideration regarding cumulative radiation dose should be considered when imaging. MRI can evaluate Crohn's disease without the ionizing radiation; however, it may not be as easily or readily available in many EDs.

Management

Crohn's disease cannot be cured; medications, such as steroids and immunosuppressants, are used to slow the progression of disease and to treat flares. Surgery, although not first-line, is employed in refractory or complicated cases. Patients with Crohn's disease are at increased risk for colorectal cancer, and regular screening is a consideration.

CASE 20

Radial Head Fracture

1. **A, D**. Prominent anterior and posterior fat pads are compatible with a large elbow joint effusion (**A**); the joint fluid distends the synovium, displacing the (intracapsular but extrasynovial) fat pads and making them visible by lateral radiographs. In the posttrauma setting, a joint effusion suggests the presence of a radial head fracture. Close inspection of the radial head in this patient reveals a cortical break/step-off—an acute radial head fracture (**D**). In many cases, the fracture itself may not be discretely visualized, and these patients are treated presumptively.
2. **C**. Standard lateral elbow radiographs are obtained in 90 degrees of flexion. These lateral views can demonstrate a small anterior fat pad extending from its position in the coronoid fossa. The normal posterior fat pad is obscured owing to the olecranon groove.
3. **A**. Distal humeral, specifically supracondylar, fractures are the most common elbow fractures in children. Conversely, radial head/neck fractures are the most common elbow fractures in adults comprising approximately 33% to 50% of injuries.
4. **C**. Statistically, a posttraumatic elbow joint effusion without identification of a fracture implies a nondisplaced, nonvisualized radial head/neck fracture. These patients are treated presumptively with immobilization. Cross-sectional imaging with either CT or MRI can increase detection of fractures that are not seen by radiography. However, these modalities are not routinely used in the immediate posttraumatic ED setting as they rarely result in management changes.

Comment

Background

Radial head and neck fractures are the most common elbow fractures in adults, frequently encountered in patients who present following a fall on out-stretched hand (FOOSH)-type injury which causes the radial head to impact on the capitellum. In reporting radial head fractures, the Mason-Johnston system is most commonly referenced in radiology literature. It relies on the degree of fracture displacement, the extent of articular surface involvement, and the presence of comminution or associated elbow dislocation.

Diagnosis

Positioning the patient in 90 degrees of flexion and obtaining a true lateral view are essential for diagnostic accuracy. Normal lateral elbow radiographs can demonstrate a small anterior fat pad extending from its position in the coronoid fossa while the normal posterior fat pad is obscured owing to the olecranon groove. The vast majority of elbow fractures are accompanied by an elbow joint effusion. A posttraumatic joint effusion distends the synovium and the joint capsule; this displaces the perisynovial fat pads (both anterior and posterior) outward, resulting in a prominent anterior fat pad and a visible posterior fat pad.

Pitfalls

Occasionally fractures of the radial neck and medial epicondyle present without an elbow joint effusion and detailed inspection of these areas is warranted. An oblique radiographic view can improve assessment of the radial head and neck. Associated injuries, which can be subtle, include coronoid process fractures, osteochondral injuries to the capitellum, and medial collateral ligamentous injury (which can present with widening of the medial joint space). If there is clinical concern for Essex-Lopresti fracture-dislocation, dedicated radiograph views of the wrist should be obtained.

CASE 21

Small Bowel Obstruction

1. **A**. In small bowel obstruction (SBO), the small bowel is usually dilated out of proportion to the distal bowel beyond its transition point as demonstrated in this case.
2. **A**. Adhesions are the most common cause of SBO.
3. **D**. CT may be helpful in determining SBO complications, transition point, and etiology.
4. **D**. All statements are true.

Comment

Background

Small bowel obstruction is a partial or complete blockage of the small bowel lumen. Patients may present with nonspecific complaints such as bloating, abdominal pain, anorexia, nausea, vomiting, obstipation, constipation, or cramps. Symptomatology may depend on the location and duration. Causes of obstruction include adhesions, volvulus, intussusception, tumor, gallstones, foreign bodies, hernias, impacted stool, and inflammation.

Diagnosis
Radiographs

Radiography is usually the first-line imaging obtained in evaluating patients suspected with SBO. Usually small bowel is more centrally located and contains valvulae conniventes. SBO is suggested when the small bowel is dilated with decompression distally. Small bowel is considered dilated when it measures greater than 3 cm. Some signs of SBO on upright or left lateral decubitus films include multiple air fluid levels, air fluid levels measuring more than 2.5 cm in length, and unequal heights of air fluid levels within the same loop of small bowel. SBO may present as a nonspecific gasless abdomen.

CT

Computed tomography is often obtained to help determine the cause of obstruction, location of transition point, and associated complications. Small bowel greater than 2.5 cm in caliber with decompressed distal bowel is a sign of SBO on CT. If present, the small bowel feces sign is helpful in determining the level of the transition point given that the small bowel feces sign is usually seen proximal to the transition point. Small bowel feces sign is demonstrated when air and particulate matter are seen in loops of small bowel that resemble feces, which may occur when there is increased bowel transit time. Oral contrast is not needed in diagnosing SBO. The retained intraluminal fluid in SBO provides negative contrast enhancement. Furthermore, patients often present with nausea and vomiting associated with SBO, and they may vomit and aspirate oral contrast. CT IV contrast is helpful in evaluating associated complications of SBO.

Ischemia in SBO

Associated ischemia increases the morbidity and mortality in SBO, and urgent surgery is needed to avoid necrosis and subsequent perforation. CT signs of small bowel ischemia may include bowel wall edema or hemorrhage, interloop fluid or fat stranding, pneumatosis, and portal venous gas. In early small bowel ischemia, the wall may demonstrate hyperenhancement, and later show decreased or absent enhancement. It is important to identify SBO caused by internal hernias, obstructing masses, intussusception with a fixed lead point, closed loop obstruction, and volvulus. These conditions are associated with ischemia. Closed loop obstruction occurs when a loop of small bowel has proximal and distal transition points. The closed loop of small bowel may rotate around its mesenteric axis causing a volvulus with the associated appearance of swirling of the mesenteric vessels.

Management
Low-grade or uncomplicated SBO may be amenable to decompression with orogastric tube suction and bowel rest. High-grade or complicated SBO may require surgery. Underlying causes of SBO should be identified, when possible, to help gauge management.

CASE 22

Right Mainstem Bronchial Intubation

1. **A, D.** Both unilateral bronchial intubation and mucous plugs can lead to hypoxia and secondary altered mental status (AMS) after emergent intubation. In this setting, the most common cause of lung collapse, increased difficulty breathing, and deterioration post emergency intubation is a bronchial intubation. The right mainstem bronchus is most commonly intubated owing to its more vertical orientation. **C** is much less likely given the acute presentation. There is no radiographic evidence of pneumothorax.
2. **B.** Radiographic verification of tube placement is the ideal cost-effective and rapid way of identifying an improperly placed endotracheal tube (ETT). CT is neither cost- nor time-effective in an emergency situation. Auscultation can be susceptible to operator error and does not allow direct visualization. CO_2 capnography can provide feedback of proper tube placement in the trachea and pulmonary system, but will not differentiate between a properly placed ETT and a mainstem intubation.
3. **B.** Ideally, ETT tip position is below the clavicular line and approximately 2 cm above the carina. This allows for tube tip movement when the neck is moved; when the chin is depressed, the tube tip will move downward, and when the chin is lifted, the tube tip will move upward.
4. **A.** If the tube is inserted deep into the right main bronchus, the right upper lobe bronchus can be obstructed. This results in collapse of the left lung and the right upper lobe. Pericardial effusion and jugular venous distention can be signs of a cardiac tamponade forming. Pulmonary edema and Curly's B lines are signs of congestive heart failure and fluid overload in a patient. Inferior vena cava collapse on ultrasound with inspiration is a sign of dehydration and decreased fluid volume in a patient.

Comment

Background
Mainstem bronchial intubations occur frequently in emergency situations when an airway needs to be established rapidly and several factors contribute to excessively caudal tube placement. This is a relatively benign complication if identified rapidly after intubation and corrected immediately. Because many patients who are initially intubated are intubated because of their deteriorating respiratory status, this complication can actually further worsen their situation. Any patient who is not improving clinically after intubation must be checked for a mainstem intubation and must be reevaluated immediately. Longstanding physiologic sequelae of endobronchial intubation include barotrauma secondary to ventilation of a solitary lung with higher pressures than normal. Hemothorax and pneumothorax may also occur. Finally, if

endobronchial intubation is not reversed in a timely manner, altered mental status and cerebral hypoxia may result.

Diagnosis
Portable chest radiography is an accessible, rapid, low-radiation, and inexpensive tool.

Management
Routine radiographic confirmation of ETT placement. Reposition and confirm as necessary.

CASE 23

Pulmonary Edema

1. **B, D.** Dyspnea, pleuritic chest pain, and cough may reflect a pulmonary edema and can occur in many underlying conditions. Confirming the diagnosis may rely on the clinical circumstances and typical radiographic findings. Indistinct pulmonary vasculature, perihilar opacification, pleural effusions, and cardiomegaly are characteristic of pulmonary edema. Toxin inhalation, although noncardiogenic, would result in an intense irritation of the small airways and alveoli, leading to fluid accumulation.
2. **A,B, D.** See below.
3. **A.** Kerley lines are best visualized at the costophrenic angle and become smaller as you move toward the hilum. They may be difficult to visualize as edema enters the alveolar space. Diffuse lung haziness may be difficult to differentiate from bronchopneumonia; however, the patient's history should help in distinguishing the two.

Comment

Background
Pulmonary edema is defined as excess fluid around the capillary bed and in alveoli of the lungs. It is a condition caused by excess fluid outflow into the interstitium caused by changes in Starling forces. Increased capillary pressure (heart failure) and increased capillary permeability (by toxins) are two of the major causes, respectively.

Cardiogenic pulmonary edema (CPE) should be differentiated into two basic types: CPE and noncardiogenic (NCPE). CPE is defined as pulmonary edema owing to increased capillary hydrostatic pressure secondary to elevated pulmonary venous pressure. NCPE is caused by either altered capillary membrane permeability or decreased plasma oncotic pressure. Inciting causes include inhaled toxins, near-drowning, oxygen therapy, transfusion or trauma, central nervous system (CNS) disorder, acute respiratory distress syndrome (ARDS), aspiration, altitude sickness, renal disorder, resuscitation, drugs, allergic alveolitis, contrast, or contusion.

Diagnosis
Cardiogenic pulmonary edema can show cardiomegaly with bilateral perihilar alveolar opacification producing a characteristic butterfly pattern and bilateral pleural effusions. Other signs include loss of diaphragmatic appreciation and Kerley lines.

CASE 24

Tension Pneumothorax

1. **B, C.** Spontaneous pneumothorax demonstrates pleural translucency and can lead to tension pneumothorax. Right upper lobe collapse owing to endobronchial intubation can include deviation of the mediastinum. Bilateral tension pneumothorax will show translucency on both sides. Pleural effusion will show fluid accumulation.

2. **C.** A visible pleural translucency with absent vascular markings is indicative of a pneumothorax, but not of a tension pneumothorax specifically. Mediastinal shift to the contralateral side, depression of the affected hemidiaphragm, and increased intracostal space are associated with tension pneumothorax. There is no left diaphragmatic depression. Presence of a small bleb is indicative of spontaneous pneumothorax, not present in this image.

3. **C.** Dysphasia and tachycardia can be found in tension pneumothorax. Decreased diaphragmatic excursion is common to pneumothorax owing to restricted lung expansion. Paradoxic chest movement would indicate flail chest.

4. **A.** Trauma or wound will cause iatrogenic pneumothorax. Positive pressure in intracellular space causes tension pneumothorax. Ruptured subpleural bleb causes primary spontaneous pneumothorax. Secondary spontaneous pneumothorax is usually caused by compromised alveoli caused by underlying lung disease.

Comment

Background
Pneumothorax is defined as the presence of air within the pleural cavity that can lead to impaired ventilation and oxygenation. The clinical presence is dependent on the degree of collapse of the affected lung. If the pneumothorax is severe, it can affect hemodynamic stability and cause a shift in the mediastinum. A spontaneous pneumothorax can occur when air enters the intrapleural space. In the absence of underlying lung disease, this is known as a primary spontaneous pneumothorax. In patients with a lung disease, air will enter the intrapleural space owing to damaged or compromised alveoli, which is referred to as a secondary spontaneous pneumothorax. In a tension pneumothorax, air trapped in the pleural space will create positive pressure that will displace the mediastinal and intrathoracic structures. Clinical presentations of hypoxia or chest pain, paired with a shifted mediastinum, as seen in this case, can confirm a diagnosis of a tension pneumothorax.

Diagnosis
Clinical presentation of a tension pneumothorax may include hypotension, hypoxia, chest pain, or dyspnea. Additionally, on examination, breath sounds are absent on the affected hemithorax. There may be distention in the jugular vein. Clinical presentation is used as the primary diagnosis in a tension pneumothorax. As tension pneumothorax requires immediate treatment, radiography should be ordered only when there is doubt regarding the clinical diagnosis, and the patient's clinical condition is hemodynamically stable. Radiographic findings of tension pneumothorax include contralateral mediastinal shift, diaphragmatic depression, and ipsilateral increased intercostal spaces. If a chest radiograph fails to show presence of a pneumothorax, a CT scan may be helpful for diagnosis.

Management
Decompression of the pleural space with chest tube allows for lung reexpansion.

CASE 25

Dural Venous Thrombosis

1. **C.** Dural venous thrombosis demonstrates hyperattenuation in the superior sagittal sinuses on the noncontrast CT. On CT venogram, filing defects are noted in the superior sagittal and straight sinuses. Venous infarct may be caused by dural venous sinus thrombosis and may demonstrate abnormal parenchymal attenuation.

2. **A.** Hypertension is not a known risk factor.

3. **C.** Headache is seen in 75% to 95% of cases. Female-to-male ratio is nearly 3:1. Dural venous thrombosis is most common in the superior sagittal sinus. Dural venous thrombosis is most commonly seen in neonates.

4. **C.** It is seen on contrast enhanced CT (CECT) or enhanced MRI. It is only seen in the superior sagittal sinus during the subacute phase (5 d–2 m).

Comment

Background
Dural venous sinus thrombosis is rare, with an incidence of three to four cases per million. It is most commonly seen in neonates and decreases in incidence with age, with a mean age of 39 years. Dural venous thrombosis is more common in women than men with a ratio of 3:1. Risk factors include prothrombotic conditions, such as pregnancy and the use or oral contraceptives, infection, malignancy, and trauma.

Diagnosis
The most common CT finding is the empty delta sign, seen within the superior sagittal sinus on CECT or post-contrast MRI. Increased density may be appreciated within the sinus on non enhanced CT (NECT). CT venography (Figure 25-3) may demonstrate a filling defect and is the examination of choice, with a reported sensitivity of 95%. On MRI, acute clot (0–5 days) is iso-intense on T1 and hypointense on T2 with subacute clot (5 d–1 mo) becoming hyperintense on T1/T2 and FLAIR. MR venography (MRV) may demonstrate lack of flow in the effected sinus.

Occlusion of a cerebral vein causes a backup of pressure and results in ischemia and infarction with or without hemorrhage. These infarcts are most commonly hemorrhagic, and tend to have a nonarterial distribution. The increased pressure from the thrombosed sinus blocks circulation and absorption of cerebrospinal fluid (CSF), thus resulting in intracranial hypertension. The superior sagittal sinus is most commonly affected, followed by the transverse sinus. Patients will most commonly experience headaches as the presenting symptom, but the clinical presentation is otherwise nonspecific, making clinical diagnosis difficult.

Management
Proper anticoagulation therapy is the mainstay of therapy in the acute setting. Elevated intracranial pressures may lead to secondary cerebral damage, so treatment should be aimed at normalizing the pressure. Medical treatment includes diuretics, but surgical interventions, such as external ventricular drainage and CSF shunts, are often needed.

CASE 26

Subarachnoid Hemorrhage (Ruptured Brain Aneurysm)

1. **A, D.** The patient had a subarachnoid hemorrhage from a ruptured aneurysm. The CT characteristics can look similar to an intraparenchymal hemorrhage and must also be on the differential. An epidural hematoma looks like a convex hyperdensity on CT that does not expand across the skull sutures. Subdural hematomas, on the other hand, appear crescent shape and cross sutures.

2. **B.** As imaging shows, the patient likely has a subarachnoid hemorrhage secondary to an aneurysm. The most likely cause of a subarachnoid hemorrhage is a ruptured aneurysm and often presents as "worst headache of my life." The other choices can cause an intraparenchymal hemorrhage and are unlikely in a subarachnoid hemorrhage.

3. **C.** A noncontrast CT is always indicated in a patient with suspected hemorrhage in the brain. The sensitivity of a head CT

within 12 hours of a hemorrhage is 98% to 100% and remains the gold standard imaging for suspected acute bleeds in the brain.

4. **A.** Hydrocephalus is divided into two categories: communicating and noncommunicating. Communicating hydrocephalus is a condition where CSF is unable to be reabsorbed from the subarachnoid space and into the venous system. Noncommunicating hydrocephalus occurs when obstruction occurs in the path of CSF flow. Patients suffering from an intraparenchymal or subarachnoid hemorrhage will have a communicating hydrocephalus as the blood increases fluid in the arachnoid space and impedes the reabsorption of fluid back into the venous system.

Comment

Background
Annually, there are about 30,000 new cases of subarachnoid hemorrhage (SAH) in the United States. A common presentation is a patient reporting to the ED with "the worst headache of my life." However, studies have shown that only 20% of patients with a confirmed SAH reported experiencing a headache. Therefore, suspicions should remain high if a hemorrhage is suspected. SAH risk factors include hypertension, female sex, smoking, alcohol use, and drug use. Although the most common cause of a subarachnoid hemorrhage is a ruptured aneurysm, other causes include vasculitides, vascular malformations, and rarely vessel dissections.

Diagnosis
The best imaging to detect a hemorrhage is an NECT of the head. The sensitivity is close to 100% within the first 12 hours. An inconclusive study can be followed up by a lumbar puncture. If this yields a xanthochromic fluid, then the diagnosis of SAH can be confirmed. Common locations include the most dependent areas of the CSF space: the suprasellar cistern, the deep sulci adjacent to the interhemispheric fissure, the interpeduncular cistern, and the Sylvian fissure.

Management
Complications of an SAH include communicating hydrocephalus, brain ischemia secondary to vasospasm, and rebleeding. A communicating hydrocephalus occurs because CSF fails to drain adequately into the venous system owing to the hemorrhage. Vasospasms are thought to occur from the oxidative effects of the hemorrhaged red blood cells. The Fischer scale can be used to determine the likelihood of a vasospasm in patients presenting with SAH and is outlined below. A score greater than 2 puts the patient at risk for a vasospasm.

Grade	Computed Tomography Appearance
1	No blood is visualized
2	Visualized layer of blood is <1 mm thick
3	Visualized layer or focal clot >1 mm thick
4	Thickness with intraventricular/intraparenchymal hemorrhage

Mortality rates range from 8% to 67%, so early treatment is indicated.

CASE 27

Orbital Floor Fracture

1. **B.** Selected CT images demonstrate a fractured left orbital floor. Zygomatic fracture may be included in the differential of a patient having blunt trauma to the eye, but is unlikely given the imaging in this case. The mandible and retina are not in the field of view on the selected images.

2. **A.** Because the orbital floor is fractured, entrapment of the extraocular muscles is possible (present in this case) and

therefore may present with eye movement deficits. This is an indication for surgery.

3. **B.** Indications for surgery include enophthalmos (posterior dislocation of the globe, present in this case) greater than 2 mm on imaging, double vision, and extraocular muscle entrapment.

4. **A.** The orbital floor is the weakest point of the orbit, and fractures here can lead to contents dislocating into the maxillary sinus (present in this case).

Comment

Background
Orbital fractures classically present following blunt trauma to the eye. The weakest point of the orbit is in the inferior orbital wall. Orbital soft tissue herniates into the maxillary sinus. A common consequence of this fracture is muscle entrapment, which leads to vision changes, such as double vision.

Diagnosis
On CT, the inferior rectus may be seen extending into this space, as well as hyperintense blood products (present in this case).

Management
Surgery is indicated for patients who have such complications. Another complication of this fracture is enophthalmos, or posterior dislocation of the eyeball within the orbit (present in this case). This will present with vision changes. When evaluating such fractures, it is important to consider the sagittal view to assess the convexity of the orbit, whereas a coronal view will demonstrate the integrity of the dependent orbital floor.

CASE 28

Zygomaticomaxillary Complex Fracture (ZMC)

1. **B, D.** The 3D reconstructions (Figures 28-3 and 28-4) demonstrate a zygomatic fracture. The axial images in particular (Figures 28-1 and 28-2) show a fracture on the left zygomatic arch at the zygomaticotemporal suture. The differential diagnosis for an injury like this includes a Le Fort fracture, given its close proximity to the pterygoid bone.

2. **C.** The zygoma articulates with the temporal, sphenoid, frontal, and maxillary bone. It does not, however, include the mandible.

3. **A.** All Le Fort fractures include the fracture of the pterygoid plates. Not all Le Fort fractures involve the orbit or spare the nasal bones. The different types do not occur at the same suture lines, hence the different classifications.

4. **A.** The treatment is reduction of the zygoma as well as fixation with malleable plates.

Comment

Background
Fractures of the zygoma most often occur secondary to trauma to the lateral midface. Important articulation points of the zygoma include the temporal, maxillary, sphenoid, and frontal bones. Fractures can occur along any of these articulations. An important fracture is between the maxillary and zygoma, which can involve the orbit. This is clinically significant because it may result in globe entrapment and visual changes, such as diplopia. Another complication is limited range of motion (ROM) of the jaw secondary to zygomatic arch compression of the temporalis tendon at the insertion site on the coronoid process of the mandible.

Le Fort Fractures
Fractures including the maxilla and pterygoid plates are divided into three subtypes of Le Fort fractures. Le Fort I level extends horizontally above the alveolar process of the maxilla and includes

the anterior or posterior walls of the maxillary sinus. Le Fort II level additionally involves the inferior and medial orbital rims. Le Fort III level further involves the connection between the upper face and skull base.

Management
Management of a zygomatic fracture includes reduction and fixation of the zygoma to malleable plates.

CASE 29

Mandible Fracture

1. **A.** The CT scans demonstrate fractures of the bilateral mandible. The other diagnoses involve fractures superior to the jaw.
2. **C.** Plain films have low sensitivity in diagnosing a mandible fracture because it is difficult to visualize. One should order either Panorex or CT imaging to make the diagnosis.
3. **C.** The most effective treatment for a mandible fracture is surgery, either fixation or reduction. None of the remaining options would adequately treat the patient.
4. **D.** The condyle is the most one likely to be fractured. The order from most to least fractured part of the mandible: condyle, angle, body, mental, ramus.

Comment

Background
Patients with mandibular fractures will often present with numbness of the chin or teeth, tenderness to palpation localized to the lower jaw, ecchymosis, pain when opening the jaw, and swelling in the area. Additionally, broken molars may also be present. A common complicating presentation is stridor or drooling, which may be indicative of airway difficulty. As a result, endotracheal intubation must be considered early.

Diagnosis
Diagnosis for patients is made either by Panorex or CT imaging. Panorex imaging may show a flattened or focal trough along the lower jaw or mandible. CT, which is the most sensitive and specific imaging modality, will show displacement of the mandible, with lucency at the area of the jaw.

Management
Treatment includes surgery, either reduction or fixation. Reduction simply refers to bringing the edges of the broken bones together. Fixation requires an arch bar placed on the mandibular or maxillary teeth, which are then attached to the jaw, giving it stabilization. The average healing time for such is around 4 to 6 weeks, and long-term complications include loss of sensation owing to damage to the mandibular nerve and loss of teeth.

CASE 30

Sinusitis

1. **C.** Trigeminal neuralgia and migraines would not have CT findings associated with them. An orbital fracture would be demonstrated on CT; however, all figures above show an intact orbit. The maxillary sinus (Figure 30-1) demonstrates an infectious involvement, likely viral.
2. **B.** Diagnosis of acute sinusitis is made clinically, and radiographs are not a first-line modality for diagnosis. A CT may be obtained if there is concern for malignancy or complications secondary to infection. However, the clinician should always first take a good history before proceeding to imaging modalities.

3. **D.** Patients with sinusitis can have a number of symptoms, but dysphagia is not one of them. Involvement of the esophagus is unlikely in sinusitis.
4. **A.** Bacterial causes of sinusitis are rare (2% to 10%), and most are actually caused by viruses. The patient must not be treated with antibiotics unless it is clinically suggested that a bacterial process is occurring.

Comment

Background
There are four different paranasal sinuses: ethmoid, maxillary, sphenoid, and frontal. Sinusitis refers to the symptomatic inflammation of these paranasal sinuses and nasal cavity. A majority of patients presenting with sinusitis have symptomatology caused by viruses such as rhinovirus, influenza, and parainfluenza. However, bacterial causes can range from 2% to 10% of episodes and require antibiotic therapy. Symptoms of sinusitis include purulent nasal discharge, tooth discomfort, facial pain, and pressure that is worse when bending forward. Additionally, patients may experience a cough, ear fullness, headaches, and fevers.

Diagnosis
Diagnosis is made clinically based on symptoms. Patients rarely require imaging if sinusitis is suspected. However, CT can play a role if the clinician believes the infection has spread to surrounding tissue, or worse, into the cavernous sinus. Additionally, CT can guide other suspected diagnoses, such as allergic rhinitis, which would have an absence of CT features demonstrated above.

Management
Treatment for this condition is usually supportive unless bacterial sinusitis is expected, in which case it may be treated like a pneumonia.

CASE 31

Tonsillitis

1. **B.** The patient's CT findings are consistent with tonsillitis, complicated by peritonsillar abscess. Sinusitis and orbital cellulitis would present superior, and a foreign body would not demonstrate a bilateral finding as it does in tonsillitis.
2. **A or B.** Either of these choices may work. The images show a peritonsillar abscess, likely secondary to a bacterial infection. However, most cases of simple tonsillitis are caused by a virus.
3. **A.** In this situation, the treatment is antibiotic and drainage as CT shows peritonsillar abscess. Pain relief, antiinflammatory medications, and salt water gargle is appropriate for a viral cause of tonsillitis without complication. Aspirin should never be given to a child.
4. **B.** Patients with group A streptococcus who are not properly treated may develop rheumatic fever. The sequel of rheumatic fever can be remembered by JONES criteria (J: joint arthritis; O: obvious–heart/carditits; N: subcutaneous Nodules; E: erythea marginatum; S: Sydenham's chorea).

Comment

Background
Presenting symptoms of tonsillitis include sore throat; red, swollen tonsils; pain while swallowing; fatigue; coughing; and swollen lymph nodes in the neck. The most important aspect of managing tonsillitis is correctly diagnosing the etiology. Viruses are most likely to cause tonsillitis. The most common viral pathogens include Epstein-Barr virus (EBV), cytomegalovirus (CMV), herpes simplex virus (HSV), influenza, enterovirus, and adenovirus.

The most common bacterial cause of tonsillitis is group A strepto-coccus pharyngitis. Patients between the ages of 5 and 15 should especially be screened for this pathogen because anywhere between 15% and 30% of all pharyngitis is in patients between 5 and 15 years of age. Other bacterial causes include *Mycoplasma pneumonia* and *Neisseria gonorrhea*.

Diagnosis

Diagnosis includes throat culture or rapid antigen detection test. Those with evidence of acute pharyngitis and absence of viral symptoms or children with symptoms who have been exposed to individuals with GAS should get a rapid antigen test done to exclude the possibility of group A streptococcus.

Management

Treatment for most patients with tonsillitis includes pain relief and antiinflammatory medications. Salt water gargle may also be used in order to alleviate symptoms. If a bacterial etiology is suspected, the patient should be prescribed penicillin or clindamycin if the patient is penicillin (PCN)-allergic.

CASE 32

Epiglottitis

1. **B, D.** Laryngocele often mimics epiglottitis in clinical presentation and lateral radiography of the neck. Although a rare infectious complication, laryngocele should also be included in the differential diagnosis for epiglottic enlargement seen on lateral neck x-ray. The epiglottis appears normal on lateral neck x-ray in bacterial tracheitis and retropharyngeal abscess.
2. **A.** Although rates of infection caused by *Haemophilus influenza* (Hib) have reduced significantly owing to infant vaccination, it is still a common cause of epiglottitis, even in immunized children.
3. **C.** Soft-tissue neck x-ray will show epiglottic enlargement, which is a finding in both epiglottitis and laryngocele; therefore it is not the best modality to distinguish between the two processes.
4. **C.** Presenting symptoms in **A** and **B** may be seen with epiglottitis; however, the "tripod" or "sniffing" position is a characteristic presentation. Ear pain and vomiting are typically not associated with epiglottitis.

Comment

Background

Epiglottitis is a cellulitis of the epiglottis, aryepiglottic folds, and surrounding structures secondary to direct invasion of the epithelial layer by pathogenic organisms primarily from the posterior nasopharynx. Once swelling begins, it spreads rapidly to involve the entire supraglottic larynx; subglottic areas are unaffected because swelling is blocked by epithelium at the level of the vocal cords. This swelling is what is visualized on soft-tissue neck x-rays. Swelling can become excessive enough to cause airway obstruction, which can lead to cardiopulmonary arrest and intubation.

Diagnosis

Epiglottitis is typically a clinical diagnosis and does not require imaging. Laryngoscopic visualization of the epiglottis is gold standard. Lateral neck radiographs will be abnormal in 77% to 88% of cases showing inflammation and edema of the supraglottic structures (epiglottis, aryepiglottic folds, and arytenoid cartilage).

The classic radiographic feature seen in epiglottitis is the "thumb sign," which is an enlarged epiglottis that protrudes from anterior wall of hypopharynx (Figure 32-1).

Ultrasonography in the longitudinal plane in adults will show the "alphabet P sign," which is an acoustic shadow of the swollen epiglottis and hyoid bone at the level of the thyrohyoid membrane.

CASE 33

Orbital Cellulitis

1. **B.** CT images show soft-tissue swelling surrounding in the left orbit. This points to a differential diagnosis of orbital cellulitis or associated soft-tissue inflammation. Retinal detachment is unlikely given the presentation and the age of the patient. Likewise, acute angle-closure glaucoma would not present in a 5-year-old child. Neoplasm is also unlikely because there is soft-tissue swelling, whereas a neoplasm would show a mass in conjunction with swelling.
2. **B.** CT with contrast is the appropriate first-line imaging modality in patients with suspected orbital infection.
3. **D.** Streptococcus, *Staphylococcus aureus*, and *Streptococcus pyogenes* are all bacteria that can invade orbital tissue from surrounding sinuses. Klebsiella would not cause this presentation and is a bacterium that causes infection in the elderly, diabetics, and alcoholics. It is unlikely to occur in a child.
4. **A.** The first-line treatment for a patient with orbital cellulitis is IV antibiotics. Patients should be treated for 48 hours; if no improvements are seen clinically, the patient may be referred for either endoscopic or external drainage, depending on the site and size. NSAIDs and follow up are not adequate treatment.

Comment

Background

Orbital cellulitis is the inflammation of eye tissue surrounding the orbit. Patients may face any number of ocular symptoms, such as loss of vision, diplopia, limited ROM of the extraocular muscles, and bulging of the eye. Additionally, the tarsus may become inflamed, and the patient may experience discharge. Systemic symptoms of an infection may also be present, such as fever, myalgia, and lethargy. The cause of orbital cellulitis is often an infection in the nearby sinuses, such as the ethmoid or maxillary sinus. *Staphylococcus aureus*, *Streptococcus pneumonia*, and *Streptococcus pyogenes* are common etiologic pathogens.

Diagnosis

CECT of the face/orbits is the appropriate examination. Carefully inspect the orbital contents and note preseptal, retrobulbar, intra/extraconal, globar involvement.

Management

Intravenous antibiotics targeting common pathogens, such as vancomycin, ceftriaxone, cefotaxime, and ampicillin-sulbactam, are used. Endoscopic or external drainage must be explored if IV antibiotics have not produced a clinical improvement in the patient's symptoms. The most common complications are spread of infection into the cavernous sinus as well as cavernous sinus thrombosis. Typically, patients respond to the IV antibiotics and recover with no further neurologic deficits.

CASE 34

Jefferson Fracture

1. **B.** The axial plane CT (Figure 34-2) shows most clearly that this is a Jefferson fracture. The Jefferson fracture is defined as a fracture of the C1 vertebra at the weakest points: the anterior and posterior junction of the arches, as well as the lateral masses.
2. **D.** Although Jefferson fractures are not classically associated with neurologic deficits, 50% of these fractures are associated with other C-spine injuries; 33% are associated with C2 fractures, and vertebral artery injury can be seen.

3. **C.** The Jefferson fracture is caused by spinal axial loading and fracturing of the weakest aspects of the C1 vertebrae. This results in multiple fractures in the ring, most notably the anterior and posterior junction of the arches.
4. **B.** Because the Jefferson fracture is not associated with neurologic deficit, neurologically intact patients may not need surgical intervention. However, patients should be screened for associated injuries that may require intervention. Notably, asymmetric fractures may affect blood vessels or nerves and could require surgical intervention.

Comment

Background
These fractures are normally caused by trauma to the head, which is translated down axially, and impacts the weakest points along the C1 vertebrae. This includes the anterior and posterior junction points, which are all classically fractured symmetrically, producing four breaks in the ring. Presenting symptoms include neck pain and occipital headaches. The transverse ligament may also be affected by the fracture, which can lead to instability, but this is not seen in a classic Jefferson fracture. Instead, the asymmetric Jefferson fracture involves the transverse ligament and may produce two or three breaks in the C1 vertebra instead of the four seen in a classic Jefferson fracture. To determine whether the transverse ligament is involved in this fracture, separation of the fragments must be measured. Separation greater than 5.4 mm on CT or 7 mm on radiograph indicates the ligament has been involved. This measurement is known as the Rule of Spence.

Diagnosis
Patients with axial loading injuries should receive CT spine evaluation. MR may provide greater detail regarding ligamentous injury.

Management
Immobilization versus surgical intervention depends on concommitant injuries/neurologic status. CTA may aid in the evaluation for vascular injuries.

CASE 35

Dens Fracture

1. **C.** CT demonstrates a posteriorly displaced, mildly distracted dens fracture. The fracture line extends along the base of the dens.
2. **B.** CT shows a fracture of odontoid at the base, which points to a diagnosis of a type II fracture. Type I fractures occur at the distal dens/tip. Type III fractures occur through the C2 body. Type IV dens fractures do not exist.
3. **A.** Surgical fusion is indicated for a type II dens fracture, whereas type III and I require conservative measures.
4. **B.** The primary mechanism of dens fractures is via hyperflexion of the neck. This normally occurs in MVAs and results in the odontoid process being displaced anteriorly. Hyperextension can also cause an odontoid fracture; however, it is less likely and results in the odontoid process being displaced posteriorly.

Comment

Background
Motor vehicle accidents are a common ED presentation. The decision to get a C-spine imaging in this situation is usually determined by the Canadian C-Spine rule. The criteria for this includes

* Age >65 years
* Dangerous mechanism (e.g., a high speed MVA, head on collision)
* Paresthesias in extremity

Common fractures of the cervical spine in MVAs include teardrop fractures, burst fractures, hangman fractures, and odontoid fractures.

Diagnosis
Medium and high-risk patients should be evaluated with NECT of the spine. Low-risk patients may benefit from radiographs.

Management
Three types of odontoid fractures:

* Type I: fracture occurs distal/tip
* Type II: transverse fracture at the base
* Type III: fracture through the base and extending into the body

Types III and I are generally stable and can be treated with conservative measures, whereas type II, an unstable fracture, is treated with surgical fusion.

CASE 36

Gastric Volvulus (Mesenteroaxial)

1. **C, D.** The distended viscus conforms to the shape of the stomach and is consistent with massive gastric distention, probably secondary to obstruction.
2. **D.** The CT demonstrates twisting of the stomach along its short axis, which is consistent with mesenteroaxial volvulus. This results in abnormal, upside down configuration of the stomach with the gastric antrum and pylorus located superior to the gastroesophageal (GE) junction.
3. **A.** Organoaxial volvulus is the most common type of gastric volvulus in adults and is seen in two-thirds of patients.
4. **D.** Vomiting is not included in the clinical triad of Borchardt, which is seen in about 70% of patients with gastric volvulus.

Comment

Background
The stomach is an uncommon site for volvulus in the GI tract, which occurs owing to twisting of the stomach on its mesentery. The classic clinical triad of sudden onset epigastric pain, intractable retching, and inability to pass a nasogastric tube into the stomach is described by Borchardt in 1904 and is seen in about 70% of patients. Gastric volvulus can range from being asymptomatic to being catastrophic, with delay in diagnosis leading to gastric ischemia resulting in necrosis, perforation, mediastinitis, and peritonitis.

Diagnosis
The diagnosis may be suggested on radiography and made on upper GI or cross sectional imaging.

The most commonly used classification, which was proposed by Singleton, is based on the axis along which the stomach twists.

Organoaxial volvulus: This is the most common type in adults and accounts for about two-thirds of all cases. The stomach twists along its long axis (cardiopyloric line that extends from the gastric cardia to the pylorus) resulting in superior displacement of the greater curvature and the lesser curvature located caudally. The antrum rotates anterosuperiorly and the fundus posteroinferiorly. A twist greater than 180 degrees results in complete obstruction. However, most patients have incomplete or partial obstruction with the twist less than 180 degrees. This type of volvulus is usually associated with trauma and paraesophageal hiatal hernia. Patients with redundant paraesophageal hernia can have secondary rotation of the stomach along its long axis, and when asymptomatic, it is preferable to use the term "organoaxial position" of the stomach rather than calling it volvulus. In the pediatric population, large Bochdalek hernia is usually the predisposing cause.

Mesenteroaxial volvulus: This is less common in adults, but more common than organoaxial volvulus in the pediatric population. This results from twisting of the stomach along its short axis, which is perpendicular to the cardiopyloric line. Most of these cases are partial with the twist less than 180 degrees. The gastric antrum is displaced superior to the GE junction with the stomach typically appearing "upside down" with the gastric antrum and pylorus superior to the fundus and proximal body.

Combined: Least common and a complex type with both organoaxial and mesenteroaxial components.

Management
Endoscopic or surgical intervention. Complications include ulceration, perforation, and hemorrhage.

CASE 37

Thoracolumbar Burst Fracture

1. **A, C.** A burst fracture with perched facets is present. Burst fracture is a type A3 compression fracture of the spinal column caused by high-energy axial forces. The perched facet's inferior articular process sits on the superior articular process of the vertebrae beneath it.
2. **B.** Burst fracture is a type A3 compression fracture of the spinal cord.
3. **D.** Type D2 sagittal translation results from axial compression and hyperflexion. This allows for facet perching or frank locking to occur.
4. **A.** In a classic spinal burst fracture, fragments are retropulsed from the poseterosuperior corner with the inferior endplates remaining intact.

Comment

Background
High-energy axial forces, such as a fall from a height, an MVA, or a high-intensity sports injury, result in the failure of the middle and anterior spinal columns, resulting in a specific form of a compression fracture, called a burst fracture. When this injury occurs, fragments of the posterosuperior vertebral body may retropulse into surrounding tissues and spinal canal causing potential neurologic injury to the spinal cord, conus medullaris, or cauda equina.

Burst fractures can be stable or nonstable. A stable fracture implies that the patient is neurologically intact with an intact posterior arch and less than a 50% anterior body height collapse. Unstable fractures have neurologic deficits and dislocations, with loss of greater than or equal to 50% of vertebral body height. Initially, stable injuries can become unstable.

A patient may experience acute back pain and restricted motion. There may be accompanied neurologic deficits, including motor and sensory changes. Approximately 50% of thoracolumbar burst fractures have associated neurologic deficit that are usually seen at the time of the injury.

Diagnosis
Evaluation of burst fractures solely on conventional radiography can often result in misdiagnosis. Certain signs warrant further evaluation by CT to determine the degree of spinal canal compromise, the presence of posterior element fractures, and the nature of the retropulsed fragment(s). MR can provide more detailed information about the state of the spinal cord if compromise is suspected clinically or noted on CT.

Management
Patients can receive surgical or nonsurgical treatment for these fractures. Nonoperative treatment includes analgesics, a brace, bed rest, and a cast. Operative treatment includes intervertebral fusion, with or without spinal decompression. Insufficient evidence exists that operative management is preferred to nonoperative management in fractures without a neurologic deficit.

CASE 38

Sternal Fracture

1. **A.** Sternal fractures are demonstrated on CT.
2. **B.** Bronchitis is not associated with acute sternal fractures in the setting of trauma.
3. **D.** When associated with other injuries, morbidity is 25% to 45%.
4. **A.** CT will detect rib fractures, pulmonary contusion, and pneumothorax.

Comment

Background
Sternal fractures are predominantly associated with automobile injuries and blunt anterior chest traumas. The injuries are different in those that face direct trauma versus those with indirect trauma. Direct trauma accounts for most of the cases and consists of direct impact sports, pedestrian collisions, falls, and assaults. Indirect injuries include thoracic kyphosis, osteoporosis among elderly patients, postmenopausal women, and patients on long-term steroid therapy. The morbidity rate is between 25% and 45% when associated with other injuries. In isolated cases, the morbidity rate is only 7%.

Diagnosis
Typical symptoms include crepitus, localized tenderness, hypoxemia, and respiratory insufficiency. Associated findings include rib fractures, flail chest, and sternoclavicular dislocation. CT should be considered in the proper clinical contexts. CT will also allow adjacent mediastinal, parenchymal, and thoracic evaluation.

Management
If the sternum is left fractured, there are short-term and long-term complications that can occur. Short-term complications include interfered ventilation and chest pain. Long-term complications include development of false joint and overlap deformities.

CASE 39

Pancreatitis

1. **D.** Pancreatitis presents with epigastric pain, which may be confirmed by focal enlargement on CT. Although duodenal ulcer, gastric ulcer, gastritis, and peritonitis present with epigastric pain, these conditions would not present with abnormal pancreas on imaging.
2. **B.** Because this case has two of three criteria necessary for diagnosing pancreatitis, classic pain presentation, and imaging findings, fluid resuscitation and pain management may be begun. Serum amylase and lipase would be performed with characteristic pain symptoms present and if no imaging were performed.
3. **A.** CT of the abdomen is the most appropriate imaging choice for pancreatitis because of accessibility, speed, cost, and detail. Imaging is not necessary to make the diagnosis; serum values are diagnostic in the proper clinical context. CT is helpful to evaluate for complications of pancreatitis. CT is also compatible for intervention if drainage is needed.

4. **A.** A pancreatic abscess would be the suspected complication in a patient with persistent fevers and leukocytosis, along with a localized and ill-defined collection of pus in the pancreatic region.

Comment

Background
In the United States, the most common causes of pancreatitis are gallstones and chronic alcohol use. Other causes include medicines, hypertriglyceridemia, hypercalcemia, recurrent endoscopic retrograde cholangiopancreatography (ERCP), cystic fibrosis, infections, and trauma. Rare causes are pancreas divisum, emboli, biliary cysts, complication of mumps, secondary to burns, and familial chylomicronemia syndrome.

Pancreatitis presents with mild to severe pain in the epigastric region that may radiate to the back. Eating may worsen the pain and leaning forward may reduce the pain. Nausea, vomiting, fever, and leukocytosis are usually present. Severe disease presents with tachypnea, hypoxemia, and hypotension. Hypernatremia may occur in severe pancreatitis owing to large third-space fluid loss and decreased fluid intake, causing hypovolemia. In acute necrotizing pancreatitis, secondary bacterial infection may occur. Necrosis destroying the pancreatic parenchyma may lead to decreased secretion of insulin, leading to hyperglycemia. Hypocalcemia may occur owing to precipitation of calcium soaps in the abdominal cavity. Acute pancreatitis may lead to ARDS and postcholecystectomy syndrome. Abscesses may be an early complication. Pseudocysts may occur 4 to 6 weeks after an episode of acute pancreatitis. If the pancreatitis or the cause of the pancreatitis persists, it may become chronic pancreatitis. Long-term, chronic pancreatitis (+20 years) has an increased likelihood of developing pancreatic cancer.

Diagnosis
Some patients may have chest x-ray (CXR) abnormalities, such pleural effusions (elevated amylase in pleural fluid), atelectasis, elevated hemidiaphragm, or pulmonary consolidations.

Diagnosis of pancreatitis requires two of the following criteria: acute onset of sever epigastric pain radiating to the back, increased amylase or lipase more than three times the upper limit of normal, and characteristic abdominal imaging findings of focal or diffuse pancreatic enlargement with heterogeneous enhancement with IV contrast on CT or diffusely enlarged and hypoechoic pancreas on ultrasound. Other CT findings include pseudocyst formation, peripancreatic collection, and/or fat stranding. Necrosis is visualized by the absence of enhancement on CT. A third of patients with pancreatitis have ileus, which causes difficulty in visualizing the pancreas using ultrasound. Therefore, ultrasound is used to rule out gallstones as a cause of pancreatitis, specifically in patients who have alanine aminotransferase (ALT) levels greater than 150 U/L. ERCP would be used in these cases, which decreases morbidity and mortality. ERCP is also useful to evaluate causes of recurrent pancreatitis and in draining pancreatic pseudocysts (diagnostic and therapeutic). Abdominal x-rays are usually normal or may just show ileus ("sentinel loop"), if present.

Management
Supportive measures, such as fluid resuscitation and pain control, resolve pancreatitis most of the time. Treating the underlying cause prevents recurrent attacks. Antibiotics may be necessary in some cases of necrotizing pancreatitis owing to local inflammation caused by gut bacteria. Surgery may be needed in biliary pancreatitis, necrotizing pancreatitis, and/or taking care of complications.

CASE 40

Obstructive Uropathy

Ureteral Stone With Acute Urinary Tract Obstruction

1. **C.** Only this choice would have hydroureteronephrosis and a calculus at the ureterovesicular junction (UVJ) with associated perinephric stranding indicating obstructive uropathy. Although bladder outlet obstruction and congenital megaureter may have a dilated ureter, they are not associated with ureteral calculi. The ureter is not dilated in ureteropelvic junction (UPJ) obstruction.
2. **D.** Forniceal rupture spares the kidney from further damage by releasing built-up intrapelvic pressure.
3. **A.** Organisms most commonly associated with struvite stones include Proteus, Pseudomonas, and Klebsiella species. Of patients, 25% with uric acid stones have gout. Cystine stone comprises 2% of renal calculi.
4. **D.** Low dietary intake of calcium increases gut absorption of oxalate, leading to hyperoxaluria, a risk factor for calcium–oxalate stones.

Comment

Background
Common types of stones include, in order of decreasing density, calcium (75%), struvite (15%), uric acid (6%), and cystine (2%). Calcium stones include mixed (50%), calcium oxalate (40%), and calcium phosphate/apatite (10%). Risk factors include idiopathic (85%), horseshoe kidney, hyperparathyroidism, sarcoidosis, renal tubular acidosis, immobilization, hypercalcuria, and hyperoxaluria. Struvite stones are caused by urea-splitting bacteria: Proteus, Klebsiella, and Pseudomonas. When the stones are large and branched, they are termed staghorn calculi. Uric acid stones are cause by acidic, concentrated urine, small bowel disease, gout, and cell lysis.

Diagnosis
In a patient with suspected renal obstruction as a cause for acute renal failure, ultrasound is a quick and inexpensive imaging modality to detect hydronephrosis. Although ultrasound may detect larger stones within the kidney, small stones (<3 mm) or stones close to the corticomedullary junction may be difficult to identify. Ureteral calculi are not well detected on ultrasound. If the cause is not seen on US, additional imaging may be performed with CT. NECT is the modality of choice. Typical CT findings include hydroureteronephrosis with perinephric stranding and fluid and radiopaque obstructing ureteral calculus. Asymmetric delayed renal enhancement may be seen on contrast-enhanced scans. Approximately 77% of ureteral stones are surrounded by a rim of soft tissue known as the "soft-tissue rim sign," which assists in differentiating from phleboliths.

Management
Stone size is an important predictor of spontaneous passage. Of stones, 80% measuring less than 4 mm will pass spontaneously, whereas only 20% of stones larger than 8 mm will pass spontaneously. Thus small stones with mild hydronephrosis may be treated with hydration, pain control, and observation. Patients with larger stones or intractable pain may require drainage with ureteral stent or percutaneous nephrostomy. Evidence of infected hydronephrosis requires hospital admission and prompt drainage.

CASE 41

Free Intraperitoneal Air

1. **B, C, E.** Vaginal insufflation can dilate genital organs and push air into the abdomen. Bowel perforation causes escape of GI

gases into the peritoneum. Subcutaneous emphysema, while it may be present along with pneumoperitoneum, does not cause pneumoperitoneum. A pneumoperitoneum is common after abdominal surgery; it usually resolves 3 to 6 days after surgery, although it may persist for as long as 24 days after surgery.

2. **A.** The anterior wall of the first part of the duodenum is the most common location for perforated ulcers, although they can occur posteriorly and in the pyloric channel. Duodenal ulcers are more common in males and in the 25- to 35-year age range, although gastric ulcers are much more common in older populations. Ulcers of the esophagus, stomach, and duodenum are seen with 95% accuracy with endoscopy and 75% to 80% accuracy with an upper GI series.

3. **E.** Intraperitoneal gas in the paracolic gutter is generally associated with GI perforation. Paramesenteric gutters are recesses between the colon and the root of the mesentery. Morison's pouch (also called the hepatorenal recess or subhepatic recess) is the space that separates the liver from the right kidney.

4. **D.** A and C are seen on x-ray images. B is seen on CT images. Various techniques demonstrate free abdominal air with varying sensitivities including US, CXR, abdominal radiograph (AXR), and CT. Upright CXRs are commonly used to screen for suspected free intraperitoneal air. US is very operator dependent, but can have great utility in experienced hands.

Comment

Background
Peptic ulcer disease (PUD) is the most common cause of spontaneous rupture within the abdomen. The most common location is the duodenum. Hemorrhage is the most common complication, followed by perforation and obstruction. There may be associated pancreatitis in some cases. Incidence of PUD increases with age and with increased NSAID use, smoking history, and prevalence of *Helicobacter pylori*. There has been a decrease in PUD and the associated complications over the past couple of decades owing to drug therapies.

Diagnosis
Of ulcer perforations, 80% to 85% demonstrate free intraperitoneal air on imaging (see images above). The classic presentation is an abrupt onset of severe, generalized abdominal pain with a rigid abdomen. Although posterior duodenal ulcers are more common, anterior ulcers are associated with perforation. Duodenal ulcers are rarely malignant; however, gastric ulcers are malignant 5% to 10% of the time.

Management
Up to 30% of perforated ulcers have a surgical indication. Excellent prognosis is seen with surgical correction within the first 6 hours. Surgical delay greater than 12 hours, a posterior perforation, and persistent or progressing signs of peritonitis are poor prognostic indicators. Medical management of PUD should be initiated with discontinuation of risk factors and with appropriate pharmacotherapy. Medications are aimed at reducing acid output (antacids, H2 receptor blockers, proton pump inhibitors (PPIs), increasing mucosal protection (sucralfate), and eliminating infectious agents (*H. pylori*). Any ulcer recurrence usually happens within the first 2 years after surgery.

CASE 42

Ovarian Torsion

1. **B, D, E.** Tuboovarian abscess would present as multilocular mass on US. Pyelonephritis is not typically a pelvic complaint, and sonographic findings would show enlargement of the kidney, not the ovary.

2. **D.** All of the listed findings are commonly seen on CT and US of the abdomen and pelvis. See comment below.

3. **C.** Ultrasound is less expensive than CT and MRI but has about the same diagnostic performance of both. Transvaginal and transabdominal ultrasounds should both be obtained to best visualize abdominal and pelvic structures. Pelvic x-ray would not visualize the pelvic viscera.

4. **E.** Ovarian masses are the primary risk factor for torsion. Masses 5 cm in diameter or larger are associated with increased risk of progression to torsion.

Comment

Diagnosis
In the workup of a patient with suspected ovarian torsion, pelvic US is recommended as the first-line imaging modality; both transvaginal and transabdominal sonography should be performed. Sonographic findings associated with torsion are

- Enlarged ovary ipsilateral to torsion secondary to edema and vascular and lymphatic engorgement
- Heterogenous appearance of ovarian stroma, often with multiple small peripheral follicles ("string of pearls" appearance)
- Decreased or absent Doppler flow. Because of the dual supply nature to the ovary, flow may be present in torsion. This can be distinguished by noting arterial flow during systole without flow in diastole, indicating outflow obstruction.
- "Whirlpool sign" in ovarian vessels: round hyperechoic structure with concentric hypoechoic stripes

CT and MRI findings consistent with torsion are

- Enlarged, edematous ovaries in abnormal location
- Lack on enhancement of ovary on CT
- "Whirlpool sign" showing coiled ovarian vessels

CASE 43

Fetal Demise

Intrauterine Fetal Demise

1. **D.** The lack of a fetal heart beat, as visualized by the lack of fluctuation in the M-Mode ultrasound tracings, in an embryo with a crown-rump length of 4 cm is diagnostic of intrauterine fetal demise.

2. **B.** In a normal-appearing gestational sac, the first structure visualized by ultrasound is the round, anechoic yolk-sac, which appears around 5 to 6 weeks of pregnancy.

3. **C.** Classically, a crown rump length of 5 mm was used to determine when a heartbeat should be visualized in a developing embryo; however, recent recommendations by the Society of Radiologists in Ultrasound have changed this to 7 mm in order to increase both the specificity and positive predictive value of the test.

4. **D.** Given the mean sac diameter, this pregnancy is suspicious for pregnancy failure. In a pregnancy of uncertain viability, care must be taken to determine if the pregnancy will render a viable fetus. Clinical follow-up with ultrasound would be recommended, generally around 2 weeks after the initial scan, to evaluate for an embryo with a heartbeat.

Comment

Background
Determining viability of an IUP has historically been very difficult, but over the past 30 years, two common clinical

tools—β-hCG and ultrasonography—have revolutionized management. When a pregnant female presents during the first trimester with symptoms of a pregnancy-related complication, the clinician is able to use these tools to answer an important question, "Is this a viable pregnancy?" Determining viability, as opposed to locating an ectopic pregnancy, is vital to the management algorithm. Recently, the Society of Radiologists in Ultrasound released new guidelines related to the determination of nonviability in the first-trimester pregnancy.

Diagnosis

There are fairly routine stages of development in a normal pregnancy, such that at 5 weeks of age a gestational sac is usually present within the uterus. Early on, the gestational sac may be as simple as an anechoic, round cyst located within the echogenic uterine lining, the decidua. However, the sonographic "double decidual sac sign" or "intradecidual sign" are used to describe early pregnancy, but may be absent on at least 35% of gestational sacs using transvaginal ultrasound. Between the fifth and sixth week of pregnancy, a yolk sac appears as a circular, anechoic structure measuring between 3 and 5 mm. Finally, the embryo appears at approximately 6 weeks and should be adjacent to the yolk sac. By this time, an embryonic heartbeat should be noted using M-mode sonography.

Management

Generally, viability was determined using the presence of an embryonic heartbeat when the fetal pole reached a desired crown-rump length of 5 mm. However, the current recommendation states that, at a crown-rump length of 7 mm or greater, if no heartbeat is present, nonviability is almost certain. There are, however, other criteria to consider when determining viability. The size of the gestational sac, the mean sac diameter (MSD), and presence of a fetal pole has also been used for determining viability. The current recommendation states that a MSD of 25 mm without the presence of a visible fetal pole is diagnostic of a failed pregnancy. Between 16 and 24 mm, the lack of a fetal pole is suspicious for a failed pregnancy, but it is not entirely diagnostic. If these findings were not demonstrated on the initial ultrasound, close clinical and sonographic follow-up would be recommended around 14 days after the initial ultrasound; at that point in time, if an embryo without cardiac activity is present, nonviability is certain.

CASE 44

Testicular Torsion

1. **D.** In the acute setting, ruling out testicular torsion is the most important diagnostic consideration. In this case, a lack of both color and power Doppler ultrasound is diagnostic of testicular torsion.
2. **B.** The loss of venous Doppler flow is often the earliest finding in testicular torsion.
3. **C.** Early diagnosis of testicular torsion is vital for testicle salvage, and up to 6 hours after the start of symptoms, there is close to a 100% salvage rate.
4. **B.** Testicular torsion is a surgical emergency and, in order to salvage a functional testicle, surgical exploration and orchiopexy comprise the treatment of choice, especially within the first 24 hours. If urologic intervention is not available, manual detorsion can be considered.

Comment

Background

Acute scrotal pain, in both pediatric and adult patients, is a common presentation in the emergency room; however, the differential diagnosis includes both surgically emergent and nonemergent causes. Testicular torsion is the source of acute scrotal pain in

about 25% of all cases and, as most cases of testicular torsion are in adolescent males, a rapid diagnosis is important for testicular salvage. Generally, torsion of 6 hours or less has a salvage rate of between 80% and 100%; however, by 12 hours, that rate plummets to less than 20%.

Diagnosis

Clinically, most cases present with acute, unilateral scrotal or groin pain with associated nausea and vomiting. Scrotal edema and a high riding testicle owing to shortening of the spermatic cord also may be seen. Ultrasound with both color and power Doppler imaging is the preferred imaging modality because it is often rapidly available in the emergency setting. Initially, gray-scale ultrasound may demonstrate normally appearing testicular parenchyma. Although this may indicate testicular viability, evaluation of the venous and arterial flow is absolutely vital. As such, the absence of either venous or arterial flow is a very specific finding, with the loss of venous flow occurring first before the loss of arterial flow.

Management

Once torsion is confirmed, emergent surgical exploration is indicated. Bilateral orchiopexy is usually performed, as the bell-clapper deformity, which predisposes adolescent males to torsion, is commonly found bilaterally. The bell-clapper deformity describes an anatomic variant in which the testicle is freely suspended in the scrotum via its vascular pedicle, as opposed to being attached to the scrotum by the normal tunica vaginalis. Unfortunately, the loss of arterial blood flow by Doppler with concurrent heterogeneity of the testicular parenchyma is considered 100% predictive of nonviability at surgical exploration.

CASE 45

Galeazzi Fracture

1. **A.** Galeazzi fracture
2. **C.** A type II Galeazzi fracture occurs as a result of axial loading of the forearm in pronation, which causes anterior displacement of the radius and dorsal dislocation of the distal ulna. **A** is a type I Galeazzi fracture. A type I fracture occurs as a result of axial loading of the forearm in supination, which causes dorsal displacement of the radius and volar dislocation of the distal ulna.
3. **B.** In a child, the next step in management is a closed reduction and immobilization in supination in an above-elbow cast for 4 to 6 weeks. **A** is performed only when the reduction is lost or unattainable. **C** and **D** are performed only on adults.
4. **B.** Triangular fibrocartilage complex (TFCC) primarily stabilizes the distal radioulnar joint (DRUJ). The radius and the ulna are constrained firmly by the interosseous membrane (**D**) and ligamentous structures (**A** and **C**) at the proximal and distal radioulnar joints.

Comment

Background

A Galeazzi fracture is a distal radial shaft fracture with disruption of the DRUJ. The cause of this type of fracture is most commonly a fall that results in an axial load to be placed on a hyperpronated forearm. A type I fracture causes dorsal displacement of the distal radius, and a type II causes a volar/anterior displacement of the distal radius.

Diagnosis

This fracture presents clinically with swelling and tenderness, with possible deformity over the distal forearm. Radiographic imaging is necessary for accurate diagnosis. Finding suggestive of DRUJ injury on plain radiographs include fracture of the ulnar styloid base, widening of the DRUJ on the AP view, dislocation or subluxation of the radius relative to the ulna on the true lateral view, shortening of the radius more than 5 mm relative to the distal ulna, and asymmetry compared with the uninjured contralateral DRUJ. When degree and/or assessment of injury is difficult on plain radiographs, an axial CT is recommended.

Management

Management of a Galeazzi fracture differs between children and adults. In children, the nonsurgical treatment of choice is closed reduction and immobilization in supination in an above-elbow cast for 4 to 6 weeks. If there is a loss of reduction or if the fracture is irreducible, the next step is an open reduction and internal fixation (ORIF) and immobilization in supination in an above-elbow cast for 4 to 6 weeks. In adults, owing to the high instability of the fracture, a surgical treatment is usually required for good results and to avoid further long-term injury and deformity. ORIF with plating of the radius is the treatment of choice in adults. If the reduction is unstable or irreducible, further investigation of the DRUJ and TFCC may be required.

CASE 46

Fifth Metacarpal Fracture (Boxer's)

1. **C, D.** Boxers/fifth metacarpal fractures are interchangeable terms. These are likely voluntary fractures and are commonly seen in young males as a result of improper punching technique.
2. **B.** Fracture of the fifth metacarpal neck account for 20% of all hand fractures.
3. **A.** Cefazolin (or a first generation cephalosporin) every 8 hours for three doses is one of the most commonly used antibiotics in the treatment of open fractures.
4. **B.** Apply metacarpal block, reduce fracture, apply ulnar gutter back slab, and apply high arm sling. Discharge patient home with follow-up appointment in 7 days.

Comment

Background

A fifth metacarpal neck fracture, or Boxer's fracture, is classically a transverse fracture of the neck of the fifth metacarpal bone. This hand fracture accounts for 20% of all hand fractures. Of all injury-related cases in the ED, 15% are hand injuries. Boxer's fracture typically occurs from intentional injury. Boxer's fracture is a result of a person using a closed fist to strike a hard surface, such as a wall, bone, or any immovable object. This injury can also occur if the patient has used improper punching technique. Proper punching technique is exhibited when the second and third knuckles make contact before the fourth and fifth knuckles. This injury is often seen in patients who have been in a fight or patients that have punched a hard surface out of frustration. When an improper punching form is used, the angular force created a backward bend in the metacarpal bone, thus causing a fracture with enough load.

The patient may hear a popping or snapping noise prior to fracturing the metacarpal bone. Visual scratches or cuts may be seen around the patient's hand dorsally (knuckles). Focal pain, with or without movement of hands or fingers, swelling, and tenderness in the distal third of the fifth metacarpal will be experienced with accompanying deformity or misalignment and discoloration around the affected area.

Diagnosis

Diagnosis is commonly made by a physician clinically and confirmed by a plain radiograph.

Management

Treatment is determined by whether or not the injury is a closed or open fracture with or without a rotational deformity or associated injury. A patient who has closed fracture with palmar angulation less than 50 degrees receives a high arm sling, neighbor strapping for 1 week, and will be asked to follow the rest, ice, compression, elevation (RICE) instructions. Treatment for angulation greater than 50 degrees needs to reduce the fracture and apply metacarpal block, ulnar gutter back slab, and high arm sling. Those who have undergone an open fracture will be referred to a plastics team and will need to be immunized for tetanus, receive temporary sterile dressing, intravenous antibiotics, and have a high arm sling applied until they are admitted to plastics ward.

CASE 47

Hip Dislocation

1. **C.** Radiography illustrates the displacement of the femoral head from acetabulum. Femoral neck or hip fractures are unlikely, as both appear unaffected. Slipped capital femoral epiphysis (SCFE) is a pediatric disorder and would be seen with widening of the physis and/or slip of the femoral head.
2. **A.** Hip dislocations as a result of MVAs are primarily posterior. All other options describe mechanisms of alternate conditions (i.e., anterior hip dislocation).
3. **B.** The sciatic nerve passes posterior to the acetabulum, below the piriformis, and is most commonly injured in hip dislocations. Although the femoral nerve can also be injured, it is not the most likely nerve complication for this condition.
4. **C.** Although physical therapy and resting and icing the hip are part of treatment, the first step to treating the hip dislocation is a reduction.

Comment

Background

Hip dislocation may occur in an anterior, posterior, or central direction. A classic presentation of a posterior dislocation of the hip is seen with the head of the femur in a superolateral position and dislocated from the acetabulum. It is possible that the injured femoral head appears smaller owing to the difference in distance from the radiographic plate. This type of dislocation is responsible for the majority of hip dislocations and is often the result of trauma, most commonly, MVAs in which the femur is forced out of the joint when the knee hits the dashboard. Posterior hip dislocations are likely to be seen with additional fractures in the area of the hip joint.

Anterior dislocations of the hip are much less common, only seen in 10% to 15% of all hip dislocations. Radiographs reveal the femoral head in an anteromedial position toward either the superior pubic ramus or the obturator foramen. These occur when a force is applied with the hip in an abducted and externally rotated position. Additional injuries are much less likely.

Central hip dislocations present with acetabular fractures, allowing for the femoral head to project into the pelvic cavity.

Management

Various potential complications are involved with traumatic hip dislocation. The most common complications are AVN, posttraumatic osteoarthritis, and heterotopic ossification. Sciatic nerve damage occurs in 10% to 20% of all hip dislocations, and thus the neurologic status of the patient before and after treatment must be assessed. Treatment can also be affected by the associated problems with a hip dislocation. The piriformis, gluteus maximus, ligamentum teres, capsule, labrum, or a bony fragment may prevent reduction in posterior dislocations, whereas the labrum, psoas, or the capsule may prevent reduction in anterior dislocations. To have the best outcome after a traumatic hip dislocation, it is vital to maintain follow-up with the patient.

CASE 48

Salter-Harris Fracture (Type II)

1. **B.** Salter-Harris fracture type II
2. **B.** Salter-Harris fracture type II is the most common type of Salter-Harris fracture, with an incidence of 75%. It occurs through the physis and metaphysis without involvement of the epiphysis.
3. **C.** Children 10 to 15 years of age most commonly sustain Salter-Harris fractures.
4. **D.** Sports-related injuries are the most common cause of this condition. Child abuse, genetics, injury from extreme cold, radiation and medications, neurologic disorders, and metabolic diseases are less-common causes.
5. **B.** The Tillaux fracture is a Salter-Harris type III fracture involving the anterolateral aspect of the growth plate and the epiphysis. Fusion of the growth plate begins centrally, proceeds medially, and completes laterally. The Tillaux pattern is secondary to injury after the medial distal tibial growth plate has fused. When these types of fractures are suspected, additional imaging, such as CT, is typically performed for orthopedic repair purposes.

Comment

Background
Salter-Harris fractures are fractures that occur through the epiphyseal plate or growth plate. Thus this is a common injury found in the pediatric population. There are nine types of Salter-Harris fractures, which are categorized by the involvement of the physis, metaphysis, and epiphysis.

Classification

Type I: A transverse fracture involving the physis
Type II: A fracture involving the physis and the metaphysis with no epiphyseal involvement
Type III: A fracture involving the physis and epiphysis with no metaphyseal involvement
Type IV: A fracture involving the physis, metaphysis, and epiphysis.
Type V: A compression fracture involving the physis with no metaphyseal or epiphyseal involvement
Type VI: Injury to the perichondral structures
Type VII: Isolated injury to the epiphyseal structures.
Type VIII: Isolated injury to the metaphysis, with possible impairment of endochondral ossification
Type IX: Injury of the periosteum, which may impair the intramembranous ossification
A pneumonic to remember the first five most common:
S lip of physis (I)
A bove physis (II)
L ower than physis (III)
T hrough physis (IV)
R ammed physis (V)

Diagnosis and Management
In a suspected fracture, radiography is the best initial test. If further testing is needed, a CT is the next best option for evaluation. Treatment depends on the severity of the fracture. Pain medication, in addition to cast/splint and or surgery, will be needed.

CASE 49

Patellar Dislocation

1. **B, D.** The imaging clearly illustrates the displacement of the patella. A femoral fracture is commonly associated with patellar

dislocations and should also be considered. Whereas the other conditions are possible and could be included in the differential, they are unlikely after examining the radiographs.
2. **C.** The peroneal and tibial nerves are most likely to be injured in knee dislocations. Both nerves are terminal branches of the sciatic nerve, branching above the popliteal fossa.
3. **D.** Although MRI and CT scans are both useful tools, MRIs are better able to detect soft-tissue anomalies.
4. **B.** In the Schenck classification system, KDII is described as both cruciate ligaments disrupted completely with collaterals intact.

Comment

Injuries Commonly Associated With Patellar Dislocations
Most patients enduring knee dislocations have additional complications associated with the injury. Easily missed is vascular damage, which occurs primarily in the popliteal artery. In treatment of knee dislocations, the integrity of the vasculature surrounding the knee must be assessed. Revascularization may be necessary, which can often lead to the development of a compartment syndrome. Nerve damage is also likely with injuries to the peroneal and tibial nerves being the most common. Additionally, accompanying fractures and meniscus lesions are probable. It is crucial to consider these injuries when examining and treating a patient suffering from a patellar dislocation.

Classification of Patellar Dislocations
Knee dislocations must be described using a combination of classification systems because each gives information on neurologic, vascular, and infectious complications. One method is a classification of the direction of the tibia dislocation. The possible dislocations include anterior, posterior, medial, lateral, and rotational. Rotational dislocations can be further described as anteromedial, anterolateral, posteromedial, and posterolateral. Anterior dislocations are the most common of all patellar dislocations.

Another type of classification is through the mechanism that caused the injury: high-energy mechanisms (e.g., MVAs) or low-energy mechanisms (e.g., nonmotorized sports injuries).

Schenck has created an additional classification system for the injury that separates it into five categories.

KDI: Intact posterior cruciate ligament (PCL) with variable injury to collateral ligaments
KDII: Both cruciate ligaments disrupted completely with collaterals intact
KDIII: Both cruciate ligaments disrupted completely with one collateral ligament disrupted
KDIV: Both cruciate ligaments and collateral ligaments disrupted
KDV: Dislocation with periarticular fracture

In practice, it is important to describe the condition using a variety of the above classification systems to best evaluate and treat the patient.

CASE 50

Ankle Mortise Disruption

Fracture-Disruption of Ankle Mortise

Supination External Rotation Ankle Injury
1. **B.** Images demonstrate at least a spiral fracture of the distal fibula and widening of the medial mortise, which may suggest deltoid ligament injury, and this places the injury in the

category of supination external rotation ankle injury using the Lauge-Hansen Classification.

2. **B.** Danis-Weber type B fibular fracture occurs at or crosses the tibiofibular syndesmosis.

3. **A.** Anterior tibiofibular ligament rupture is the first stage of supination external rotation ankle injury.

4. **C.** Deltoid ligament rupture or medial malleolar fracture is the last stage of supination external rotation ankle injury.

Comment

Supination External Rotation Injury

The most encountered type of mechanism for an ankle fracture is supination external rotation injury. Supination external rotation ankle injury has four stages. The first stage involves rupture of the anterior-inferior tibiofibular ligament. Rupture of the anterior-inferior tibiofibular ligament may be occult on x-ray. Widening of the tibiofibular space in supination external rotation injury may suggest rupture of the anterior-inferior tibiofibular ligament. Stage 2 is a spiral fracture of the fibula. The next stage is rupture of the posterior inferior tibiofibular ligament or fracture of the posterior malleolus of the tibia. Stage 4 involves fracture through the medial malleolus or disruption of the deltoid ligament. Deltoid ligamentous rupture may be present if there is widening of the medial mortise in a supination external rotation injury.

Lauge-Hansen Classification

Supination-adduction, supination-external rotation, pronation-abduction, and pronation-external rotation are categories under the Lauge–Hansen Classification. The first word in the Lauge–Hansen Classification is based on the position of the foot at the time of injury. The second word is the direction of the applied force. The mechanism and stage can be determine by the fibular fracture position in relation to the plafond, type of fibula fracture, type of medial malleolar fracture, presence of a posterior malleolar fracture, and signs of widening of the mortise or tibiofibular space. Knowing the mechanism allows the prediction of sequence or staging in ankle injuries. Ankle fractures usually follow an order of sequence involving bones and ligaments and do not skip the order of sequence. For example, a spiral fibular fracture at the plafond would be a supination external rotation injury. Before a spiral fibular fracture occurs in a supination external rotation injury, the anterior-inferior tibiofibular ligament ruptures.

Danis–Weber Classification

Danis–Weber classification is based on a fibular fracture occurring below the syndesmosis, at or crossing the syndesmosis, or above the syndesmosis. Higher up fibular fractures are associated with more damage to the syndesmosis. Ankle instability increases when there is more damage to the syndesmosis. Type A Danis–Weber is a fibular fracture below the syndesmosis and corresponds with a supination adduction injury. Type B Danis–Weber is a fibular fracture at or crossing the syndesmosis and corresponds with a supination-external rotation injury. Type C Danis–Weber is a fibular fracture above the syndesmosis that corresponds with a pronation external rotation injury.

CASE 51

Perianal Abscess

Anorectal Abscess

1. **A.** There is a perianal fluid collection in a patient with Crohn's disease and fever, which is suggestive of an anorectal abscess.

2. **A.** Perianal abscess is the most common type of anorectal abscess.

3. **A.** An infected anal gland is the most common cause of an anorectal abscess.

4. **C.** A supralevator abscess may be caused by superior extension of an intersphincteric abscess or inferior extension of an infectious or inflammatory process.

Comment

Background

Anorectal abscesses occur among all age groups. The median age of presentation is 40 years (range 20–60 years). Males are twice as likely to develop anorectal abscesses as are women. The majority of anorectal abscesses develop when anal glands become blocked and infected. Infection from the anal glands follow the path of least resistance and spread along one of the planes in the anorectal region to form an abscess. Other causes of anorectal abscess include STI and infected anal fissure. Risk factors include Crohn's disease or ulcerative colitis, diabetes, immunocompromise, steroid use, constipation, and diarrhea.

Anorectal abscesses are often classified as perianal, intersphincteric, ischiorectal, or supralevator abscess. Perianal is a superficial abscess that lies beneath the anal verge and does not extend across the external anal sphincter. Intersphincteric abscesses occur between the internal and external anal sphincters. An ischiorectal abscess occurs when the intersphincteric abscess goes across the external anal sphincter. Supralevator abscesses extend superiorly above the levator ani or may be related to the extension of an intraabdominal process.

Diagnosis

Usually history and physical examination can be used to diagnose an anorectal abscess with no need for imaging. Imaging may be helpful when there is a suspicion of a supralevator abscess and an abdominal pelvic source for an anorectal abscess. Imaging often can help determine the extent of an anorectal abscess and plan treatment. Imaging may reveal undrained collections and/or subtherapeutic treatment in patients with recurrent abscesses. Furthermore, imaging may help determine the extent and possible associated complication in those patients with diverticulitis, Crohn's disease, PID, anorectal malignancy receiving radiation therapy, urinary retention, and neutropenia. CT, MRI, and US have all been used in diagnosing anorectal abscesses, but CT is often used initially owing to its availability.

Management

Anorectal abscesses are often treated in the outpatient setting by incision and drainage with local anesthesia. More complex anorectal abscess may require incision and drainage in the operating room with regional or general anesthesia. Some supralevator abscesses may be treated with CT-guided drainage. Complication of anorectal abscesses include sepsis, fistula formation, and reoccurrence.

CASE 52

Sigmoid Volvulus

1. **A, B**. Cecal volvulus, sigmoid volvulus

2. **B.** Sigmoid colon is the most common site of volvulus (70%), followed by the cecum (25%) and the transverse colon (5%).

3. **D.** Doughnut is described for intussusception.

4. **C.** Rectal tube insertion is sufficient in treating 90% of cases.

Comment

Background

Volvulus is the second most common cause of large bowel obstruction following large bowel mass as the most common cause. Any segment of the colon can undergo volvulus. A segment of redundant mobile colon on a mesentery and a fixed point around which rotation can occur are the two major factors predisposing colonic volvulus. Sigmoid colon is the most common site of volvulus (70%), followed by the cecum (25%) and the transverse colon (5%). The abnormal twisting of colon results in closed loop bowel obstruction, and vascular compromise can lead to gangrene, perforation, and death. Sigmoid volvulus affects elderly patients, particularly those who are debilitated. Volvulus of sigmoid colon is not caused by a congenital defect, but rather is related to dietary and behavioral factors, including increased fiber in the diet, which increases the bulk of the stool and elongates the colon.

Diagnosis

Conventional radiographs show abnormally distended air-filled sigmoid colon looping upward from the lower abdomen. Often the tip of the loop reaches high into the abdomen; the apex of the loop usually extends above T10 vertebral level and can lie to the left or right of the midline. An opaque vertical stripe is seen along the apposed medial walls of proximal and distal limbs of sigmoid loop, which is commonly known as the "coffee bean sign." Absence of rectal gas is another radiographic sign, indicating obstruction at the level of the sigmoid colon. The differentiation of cecal volvulus from sigmoid volvulus on radiographs can sometimes be challenging. Other conditions that can mimic sigmoid volvulus on radiographs are pseudo-obstruction and distended, redundant transverse colon.

Contrast enema is another useful technique to diagnose sigmoid volvulus; however, this is infrequently performed in the emergency setting. CT is more frequently ordered in the emergent setting. A "bird beak sign" on CT indicates sharp tapering of a distended bowel lumen. Identification of two transition points and a "whirl sign" provide additional diagnostic clues and imply twisting of the sigmoid mesentery. The "X-marks-the spot sign" and "split wall sign" are other imaging signs on CT that may improve the diagnostic confidence to define large bowel volvulus. The X-marks-the-spot sign refers to a complete twist of the two limbs of a loop of bowel on itself (two crossing transition points at a single location), and the split wall sign refers to a subtle twisting of a single limb of a distal sigmoid, which causes visual separation of its walls by mesenteric fat.

Management

Rectal tube insertion is successful in treating 90% of cases. The most serious complication of untreated sigmoid volvulus is bowel ischemia. Mortality rate is 20% to 25%.

REFERENCES

Case 1

Emergency Radiology: The Requisites 1st ed, Ch 9.

Case 2

Emergency Radiology: The Requisites, 1st ed, Ch 1.
Mozaffarian D, Benjamin E, Go A, Arnett D, Blaha M, et al. Heart disease and stroke statistics—2015 update: a report from the American Heart Association. *Circulation*. 2015;131(4):e29–322.
Srinivasan A, Goyal M, Azri F, et al. State-of-the-art imaging of acute stroke. *Radiographics*. 2006;26(Suppl 1):S75–S95.
Wintermark M, et al. Imaging recommendations for acute stroke and transient ischemic attack patients: a joint statement by the American Society of Neuroradiology, the American College of Radiology and the Society of NeuroInterventional Surgery. *J Am Coll Radiol*. 2013;10(11):828–832.

Case 3

Anderson Jr FA, Wheeler H, Goldberg RJ, et al. A population-based perspective of the hospital incidence and case-fatality rates of deep vein thrombosis and pulmonary embolism: the Worcester DVT study. *Arch Intern Med*. 1991;151(5):933938. https://doi.org/10.1001/archinte.1991. 00400050081016.

Molvar C. Inferior vena cava filtration in the management of venous thromboembolism: filtering the data. *Semin Interv Radiol*. 2012;29 (3):204–217. https://doi.org/10.1055/s-0032-1326931.

Case 4

Castañer E, Gallardo X, Ballesteros E, et al. CT diagnosis of chronic pulmonary thromboembolism. *Radiographics*. 2009;29(1):31–50. https://doi. org/10.1148/rg.291085061.
Stein P, Alavi A, Athanasoulis C, et al. Tissue plasminogen activator for the treatment of acute pulmonary embolism. A collaborative study by the PIOPED Investigators. *Chest*. 1990;97(3):528–33.
Wells PS, Ginsberg JS, Anderson DR, et al. Use of a clinical model for safe management of patients with suspected pulmonary embolism. *Ann Intern Med*. 1998;129:997–1005.
Wittram C, Maher MM, Yoo AJ, et al. CT angiography of pulmonary embolism: diagnostic criteria and causes of misdiagnosis. *Radiographics*. 2004;24(5):1219–1238. https://doi.org/10.1148/rg.245045008.

Case 5

Emergency Radiology. The Requisites, 1st ed, Ch 9.
Pereira JM, Sirlin CB, Pinto PS, Jeffrey RB, Stella DL, Casola G. Disproportionate fat stranding: a helpful CT sign in patients with acute abdominal pain. *Radiographics*. 2004;24(3):703–715. https://doi.org/ 10.1148/rg.243035084.
Wilkins T, Embry K, George R. Diagnosis and management of acute diverticulitis. *Am Fam Physician*. 2013;87(9):612–620.

Case 6

Brant WE, Helms CA. *Fundamentals of Diagnostic Radiology*. Philadelphia: Lippincott Williams & Wilkins.
Greenberg MS. *Handbook of Neurosurgery*. Thieme Medical Publishers, NY; 2010.
Emergency Radiology: The Requisites, 1st ed, Ch 1.
Jallo J. *Loftus CM. Neurotrauma and Critical Care of the Brain*: Thieme Medical Publishers; 2009.
Scheld WM, Whitley RJ, Marra CM. *Infections of the Central Nervous System*. Philadelphia: Lippincott Williams & Wilkins; 2004.

Case 7

Brant WE, Helms CA. *Fundamentals of Diagnostic Radiology*. Philadelphia: Lippincott Williams & Wilkins; 2007.
Emergency Radiology: The Requisites, 1st ed, Ch 1.
Jallo J, Loftus CM. *Neurotrauma and Critical Care of the Brain*. Thieme Medical Pub; NY, 2009.

Case 8

American Thoracic Society. Guidelines for the management of adults with community-acquired pneumonia: diagnosis, assessment of severity, antimicrobial therapy, and prevention. *Am J Respir Crit Care Med*. 2001;163:1730–1754.
Lutfiyya MN, Henley E, Chang LF, Reyburn SW. Diagnosis and treatment of community-acquired pneumonia. *Am Fam Physician*. 2006; 73(3):442–450.
Niederman MS. Pneumonia, including community-acquired and nosocomial pneumonia. In: Crapo JD, et al., eds. Baum's Textbook of Pulmonary Diseases. Vol 1. 7th ed. Philadelphia: Lippincott Williams & Wilkins; 2004:424–454.
Niederman MS, Mandell LA, Anzueto A, et al.
Solensky R, Earl HS, Gruchalla RS. Clinical approach to penicillin-allergic patients: a survey. *Ann Allergy Asthma Immunol*. 2000;84:329.

Case 9

Emergency Radiology: The Requisites, 1st ed, Ch 9.
Hanbidge AE, Buckler PM, O'Malley ME, et al. From the RSNA refresher courses: imaging evaluation for acute pain in the right upper quadrant. *Radiographics*. 2004;24(4):1117–35.
Mirvis SE, Whitley NO, Miller JW. CT diagnosis of acalculous cholecystitis. *J Comput Assist Tomogr*. 1987;11(1):83–87.

Case 10

Emergency Radiology: The Requisites, 1st ed, Ch 4.
Memarsadeghi M, Breitenseher MJ, Schaefer-Prokop C, et al. Occult scaphoid fractures: comparison of multidetector CT and MR-imaging-initial experience. *Radiology*. 2006;240(1):169–176.

Case 11

Emergency Radiology: The Requisites, 1st ed, Ch 4.

Rouleau DM, Hebert-Davies J. Incidence of associated injury in posterior shoulder dislocation: systematic review of the literature. *J Orthop Trauma.* 2012;26:246–251.

Wolfson AB, Harwood-Nuss A. *Harwood-Nuss' Clinical Practice of Emergency Medicine.* 5th edition, Philiadelphia: Lippincott Williams & Wilkins; 2009. Ch 114.

Case 12

Emergency Radiology: The Requisites, 1st ed, Ch 9.

Maddu KK, Mittal P, Shuaib W, Tewari A, Ibraheem O, Khosa F. Colorectal emergencies and related complications: a comprehensive imaging review-imaging of colitis and complications. *AJR American J of Roentgenology.* 2014;203:1205–1216.

Thoeni RF, Cello JP. CT imaging of colitis. *Radiology.* 2006;240:623–638.

Case 13

Emergency Radiology: The Requisites, 1st ed, Ch 5.

Vande Berg BE, Malghem JJ, Labaisse MA, Noel HM, Maldague BE. MR imaging of avascular necrosis and transient marrow edema of the femoral head. *Radiographics.* 1993;13:501–520.

Wassenaar RP, Verburg H, Taconis WK, van der Eijken JW. Avascular osteonecrosis of the femoral head treated with a vascularize iliac bone graft: preliminary results and follow-up with radiography and MR imaging. *Radiographics.* 1996;16:585–594.

Case 14

Emergency Radiology: The Requisites, 1st ed, Ch 11.

Nienaber CA, Clough RE. Management of acute aortic dissection. *Lancet.* 2015;385(9970):800–811. https://doi.org/10.1016/S0140-6736(14)61005-9.

Case 15

Emergency Radiology: The Requisites, 1st ed, Ch 4.

Kaewlai R, Avery LL, Asrani AV, Abujudeh HH, Sacknoff R, Novelline RA. Mutidetector CT of carpal injuries: anatomy, fractures, and fracture-dislocations. *Radiographics.* 2008;28:1771–1784.

Case 16

Emergency Radiology: The Requisites, 1st ed, Ch.

Levine D. Ectopic pregnancy. *Radiology.* 2007;245(2):385–397.

Lin EP, Lin E, Bhatt S, Dogra V, et al. Diagnostic clues to ectopic pregnancy. *Radiographics.* 2008;28(6):1661–1671.

Rana P, Kazmi I, Singh R, et al. Ectopic pregnancy: a review. *Arch Gynecol Obstet.* 2013;288(4):747–757.

Case 17

Avery LL, Scheinfeld MH. Imaging of penile and scrotal emergencies. *Radiographics.* 2013;33:721–740.

Emergency Radiology: The Requisites, 1st ed, Ch 10.

Yagil Y, Naroditsky I, Milhem J, et al. Role of Doppler ultrasonography in the triage of acute scrotum in the emergency department. *J Ultrasound Med.* 2010;29:11–21.

Case 18

Ataei N, Madani A, Habibi R, Khorasani M. Evaluation of acute pyelonephritis with DMSA scans in children presenting after the age of 5 years. *Pediatr Nephrol.* 2005;20(10):1439–1444.

Craig WM, Wagner BJ, Travis MD. From the archives of the AFIP: pyelonephritis: radiologic-pathologic review. *Radiographics.* 2008;28:255–276. http://pubs.rsna.org/doi/citedby/10.1148/rg.281075171.

Nikolaidis P, Casalino DD, Remer EM, et al. ACR appropriateness criteria–acute pyelonephritis. In: *ACR Criteria.* 2012. https://acsearch.acr.org/docs/69489/Narrative/.

Roberts JA. Etiology and pathophysiology of pyelonephritis. *Am J Kidney Dis.* 1991;17(1):1–9.

Case 19

Furukawa A, Takao S, Michio Y, et al. Cross-sectional imaging in Crohn disease. *Radiographics.* 2004;24:689–702.

Peppercorn M, Kane S. Clinical manifestations, diagnosis and prognosis of Crohn disease in adults. *UpToDate.* Ed. Rutgeerts and Grover. Web. 22 Nov. 2015. http://www.uptodate.com/contents/clinical-manifestations-diagnosis-and-prognosis-of-crohn-disease-in-adults?source=search_result&search=crohn's&selectedTitle=3~150.

Weerakkody Y, Gaillard F. Crohn disease. *Radiopaedia.* Web. 23 Nov. 2015. http://radiopaedia.org/articles/crohn-disease-1.

Case 20

Emergency Radiology: The Requisites, 1st ed, Ch 4.

John SD, Wherry K, Swischuk LE, Phillips WA. Improving detection of pediatric elbow fractures by understanding their mechanics. *Radiographics.* 1996;16:1443–1460.

Singer AD, Hanna T, Jose J, Datir A. A systematic, multimodality approach to emergency elbow imaging. *Clin Imaging.* 2016;40(1):13–22.

Sheehan S, Dyer GS, Sodickson AD, Patel KI, Khurana B. Traumatic elbow injuries: what the orthopedic surgeon wants to know. *Radiographics.* 2013;33:869–888.

Case 21

Emergency Radiology: The Requisites, 1st ed, Ch 9.

Mullan CP, Siewert B, Eisenberg RL. Small bowel obstruction. *Am J Radiol.* 2015;198:105–117.

O'Malley RG, Al-Hawary MM, Kaza RK, et al. MDCT findings in small bowel obstruction: implications of the cause and presence of complications on treatment decisions. *Abdom Imaging.* 2015;40:2248–2262.

Paulson E, Thompson W. Review of small bowel obstruction: the diagnosis and when to worry. *Radiology.* 2015;275:332–342.

Case 22

Brunel W, Coleman DL, Schwartz DE, et al. Assessment of routine chest roentgenograms and the physical examination to confirm endotracheal tube position. *Chest.* 1989;96(5):1043–1045.

Conrardy PA, Goodman LR, Lainge F, et al. Alteration of endotracheal tube position: flexion and extension of the neck. *Crit Care Med.* 1976;4(1):7–12.

Frank G, Knipe H. Endobronchial intubation. *Radiopedia.org.* UMB Medica Network. Web. 8 November 2015.

Case 23

Gay SB, Olazagasti J, Higginbotham JW, et al. Introduction to Chest Radiology. University of Virginia Health Sciences Center, Department of Radiology. Web. 18 Nov. 2015. https://www.med-ed.virginia.edu/courses/rad/cxr/pathology2chest.html.

Case 24

Emergency Radiology: The Requisites, 1st ed, Ch 8.

Roberts DJ, Leigh-Smith S, Faris PD, et al. Clinical manifestations of tension pneumothorax: protocol for a systematic review and meta-analysis. *Systematic Reviews.* 2014;3:3.

Case 25

Emergency Radiology: The Requisites, 1st ed, Ch 1.

Schell CL, Rathe RJ. Superior sagittal sinus thrombosis: still a killer. *West J Med.* 1988;149(3):304–307.

Case 26

Emergency Radiology: The Requisites, 1st ed, Ch 1.

Mirvis SE, Kubal W, Shanmuganathan K, et al., eds. *Problem Solving in Emergency Radiology.* Philadelphia, PA: Elsevier; 2015.

Case 27

Abujudeh HH. *Emergency Radiology Cases.* NY: Oxford Press; 2014.

Emergency Radiology: The Requisites, 1st ed, Ch 1.

Mirvis SE, Kubal W, Shanmuganathan K, et al., eds. *Problem Solving in Emergency Radiology.* Philadelphia, PA: Elsevier; PA; 2015.

Case 28

Abujudeh HH. *Emergency Radiology Cases.* NY: Oxford Press; 2014:34–40.

Emergency Radiology: The Requisites, 1st ed, Ch 1.

Case 29

Emergency Radiology: The Requisites, 1st ed, Ch 1.

Kyrgidis A, Koloutsos G, Kommata A, et al. Incidence, aetiology, treatment outcome and complications of maxillofacial fractures: a retrospective study from Northern Greece. *J Craniomaxillofac Surg.* 2013;41(7):637–643.

Nair MK, Nair UP. Imaging of mandibular trauma: ROC analysis. *Acad Emerg Med.* 2001;8(7):689–95.

Case 30

Ah-See KW, Evans AS. Sinusitis and its management. *BMJ.* 2007;334 (7589):358–361. https://doi.org/10.1136/bmj.39092.679722.BE.

Emergency Radiology: The Requisites, 1st ed, Ch 1.

Gwaltney JM. Acute community-acquired sinusitis. *Clin Infect Dis.* 1996;23 (6):1209–1225. https://doi.org/10.1093/clinids/23.6.1209.

Case 31

Emergency Radiology: The Requisites, 1st ed, Ch 1.
Gerber MA, Baltimore RS, Eaton CB, et al. Prevention of rheumatic fever and diagnosis and treatment of acute streptococcal pharyngitis. *Circulation*. 2009;119(11):1541.
Shulman ST, Bisno AL, Clegg HW, et al. Clinical practice guideline for the diagnosis and management of group A streptococcal pharyngitis: 2012 update by the infectious diseases society of America. *Clin Infect Dis*. 2012;55(10):86–102.

Case 32

Emergency Radiology: The Requisites, 1st ed, Ch 1.
Li SF, Siegel B, Hidalgo I, et al. Laryngopyocoele: An unusual cause of a sore throat. *Am J Emerg Med*. Web 8 Nov 2015. http://www.sciencedirect.com/science/article/pii/S0735675711003354.
Woods CR. Epiglottitis (supraglottitis): clinical features and diagnosis. *UpToDate*. Web. 23 June 2015. https://www.uptodate.com/contents/epiglottitis-supraglottitis-clinical-features-and-diagnosis.

Case 33

Abujudeh HH. *Emergency Radiology Cases*. Oxford Press; 2014;215–220.
Emergency Radiology: The Requisites, 1st ed, Ch 1.

Case 34

Emergency Radiology: The Requisites, 1st ed, Ch 1.
Mirvis S, et al. ed. problem Solving in Emergency Radiology. Elsevier; 2015.

Case 35

Greenspan A, Beltran J. Chapter 4. In: *Orthopedic Imaging*: A Practical Approach, 6th ed. Philadelphia, PA: Lippincott Williams & Wilkins; 2015, Nigel R. Chapter 11. In: *Accident and Emergency Radiology: A Survival Guide*. 3rd ed. Philadelphia, PA: Elsevier; 2015.

Case 36

Eisenberg R, Levine M. Miscellaneous abnormalities of the stomach and duodenum. In: Gore RM, Levine MS, eds. *Textbook of Gastrointestinal Radiology*. 2nd ed. Philadelphia, PA: Saunders; 2000.
Emergency Radiology: The Requisites, 1st ed, Ch 9.
Peterson CM, Anderson JS, Hara AK, et al. Volvulus of the gastrointestinal tract: appearances at multimodality imaging. *Radiographics*. 2009;29:1281–1293.

Case 37

Atlas SW, Regenbogen V, Rogers LF, Kim KS. The radiographic characterization of burst fractures of the spine. *AJR Am J Roentgenol*. 1986; 147(3):575–582.
Emergency Radiology: The Requisites, 1st ed, Ch 7.
Gnanenthiran SR, Adie S, Harris IA. Nonoperative versus operative treatment for thoracolumbar burst fractures without neurologic deficit: a meta-analysis. *Clin Orthop*. 2012;470(2):567–577.

Case 38

Brookes JG, Dunn RJ, Rogers IR. Sternal fractures: a retrospective analysis of 272 cases. *J Trauma*. 1993;35:46–54.
de Oliveira M, Hassan TB, Sebewufu R. Long-term morbidity in patients suffering a sternal fracture following discharge from the A and E department. *Injury*. 1998;29(8):609–612.
Emergency Radiology: The Requisites, 1st ed, Ch 7.
Khoriati A, Rajakulasingam R, Shah R. Sternal fractures and their management. *Journal of Emergency Trauma Shock*. 2013;6(2):113–6. https://doi.org/10.4103/0974-2700.110763
Saab M, Kurdy NM, Birkinshaw R. Widening of the mediastinum following a sternal fracture. *Int J Clin Pract*. 1997;51:256–257.

Case 39

Emergency Radiology: The Requisites, 1st edition Ch 9.
Tenner S, Baillie J, DeWitt J, Vege SS. American college of gastroenterology guideline: management of acute pancreatitis. *Am J Gastroenterol*. 2013;108(9):1400–15;1416. doi: 10.1038/ajg.2013.218
Yadav D, Lowenfels AB. The epidemiology of pancreatitis and pancreatic cancer. *Gastroenterology*. 2013;144(6):1252–1261. https://doi.org/10.1053/j.gastro.2013.01.068.

Case 40

Dalrymple NC, Casford B, Raiken D, et al. Pearls and pitfalls in the diagnosis of ureterolisthiasis with unenhanced helical CT. *Radiographics*. 2000;20(2):439–447.
Emergency Radiology: The Requisites, 1st ed, Ch 9.

Case 41

Chapter 25. In: *The Mont Reid Surgical Handbook: Mobile Medicine Series*. 6 ed. St. Louis, MO: Mosby; 2008.
Coppolino F, Gatta G, Di Grezia G, et al. Gastrointestinal perforation: ultrasonographic diagnosis. *Crit Ultrasound J*. 2013;5(Suppl 1):S4. https://doi.org/10.1186/2036-7902-5-S1-S4.
Emergency Radiology: The Requisites, 1st ed, Ch 9.
Kasznia-Brown J, Cook C, et al. Radiological signs of pneumoperitoneum: a pictorial review. *Br J Hosp Med*. 2006;67(12):634–639.

Case 42

Emergency Radiology: The Requisites, 1st ed, Ch 10.
Grown WB, Lauder MR. Ovarian and Fallopian Tube Torsion. *UpToDate*. Web. 18 Nov 2015. http://www.uptodate.com/contents/ovarian-and-fallopian-tube-torsion.
Skandhan AK, Dixon A. Ovarian torsion. *Radiopaedia*. Web. 18 Nov. 2015. https://radiopaedia.org/articles/ovarian-torsion.

Case 43

Doubilet PM, et al. Diagnostic criteria for nonviable pregnancy early in the first trimester. *N Engl J Med*. 2013;369(15):1443–1451.
Emergency Radiology: The Requisites, 1st ed, Ch 10.

Case 44

Dogra VS, Gottlieb R, Oka M, et al. Sonography of the scrotum. *Radiology*. 2003;227(1):18–36.
Drlik M, Kocvara R. Torsion of spermatic cord in children: a review. *J Pediatr Urol*. 2013;9(3):259–266.
Emergency Radiology: The Requisites, 1st ed, Ch 10.
Sung EK, et al. Sonography of the pediatric scrotum: emphasis on the Ts–torsion, trauma, and tumors. *AJR Am J Roentgenol*. 2012;198(5): 996–1003.

Case 45

Atesok KI, Jupiter JB, Weiss AP. Galeazzi fracture. *J Am Acad Orthop Surg*. 2011;19(10):623–33. PubMed PMID: 21980027
Emergency Radiology: The Requisites, 1st ed, Ch 4.

Case 46

Eldridge J, Apau D. Boxer's fracture: management and outcomes. *Emerg Nurse*. 2015;23(4):24–30. https://doi.org/10.7748/en.23.4.24.e1438.
Emergency Radiology: The Requisites, 1st ed, Ch 4.
Halawi M, Morwood M. Acute management of open fractures: an evidence-based review. *Orthopedics*. 2015;38:e1025–e1033.

Case 47

Obakponovwe O, Morrell D, Ahmad M, et al. *Orthopaedics and Trauma*. 2011;25(3)3:214–22.
Singh A, Rathachai K. Chapter 4: In: *Emergency Radiology: The Requisites*. 2009;112–161.

Case 48

Dahnert W. *Radiology Review Manual*. 6th ed. Philadelphia: Lippincott Williams Wilkins; 2007.
Emergency Radiology: The Requisites, 1st ed, Ch.

Case 49

Johnson D, Pedowitz R. *Practical Orthopaedic Sports Medicine & Arthroscopy*. 641–655. Philadelphia, PA: Lippincott Williams and Wilkins; 2006.
Browner BD, Jupiter JB, Krettek C, et al. *Skeletal Trauma: Basic Science, Management, and Reconstruction*. 5th ed. Phildaelphia, PA: Elsevier; 1907–1936; 2014.

Case 50

Emergency Radiology: The Requisites, 1st ed, Ch 4.
Okanobo H, Khurana B, Sheehan S, et al. Simplified diagnostic algorithm for Lauge-Hansen Classification of Ankle Injuries. *Radiographics*. 2012;32: E71–E84.

Wilson A, Harris J Jr. Ankle. In: Pope T Jr, Harris John Jr, eds: *Radiology of Emergency Medicine*. 5th ed. Philadelphia: Lippincott Williams and Wilkins; 2013:905–45.

Case 51

Cowan M, Singer M. Anorectal emergencies. In: Moore LJ, Turner KL, Todd SR, eds. *Common Problems in Acute Surgery*. New York: Springer; 2013:383–397.
Emergency Radiology: The Requisites, 1st ed, Ch 9.
Ortega AE, Lugo-Colon H, Diaz-Carranza A, et al., Computed tomography and magnetic resonance imaging in abscess and anal fistula. In: Pescatori M, Regadas FS, Regadas FM, et al., eds. *Imaging Atlas of the Pelvic Floor and Anorectal Diseases*. Rome: Springer; 2008:63–80.
Sneider EB, Maykel JA. Anal abscess and fistula. *Gastroenterol Clin N Am*. 2013;42:773–784.

Case 52

Emergency Radiology: The Requisites, 1st ed, Ch 9.
Levsky JM, Den EI, DuBrow RA, Wolf EL, Rozenblit AM. CT findings of sigmoid volvulus. *AJR Am J Roentgenol*. 2010;194:136–143.
Maddu KK, Mittal P, Arepalli CD, Shuaib W, Tewari A, Khosa F. Colorectal emergencies and related complications: a comprehensive imaging review-noninfectious and noninflammatory emergencies of colon. *AJR Am J Roentgenol*. 2014;203:1217–1229.

Fair Game

CASE 53

Diffuse Axonal Injury (DAI)

1. **B**. Although concussion and epidural hematoma may result from the above history, diffuse axonal injury is most likely.
2. **B**. Magnetic resonance imaging (MRI) is the most accurate test. Computed tomography (CT) is offers easy accessibility and rapid acquisition.
3. **C**. Hematomas are not seen in diffuse axonal injury. Atrophy, edema, and multiple petechial hemorrhages may be seen on MRI or CT.
4. **D**. Approximately 50% of severe head trauma involved DAI. About 90% of patients with severe DAI end up in a persistent vegetative state.

Comment

Background
Brain injury in diffuse axonal injury occurs owing to multiple mechanisms. Diffuse axonal injury is seen in almost 50% of severe head traumas, although it may be seen in any head injury. Diffuse axonal injuries may occur in automobile accidents, falls, sports injuries, or shaken baby syndrome. As the name implies, axons are damaged throughout a large portion of the brain. Injuries to the axons occur from rapid acceleration and/or deceleration. This results in a shearing-type injury as brain tissues slide over each other owing to rotational forces or severe deceleration. Most lesions occur at the gray-white matter junction, even though white matter is mostly affected. Lesions are more likely to occur in areas of differing densities, such as the cerebral hemispheres, corpus callosum, and brainstem. Swelling of brain cells occurs owing to brain cells dying. This swelling in turn leads to decreased blood flow, and the release of chemicals caused by brain injury leads to further injury. Loss of consciousness is the major manifestation. Patients with minor diffuse axonal injury and intact consciousness will show signs of affected brain areas

Diagnosis
Neuroimaging is recommended for any patient with a closed head injury. Diffuse axonal injury should be suspected in any patient presenting with unconsciousness and head trauma. White matter lesions can measure anywhere from between 1 and 15 mm. Although CT is a mainstay of acute head trauma investigation, 50% to 80% of patients with DAI will have normal head CTs. Delayed imaging may be helpful in identifying findings such as edema or atrophy. Petechial hemorrhaging at the gray-white matter junction, corpus callosum, and brainstem are common.

MRI is the preferred modality (gradient echo sequences). MRI is more accurate than CT for chronic injuries. MRI uses edema to identify injury, which may not be present at the time of imaging. Diffusion tensor imaging can demonstrate injury when MRI is negative.

Management
Primary treatment of diffuse axonal injury revolves around preventing further damage and decreasing intracranial pressure. Corticosteroids are used to reduce inflammation. Management also includes a multidisciplinary approach to maximize a patient's function.

CASE 54

Burst Fracture With Spinal Cord Contusion

1. **C, D**. The entire pelvic ring is not included in the selected images; however, SI joint are normal. The femoral heads articulate normally with the acetabula. A complex fracture involving anterior, middle, and posterior elements of L1 are present. A right intertrochanteric fracture is noted.
2. **D**. All of the above.
3. **B**. Although radiography is likely to show spinal bony abnormalities, the degree and extent of injury are often underestimated, and spinal cord injuries are not appreciated. CT more accurately delineates fracture details. MR is sensitive for evaluation of cord injuries.
4. **C**. Burst fractures are a high-energy compressive (axial loading) injury. The retropulsion of bony fragments into the spinal canal are associated with neurologic deficits. Intraabdominal injuries, especially of the duodenum and pancreas, are associated. The majority of these injuries occur at L1.

Comment

Background
Burst fractures are high-energy compression injuries with axial loading forces (fall from height onto feet or motor vehicle accident [MVA]). This results in disruption of the posterior vertebral body cortex and retropulsion into the spinal canal. An estimated 90% of burst fractures occur at L1 with the majority occurring at T9 to L5. A single level burst fracture is more common than a two level burst complex.

Diagnosis
Lateral view on radiography with loss of vertebral height with anterior portion is more likely to be affected. The fracture involves the posterior vertebral body cortex, which may be difficult to appreciate on radiography. CT will provide greater bony detail and should be performed when fracture is suspected. CT also provides an opportunity to evaluate for associated intraabdominal injuries. The duodenum and pancreas are commonly injured. Retropulsed fragment involvement of the spinal canal and associated cord injury should be evaluated. MR is sensitive for evaluating the spinal cord.

Management
Surgical intervention.

CASE 55

Caecal Volvulus

1. **A, B**. There is an abnormal dilated bowel loop in the mid abdomen, which on close observation has haustral markings and represents a dilated cecum as the terminal ileum is noted laterally. Multiple dilated small bowel loops are present along with gaseous distention of the stomach. No pneumoperitoneum is visualized. This is not ileus because the rest of the large bowel is not dilated.
2. **C**. CT images confirm the abnormally dilated bowel loop to be cecum, which is twisted and flipped from its normal position in the right lower quadrant to rest in the mid abdomen. Note the

paucity of colon in the right lower quadrant and twisting of the mesentery and the distal ileum "whirl sign" with mesenteric haziness representing edema.

3. **D.** Cecal bascule is a variant of cecal volvulus where the cecum folds on itself without actual "twisting."
4. **A.** Sigmoid colon is the most common site; it accounts for about 60% to 75% of all colonic volvulus.

Comment

Background
Cecal volvulus is torsion of the cecum along its mesentery. It accounts for about 1% of the cases of intestinal obstruction and 25% to 40% of all cases of colonic volvulus. The incidence of cecal volvulus is more common in the younger population; sigmoid volvulus is more common among the 30- to 60-year-old age group. The most common cause is abnormal fixation of the right colon to the retroperitoneum, which allows for abnormal mobility. Alternately, any condition that causes restriction of bowel at a fixed point serves as a fulcrum for rotation. These conditions include adhesions, abdominal mass, scarring, and so forth.

Diagnosis
Radiography may suggest the diagnosis. CT often provides better anatomic detail to increase confidence of the diagnosis.

Axial type ($\approx$50%): Cecum rotates clockwise or counter-clockwise around its long axis, appearing in the right lower quadrant.
Loop type ($\approx$50%): Cecum both twists and inverts, typically occupying the left upper quadrant. The terminal ileum is usually twisted along with the cecum.
Cecal bascule: A variant of cecal volvulus. The cecum folds on itself without twisting and lies in the mid abdomen. This occurs when the cecum is loosely attached to its mesentery.

Management
Endoscopic or surgical intervention. Complications include ischemia and perforation.

CASE 56

Herpes Simplex Virus Encephalitis

1. **A, B, C.** Although A, B, C could have these findings, the bilateral hypoattenuation corresponding to the signal abnormalities on MR are characteristic for herpes simplex virus (HSV) encephalitis. The temporal lobe involvement is not characteristic of ischemic small vessel disease.
2. **B, C.**
3. **C.**
4. **D.** Hemorrhage is more common in older patients and would be best appreciated on gradient echo sequences. Edema is common. Enhancement is usually absent in the early phases of disease, but variable pattern enhancement occurs later in the disease. Diffuse-weighted imaging (DWI) is more sensitive than T2-weighted images.

Comment

Background
Herpes simplex virus encephalitis is a common viral encephalitis with two distinct subtypes—neonatal and childhood/adult. The majority (90%) of childhood and adult cases are caused by HSV-1; the remaining cases are related to HSV-2. HSV-1 can be reactivated in the case of immunosuppression, trauma, or other stress states. In immunocompetent adults, HSV encephalitis can result in fulminant hemorrhagic necrotizing encephalitis.

Diagnosis
Typical involvement includes the bilateral limbic system, medial temporal lobes, insular cortices, and inferolateral frontal lobes, with typical sparing of the basal ganglia. In children and immunocompromised patients, extra-limbic involvement is more common. CT may be normal or demonstrate hypoattenuation in the anterior and medial temporal lobes. Hemorrhage may be noted late in the disease. Contrast enhancement is uncommon early, but patchy enhancement may be seen later. MR will show edema in the affected area. Hemorrhage may be present. Post contrast images may demonstrate variable enhancement pattern beyond the early phase. Restricted diffusion is common but is less intense than restriction noted in the setting of infarction.

Management
Intravenous antivirals. Mortality ranges depend on the timing of intervention. Overall mortality is 70% with only 2.5% of patients fully recovering.

CASE 57

Fungal Globe

1. **B, C.** Although there is cloudiness of the vitrea, no history of trauma is present, and the globe is intact. Preseptal inflammation is present. The retrobulbar tissues are normal.
2. **D.**
3. **A.**
4. **A.** Fungal isolation from anywhere on the body and typical intraocular findings can yield a presumptive diagnosis. Amphotericin has good system coverage but poor vitreal penetration. Complications include sight loss. This entity has a male preponderance.

Comment

Background
Endophthalmitis is an intraocular inflammation involving the vitreous and anterior chamber of the eye. Infection is the most common cause, although noninfectious etiologies can occur. Fungal endophthalmitis can be exogenous (trauma, surgery) or endogenous (spread of systemic infection). Risk factors for endogenous spread include immunosuppression, intravenous (IV) drug abuse, diabetes, and sepsis. An estimated 9% to 37% of hospitalized patients with candidemia developed candida endophthalmitis. Patients present with ocular pain and blurred vision.

Diagnosis
Diagnosis is usually made clinically. CT may be performed to evaluate the extent of involvement of orbital inflammation. CT findings include hyperdensity of the vitreous humor, proptosis, intraorbital fat stranding, and scleral thickening. MR findings include T1 iso- or hyperintensity of the vitreous, restricted diffusion, and surrounding edema.

Management
Endophthalmitis is sight risking. Systemic and intravitreal therapy are mainstays. Severe cases may require surgery.

CASE 58

Acromioclavicular/Coracoclavicular (AC/CC) Separation

1. **D.** AC/CC separations are present.
2. **C, D.** AC/CC separation is associated with a direct blow or fall on adducted arm.

3. **A, B, C.** Multiple classifications systems exist and include all except Clinton.
4. **A.** Radiography sufficient to make the diagnosis.

Comment

Background
Acromioclavicular/coracoclavicular separation usually occurs from direct flow or a fall onto the shoulder with an adducted arm. These mechanisms force the acromion inferiorly and medially with respect to the clavicle. Multiple classification systems have been used, including Rockwood, Tossy, and Allman.

Diagnosis
Radiography is usually sufficient for diagnosing AC/CC separation. Stress views may be useful if initial radiographs are normal but clinical suspicion is high. CT/MR may be helpful in further evaluation if there is clinical suspicion that radiographs have underestimated the injury.

Widening of the AC joint greater than 8 mm and CC joint greater than 12 mm is diagnostic.

Management
Grade I: Sprain of the AC ligaments. Normal radiographs. Clinical diagnosis.
Grade II: Rupture of the AC ligaments. CC ligaments intact. Lateral clavicle is elevated.
Grade III: Disruption of the AC/CC ligaments. Widening of the joint spaces.
Grade IV: Clavicle is displaced posteriorly on the axillary view.
Grade V: Exaggerated AC/CC separation with increased distances.
Grade VI: Inferior displacement of the clavicle. Urgent chole cystectomy. Complications.

Treatment depends on severity of the injury, age, and lifestyle of the patient. The transition between conservative/surgical therapy is usually grade III.

CASE 59

Osteomyelitis Discitis

Infective Spondylitis

1. **B, E.** Abnormal signal and erosive changes involving the adjacent endplates of L3-L4 and the intervening disk with enhancing ventral epidural soft tissue causing compression on the thecal sac are compatible with infective spondylitis. Contiguous involvement of the vertebral endplates and disk is less suggestive of metastases or trauma.
2. **A.** Pyogenic spondylitis, although difficult to differentiate from other causes of infective spondylitis, commonly involves the lumbar spine and typically involves one spinal segment that consists of two lumbar vertebra and the intervening disc. It can be associated with paravertebral and epidural abscess or phlegmon. The involved vertebrae and the disk typically demonstrate low signal on T1 and high signal on T2, with post contrast enhancement.
3. **B.** Disk involvement is typically late in tuberculosis (TB) spondylitis. Lack of proteolytic enzymes in mycobacterial infection contributes to late disk involvement and subligamentous spread.
4. **E.** None of these conditions are usually associated with a soft-tissue component.

Modic type 1 degenerative endplate changes: May mimic infectious spondylitis because of marrow edema, which may sometimes enhance on post contrast images. However, lack of abnormal disk T2 hyperintensity, absent associated soft-tissue component, and clinical findings aid in differentiation.

Acute cartilaginous node: Concentric ring of high signal intensity around the node on T2 images, involvement of only one endplate, no diffuse signal intensity abnormality of the disk help differentiate from infectious spondylitis.

SAPHO syndrome: Refers to a combination of synovitis, acne, pustulosis, hyperostosis, and osteitis. Typically has anterior vertebral corner erosion, multilevel abnormalities, and no paravertebral or epidural abscess.

Andersson lesion: Refers to inflammatory involvement of the disk in spondylarthritides like ankylosing spondylitis. On MRI, these lesions are depicted as disk-related, signal-intensity abnormalities of one or both vertebral halves of a discovertebral unit and appear hyperintense on STIR and hypointense on T1-weighted images. Lines of increased signal intensity may be seen at the interface between the annulus fibrosis and nucleus pulposus. No soft-tissue component.

Comment

Background
Spinal infections result from hematogenous spread from distal septic foci, direct inoculation from spinal surgery or penetrating trauma, or direct extension from adjacent septic foci. *Staphylococcus aureus* is the most common infecting organism, contributing to 55% to 90% of cases. Other types of spondylitis include the following:

Tuberculous (TB) spondylitis: Preferentially involves the thoracic spine. Multiple vertebral or whole vertebral body involvement, subligamentous spread of infection, skip lesions, large paravertebral abscesses, and preferential involvement of the thoracic spine may suggest TB. It is insidious in progression.

Brucella spondylitis: Brucellosis is a zoonotic infection contracted by handling animal products and consuming dairy products made from unpasteurized milk. Predilection for the lower lumbar spine, preserved vertebral architecture despite diffuse involvement, marked hyperintensity of the disk on T2, and contrast and facet joint involvement may suggest brucella spondylitis. It may be differentiated from TB as it has smaller paravertebral abscesses, and gibbus deformities are rare.

Aspergillus spondylitis: Commonly seen in immunocompromised patients. Absence of hyperintensity within the disk with preservation of the nuclear cleft within the fungi suggest Aspergillus spondylitis.

Diagnosis
Magnetic resonance imaging is the imaging modality of choice. Involvement of two consecutive vertebrae and the intervening disk on MRI is virtually diagnostic of infective spondylitis. Infection commonly starts in the anterior portion of vertebral body where the vascular supply is rich. Lumbar spine (50%) is most commonly affected, followed by thoracic (35%) and cervical spine.

The involved vertebrae and the disk typically demonstrate low signal on T1 and high signal on T2 with variable patterns of post contrast enhancement. There can be associated paravertebral and epidural abscess or phlegmon.

Management
Most cases are managed conservatively with antibiotics and spinal brace. Surgery is indicated in the presence of neurologic signs, cauda equina syndrome, vertebral collapse, progressive spinal deformity/instability, and refractory abscesses.

CASE 60

Foreign Body Aspiration

1. **B.** Atelectasis in this case can be caused by a mucus plug, foreign body, or an intrabronchial mass. With additional history of

cough developed after eating peanuts, these images are compatible with peanut aspiration.
2. **C.** Tracheobronchial foreign bodies more often lodge in the right mainstem bronchus in older children and adults owing to the right mainstem bronchus being larger and more vertical than the left mainstem bronchus. Younger children have smaller trachea diameters, and foreign bodies may be found more proximal than the right or left mainstem bronchus.
3. **D.** Atelectasis, air trapping, and postobstructive pneumonia can all be seen in tracheobronchial aspiration.
4. **A.** Radiography is the first-line imaging modality when foreign body aspiration is suspected.

Comment

Background
Foreign body aspiration occurs more often in younger children than in adults. The peak incidence in children is 1 to 2 years of age. Younger children are more susceptible to aspiration because of their poor chewing capability and placing foreign bodies in their mouth. In adults, foreign body aspiration is uncommon but increases after the sixth decade of life. Foreign body aspiration may present more frequently in adults with swallowing impairment or with cough. The most common presentation is a sudden onset of choking with intractable cough with or without vomiting. In addition to cough, patients may present with wheezing, fever, and/or breathlessness. Patient presentation of symptoms may be related to the foreign body size, shape, and composition. The longer the foreign body is present, the more likely the patient may present with associated complications. Recurrent pneumonia, bronchiectasis, inflammatory granulation tissue, empyema, abscess, bronchial stricture, and hemoptysis are some of the late complications that may be seen in aspiration of foreign bodies. A foreign body aspiration event may not be recalled or witnessed, especially in young children or impaired adults. Therefore foreign body aspiration should be in the differential diagnosis when patients present with sudden onset of cough or wheeze or some of the later complications previously mentioned.

Diagnosis
Frontal and lateral plain radiographs of the chest and neck are often the first type of imaging obtained. Radiography can assess the location of foreign bodies and detect possible associated complications. Stone, teeth, and metal, with the exception of aluminum, are usually radiopaque on chest x-ray. Plastic, wood, thin fish bones, chicken bones, nuts and seeds, and glass are usually radiolucent, resulting in a negative radiograph for a foreign body. Air trapping may be an early secondary sign of foreign body aspiration. When foreign body aspiration involves a unilateral mainstem bronchus, the involved side fails to collapse on the expiratory or decubitus view. If the foreign body is located in the trachea, both lungs may not collapse. Late manifestations include atelectasis and postobstructive pneumonia.

CT may be used as a secondary modality when patients are clinically stable and radiographs are negative. CT may differentiate foreign body aspiration from other conditions that may present with similar symptoms.

Management
Bronchoscopy can be diagnostic and therapeutic. It should not be delayed in unstable patients.

CASE 61

Lens Dislocation (Ectopia Lentis)

1. **B, D.** There is complete posterior dislocation of the left lens, which is seen lying in the dependent portion of the vitreous.

The right lens is posteriorly subluxed without frank dislocation from partial disruption of the zonular fibers that hold the lens in its normal position.
2. **D.** Trauma is the most common cause of lens dislocation; it accounts for more than 50% of all cases. Nontraumatic lens dislocation is usually associated with connective tissue disorders such as Marfan, Ehlers–Danlos, homocystinuria, and so forth.
3. **B.** Posterior dislocations are more common than anterior dislocations as the iris impedes anterior subluxation of the lens. Marfan disease is usually associated with superotemporal lens dislocation. Homocystinuria is associated with inferonasal lens dislocation.
4. **C.** Noncontrast multidetector computed tomography multidetector CT (MDCT) is the imaging modality of choice for orbital trauma, which helps in evaluating the orbit as well as the globe in a swollen shut eye where funduscopic examination is very difficult. Ultrasound (US) is very useful in evaluating the globe and its contents, but is contraindicated in globe rupture. MRI may be difficult to perform emergently and is contraindicated when a metallic intraorbital foreign body is suspected.

Comment

Background
Trauma, the most common cause of lens dislocation, accounts for more than 50% of cases. Blunt trauma to the eye deforms the globe and typically displaces the cornea and sclera posteriorly. The globe expands in the equatorial direction causing the zonular fibers that hold the lens in position to stretch and tear, either partially or completely, resulting in subluxation or dislocation of the lens. Traumatic lens dislocation is usually unilateral. If bilateral, the radiologist should alert the clinician to evaluate for any underlying systemic cause.

Nontraumatic lens dislocations are usually bilateral and symmetric. They are associated with systemic connective tissue disorders. Marfan, homocystinuria, and Weill-Marchesani syndromes account for more than 95% cases of nontraumatic lens dislocations. Marfan is the most common cause of hereditary ectopia lentis. Lens dislocation occurs in about 75% of patients with Marfan and is usually a superotemporal dislocation. Homocystinuria, the second most common cause of hereditary ectopia lentis, is seen in about 90% of the patients, with the lens usually dislocating inferonasally.

Diagnosis
In the acute traumatic setting, MDCT can be readily available and can evaluate the globe and its contents. Fundoscopy may be difficult to perform in the immediate aftermath of orbital trauma with other injuries. US can be used to evaluate the globe but is contraindicated in the setting of rupture. MR should be avoided if a metallic foreign body is suspected.

Management
Complications from lens dislocation include secondary glaucoma, retinal detachment, chorioretinal degeneration, uveitis, and poor vision. Anterior dislocations are associated with greater rates of complications including acute glaucoma, and corneal and iridial injuries. Posterior dislocations are usually well tolerated, with the eye usually maintaining correctable vision without development of glaucoma.

CASE 62

Globe Rupture

1. **D.** Loss of normal globar contour with flattening and irregularity of the posterior globe. This is a great example of the *flat tire sign*.
2. **A.** The orbital region is very sensitive in globar rupture. Tonometry is a test for intraocular pressure and should not be performed in a potential globar rupture because it may cause further damage.

3. **B, C.** Intraocular air or a foreign body, as well as orbital fractures, may be seen on radiography.
4. **A.** Globar rupture, an ophthalmologic emergency, most commonly occurs in the setting of orbital trauma.

Comment

Background

Globe rupture occurs in the setting of traumatic compression to the globe. Tearing of the sclera is characteristic and occurs most commonly in areas where the sclera is the thinnest.

Diagnosis

Computed tomography scans are the most useful diagnostic imaging technique for globe injuries. Radiographic images are not particularly useful. MRI should be performed with discretion because foreign metallic bodies that may be present.

Management

Minor injuries can be treated by nonophthalmologists. However, serious injuries should be evaluated by an ophthalmologist. Irritation should be avoided. Additionally, the eye should be kept stable without applying any additional pressure. Any foreign bodies that may be present in the globe should be left alone until consultation with an ophthalmologist. Surgery may be required. Antibiotics may be given at presentation because infection is a common association with globe rupture.

CASE 63

Osteomyelitis

1. **A, B, C, D.**
2. **B, C.**
3. **D.**
4. **D.** Group B streptococci infections are associated with neonatal osteomyelitis

Comment

Background

Osteomyelitis is the inflammation of bone associated with infection, usually bacterial; however, nonpyogenic forms exist (tubercular, fungal). Bony infection can occur at any age. *Staphylococcus aureus* is isolated in 80% to 90% of cases; however, organisms may not be recovered in up to 50% of cases. Organisms, such as *Escherichia Coli*, are seen in particular patient populations or conditions (IV drug users and genitourinary infection) Osteomyelitis is a common complication of diabetic foot ulcers. It is frequently missed and underdiagnosed.

Diagnosis

Radiography is insensitive in the early stages. Finding may include overlying soft-tissue changes (ulcerations). Cortical changes, regional osteopenia, and periosteal reaction may be seen. Radiographs are often normal. If a high level of suspicion exists, additional investigation may be fruitful. Bone scintigraphy is highly sensitive, but not specific. Increased osteoplastic activity results in increased radiotracer uptake in the surrounding infected bone in both blood-poor and delayed images. MRI is sensitive and specific; it is able to identify soft-tissue and joint complications. Marrow edema and soft-tissue fluid/inflammation are noted. Post contrast enhancement of the marrow, periosteum, and soft tissues will be present.

Management

Intravenous antibiotics are used. If a collection is present, drainage may be considered. Surgical debridement may be necessary. Amputation may be considered if medial therapy fails.

CASE 64

Hepatic Abscess

1. **C.** The abdominal aorta is normal in caliber. The pancreas is not inflamed. The appendix is not in the field of view. The heterogeneous collection in the left hepatic lobe is compatible with hepatic abscess.
2. **B.** Biliary disease is the most common cause of hepatic abscesses in North America. Abscesses can also develop from hematogenous spread in intestinal diseases, such as inflammatory bowel disease, diverticulitis, and appendicitis. Even trauma has been shown to result in hepatic abscesses. A great number of abscesses can also develop without a source ever being identified. These are known as cryptogenic abscesses.
3. **D.** *Shigella flexneri* is not a common pathogen associated with hepatic abscess; it is associated with bloody diarrhea. Its presence can be confirmed with Shiga toxin presence on stool culture. **A, C, B** are associated with hepatic abscess formation.
4. **A.** Although smoking has many detrimental correlations to health, including pulmonary deterioration, cancer, and vascular pathology, it is not as common a risk factor for hepatic abscess formation.

Comment

Background

Although hepatic abscess can have parasitic and fungal origin, bacterial etiology remains most common in North America. In developing countries, parasitic abscesses are most common. Patients suffering from diabetes, alcoholism, immunocompromise, IV drug abuse, or recovering from gastrointestinal (GI) and abdominal surgeries are at increased risk for hepatic abscess formation. *Escherichia coli* and *Klebsiella* sp. are commonly isolated from cultures of hepatic abscess in patients in North America. Of cases, 15% may be cryptogenic. Generally, patients with a hepatic abscess present with vague constitutional symptoms such as fevers, abdominal pain, nausea, and vomiting.

Diagnosis

Radiography is insensitive for evaluating liver abscesses. Gas within an abscess or biliary tree may be present. Ultrasound appearance is variable (hyperechoic with internal echoes to hyperechoic and with central color Doppler perfusion). CT findings may vary; however, they generally include peripherally enhancing, centrally hyperattenuating lesions. Gas may be seen in approximately 20% of cases. MRI is not often the first-line modality in the emergent setting. Abscesses have characteristic signals on T1 (heterogeneous signal with central hypointensity), T2 (hyperintense), post contrast (enhanced capsule), DWI (hyperintense), and apparent diffusion coefficient (ADC), (hypointense).

Management

Medical antimicrobial therapy is warranted in all cases. CT- or US-guided drainage plays a major role in management. Imaging can help plan and assess the effectiveness of percutaneous drainage.

CASE 65

Odontogenic Abscess

1. **B, D.** The tonsillar tissue is normal. Periapical cysts are not associated with inflammatory response.
2. **A, B, C.** Each represent possible complications.
3. **B.**
4. **B, D.**

Comment

Background

Odontogenic abscess is a point in a spectrum of infection beginning with dental caries and periapical abscess. Caries result in damage to tooth enamel allowing bacteria to access the dental pulp. It spreads to the root canal and the apical foramen, resulting in a periapical abscess. Contiguous spread results in a local abscess. Osteomyelitis may occur. More fulminant disease in the floor of the mouth is Ludwig angina. Extension can spread in the deep neck space. Odontogenic abscess commonly (80%) affects the submandibular space. Sinusitis, meningitis, and cerebral abscess may relate to more distal spread.

Diagnosis

Early dental abscess may not have routine radiographic features. Panorex or CT may show well-defined lucencies involving the tooth (caries) or apical roots (periapical abscess). Evaluation of the bony structures may demonstrate disruption of the tooth socket and local abscess.

Management

Antibiotics. Surgical intervention.

CASE 66

Acute Type B Intramural Hematoma (IMH)

1. **A, B.** The hyperattenuating region on non-contrast CT suggests A or B as possibilities.
2. **C.** Unenhanced CT scans can provide information regarding the presence of IMH, mediastinal hemorrhage, or hemorrhagic pericardial effusion and calcification.
3. **B.** Aortic dissection is the most common (62% to 88%) followed by IMH (10% to 30%) and penetrating atherosclerotic ulcer (PAU) (2% to 8%).
4. **C.** Medical management plays a role treatment of acute aortic syndrome (AAS). Each form of AAS may be managed medically using IV beta blockade and then vasodilators (given in that order to prevent reflex tachycardia) to reduce the shearing forces of high blood pressure. In addition to medical management, Sanford type A lesions require surgical or endovascular intervention.

Comment

Background

Acute aortic syndrome encompasses three interrelated conditions: aortic IMH, acute aortic dissection (AD), and (PAU). The common clinical presentation of these entities is sudden onset of chest pain. There is an inherent risk of imminent aortic rupture necessitating early identification and intervention of AAS. Disruption of the media layer of the aorta is the common feature to the pathologic entities of AAS. IMH is defined as acute hemorrhage contained within the layers of the aortic wall, thus creating a false lumen. IMH may originate spontaneously as a consequence of a PAU or after thoracic trauma. Many investigators have reported an overlap between classic AD and IMH and suggest that the intramural bleeding results from microscopic tears in the aortic intima, which is contrary to the early belief that it results from rupture of vasa vasorum. Aortic wall hemorrhage can lead to aortic wall infarction, which is believed to be the precursor of acute AD. Acute IMH accounts for 5% to 15% of all cases of AAS.

Diagnosis

Approximately half of all patients with AAS have normal findings on a chest x-ray, and approximately one-third of patients have a widened mediastinum. CT, echocardiography, and MRI are diagnostic options for the evaluation of AAS in clinical practice. CT is readily available, and images are quickly acquired. Unenhanced CT provides information regarding the presence of IMH, mediastinal hemorrhage, hemorrhagic pericardial effusion, and calcification. A hyperdense crescent on unenhanced CT is the most common finding of IMH. The absence of an obvious communication between the true and false lumina explains the absence of flow on color Doppler examination and the lack of enhancement with contrast administration on CT, MRI, or angiography. IMH maintains a constant circumferential relationship with the aortic wall, whereas a dissection tends to spiral longitudinally. MRI should be the modality of choice for pregnant patients or those with renal failure.

Management

Each form of AAS may be managed medically using IV beta blockade and then vasodilators (given in that order to prevent reflex tachycardia) to reduce the shearing forces of high blood pressure. Stanford type A aortic dissections and IMH require prompt surgical intervention, whereas Stanford type B aortic dissections and IMH may be managed medically in the absence of distal ischemia or rapid disease progression.

Course of Intramural Hematoma

Prognosis of IMH is variable. Spontaneous regression can occur in 10% of patients. Progression to classic aortic dissection is seen in 28% to 47% and risk of aortic rupture is seen in 20% to 45% of IMH cases.

CASE 67

Occipitocervical Distraction (OCD)

1. **C.** Both the radiograph and CT demonstrate distraction at the craniocervical junction.
2. **B.** High energy trauma is an association.
3. **A, B, C.** Although radiography is often used in the initial phases of trauma evaluation, it is often of limited value and relatively insensitive as many of the anatomic markers may be poorly visualized. CT provides better bony evaluation. MR provides better evaluation of the cervical soft tissues and spinal cord.
4. **B.** This injury is three times more common in children than adults.

Comment

Background

Occipitocervical distraction injury results from ligamentous injury to the craniocervical junction. These ligaments stabilize the skull base to the spine. High force is required to disrupt this complex, and it is associated with high fatality in the prehospital setting. Hyperextension, hyperflexion, and lateral flexion in combination or alone can result in OCD. This injury is three times more common in children than adults.

Diagnosis

Although radiography is often a first-line imaging tool in the trauma imaging evaluation, suboptimal visualization of the entire cervical spine is common. CT is widely available, provides better osseous evaluation, and is the modality of choice. The occipitocervical joints and their intervals can be better assessed. MR provides superior evaluation of soft tissues and the spinal cord.

Management

Stabilization. Surgical intervention.

CASE 68

Atlanto-Axial Rotary Fixation (AARF)

1. **C.** Grisel syndrome is a rare cause of torticollis that involves subluxation of the atlanto-axial joint from inflammatory ligamentous laxity following an infectious process in the head and neck, usually a retropharyngeal abscess.
2. **B.** Asymmetry of the lateral masses can be normal in patients. With AARF, rotating the head will not change the asymmetric relationship. Torticollis will maintain symmetry.
3. **D.** Injury to the cervical vertebrate can cause injury to any part of the body. Impairment in control of trunk muscles but normal upper-body movement is likely an injury to the thoracic vertebra.
4. **A.** Radiographs of AARF will show C1 not oriented in line with the head. Additionally, C2 may move in conjunction with C1. Fractures are not generally present in rotary fixation. Excess of keratin sulphate is characteristic of Morquio syndrome. Absence of an X chromosome is characteristic of Turner syndrome.

Comment

Background
The most common acquired causes of AARF are trauma and upper respiratory tract infections. AARF can be caused by Grisel syndrome. This occurs when an infection or surgery affects the C1/C2 ligaments, resulting in subluxation of the atlanto-axial joint. Various arthritides (rheumatoid, psoriasis, lupus) and congenital (Down syndrome, Marfan disease, osteogenesis imperfecta) can cause AARF.

The subluxation can occur—anterior, posterior, rotary, vertical, or lateral. Rotary-type AARF is generally classified into four categories based on the presence and extent of anterior displacement of the atlas. Category 1: Rotary fixation without anterior displacement of the atlas. Category 2: Rotary fixation with anterior displacement of the atlas of 3 to 5 mm. Category 3: Rotary fixation with anterior displacement of more than 5 mm. Category 4: Rotary fixation with posterior displacement of the atlas.

Diagnosis
Clinical features, such as restriction of neck movements, prominence of the axial spinous process opposite the side of the dislocation, and spasms of the sternocleidomastoid muscles, are indicative. Radiography and CT are helpful tools.

Management
Management is based on duration of symptoms and clinical presentation. Symptoms of less than a week may be treated conservatively with soft collar, physical therapy, and pain relief. Cases of longer duration may require halo traction, immobilization, or open reduction with spinal fixation.

CASE 69

Traumatic Spondylolisthesis of the Axis—Hangman Fracture

1. **D.** A C2 fracture is present.
2. **A, D.**
3. **A.**
4. **B, D.**

Comment

Background
Somewhat of a misnomer, Hangman fracture, refers to a traumatic spondylolisthesis of the axis that involves the bilateral interarticularis, usually the result of a hyperextension and distraction injury. Most commonly patients present with neck pain after a high-energy injury, such as an MVA. This injury is rarely associated with suicidal hangings.

Diagnosis
Radiographic and CT imaging demonstrates bilateral lamina and pedicle fractures at C2. Associated anterolisthesis of C2 on C3. Extension of the fracture of the transverse foramina should raise the possibility of vertebral artery injury, and CTA may further evaluate vascular injury.

Management
Stabilization. Surgical fixation.

CASE 70

Lipohemarthrosis

1. **C.** Only this choice demonstrates a fat/fluid level within the joint.
2. **B.** Lipohemarthrosis results from an intraarticular fracture with escape of fat and blood from the bone marrow into the joint.
3. **A.** It is seen on all three modalities as well as US.
4. **D.** The only clinical significance of a lipohemarthrosis is that it indicates the presence of an intraarticular fracture. It does not reflect injury severity nor prognosis.

Comment

Background
Lipohemarthrosis results from an intraarticular fracture with escape of fat and blood from the bone marrow into the joint. The fatty marrow separates from the joint fluid and blood and layers above it, forming a fat-fluid level that can be seen on all modalities. It is most frequently seen in the knee, associated with a tibial plateau fracture or distal femoral fracture. It has also been described in the hip, shoulder, and elbow.

Diagnosis
The fat-fluid level is seen on any horizontal beam radiograph, as the beam is tangential to the fat–blood interface. In the knee, this is best achieved with a cross-table horizontal lateral view, where a long horizontal line is seen in the suprapatellar bursa indicating the fat/fluid level. CT and MRI may demonstrate a third layer owing to the greater sensitivity in detecting different densities and fluid composition. The three visible layers consist of fat above, serum/synovial fluid in the middle, and red blood cells settling below.

Management
Presence of a lipohemarthrosis is nearly diagnostic of a fracture, even when that fracture is radiographically occult. However, it is not seen in all cases of intraarticular fracture, thus absence of a lipohemarthrosis does not exclude an intraarticular fracture. It may take up to 3 hours after trauma to appear. The suprapatellar fat pad may be confused for a fat/fluid level, but will not change on repositioning, thus aiding in differentiating it. The underlying fracture should be treated.

CASE 71

Bilateral Jumped Facets

Bilateral Cervical Facet Dislocation

1. **C, D.** There are bilateral C6-C7 facet dislocations resulting in bilateral locked facets. Midsagittal image demonstrates more

than 50% anterior subluxation of C6 on C7. On the parasagittal images, there is reversal of the normal alignment of the facets with the inferior facets of C6 positioned anterior to the superior facets of C7. Axial image confirms the same and demonstrates bilateral *inverted hamburger sign*. Bilateral facet dislocation results in disruption of the discoligamentous complex (DLC).

2. **B.** Typically, unilateral facet dislocation results in anterior subluxation of the upper vertebral body by about 25% of the anteroposterior (AP) diameter of the vertebral body. Anterior translation in bilateral facet dislocation is typically more than 50%.

3. **D.** Rotation-translation morphology, according to the sub-axial cervical spine injury classification system (SLIC) classification, includes unilateral and bilateral facet fractures—dislocations, fracture separation lateral mass (floating lateral mass), and bilateral pedicle fractures. This represents horizontal displacement of one vertebra with respect to the other.

4. **D.** SLIC classification assesses the morphology of the injury, integrity of the DLC, and neurologic status to determine the prognosis and treatment options.

Comment

Background
Cervical facet dislocations are flexion injuries. Excessive flexion forces cause disruption of the ligamentous complex that stabilizes the facet joint. As a result, the superior vertebra undergoes forward subluxation, with anterior displacement of the corresponding inferior articulating facet on the superior articulating facet of the vertebra below. This results in uncovering of the articulating facet surfaces. The degree of facet uncovering could be partial (subluxed facets) or complete (perched facets). Further flexion forces can transform perched facets into a jumped facet or facet lock. Dislocations can be unilateral or bilateral. They can be associated with vascular and spinal cord injuries.

Unilateral facet dislocation is considered a stable injury. Associated neurologic deficit can be seen in about 30% of patients. Radiographic signs can be subtle and usually include hyperflexion with widening of the intraspinous distance. Findings include approximately 25% anterior translation of the vertebral body relative to the one below and malalignment of the spinous process on the AP view with the involved process pointing toward the involved side.

Bilateral facet dislocation results in complete disruption of the posterior ligament complex, posterior longitudinal ligament, intervertebral disk, and usually the anterior longitudinal ligament. There is usually more than 50% anterior translation of the vertebra. The vast majority (80%) of these cases are associated with cord injury.

Diagnosis
Computed tomography is diagnostic. Further imaging with MRI and CT angiogram are performed to exclude cord and vascular injuries.

Management
These dislocations are usually reduced under fluoroscopic guidance by applying progressive cervical traction.

SLIC (Sub-axial Cervical Spine Injury Classification System)
This is a newer classification system proposed by Vaccaro et al. for evaluating subinjuries of the cervical spine. This system helps in determining the injury pattern and severity along with treatment considerations and prognosis.

The parameters included are morphology, DLC, and neurologic status.

TABLE 71.1

Characteristic	Points
MORPHOLOGY	
No abnormality	0
Compression	1
Burst	2
Distraction (e.g., facet perch, hyperextension)	3
Rotation/translation (e.g., facet dislocation, unstable teardrop, or advanced-stage flexion compression injury)	4
DISCOLIGAMENTOUS COMPLEX (DLC)	
Intact	0
Indeterminate (e.g., isolated intraspinous widening, MRI signal change only)	1
Disrupted (e.g., widening of disk space, facet perch, or dislocation)	2
NEUROLOGIC STATUS	
Intact	0
Root injury	1
Complete cord injury	2
Incomplete cord injury	3
Continuous cord compression in setting of neurologic deficit (neuro modifier)	1

TABLE 71.2

Interpretation of Sub-axial Cervical Spine Injury Classification System (SLIC) Scoring Score	Interpretation
< 4	Nonoperative treatment
4	Operative versus nonoperative
≥5	Operative treatment

CASE 72

Pneumomediastinum

1. **A, D.** Although it may be difficult to identify all the spaces involved on radiography, CT easily delineates the involved compartments.

2. **A, B, C, D.** Each of these choices can cause pneumomediastinum.

3. **B.** An isoattenuating esophageal foreign body is present. The visualized portions of the trachea are intact. Extensive subcutaneous gas is noted and has likely traveled from mediastinal space related to barotrauma in the setting of violent coughing secondary to esophageal foreign body. Concern for intrinsic esophageal injury is warranted. There is no tension pneumothorax.

4. **D.** Removal of foreign body and treatment of underlying injury.

Comment

Background
Pneumomediastinum is the presence of mediastinal air that may originate from the tracheobronchial tree, lungs, or esophagus. The gas can extend into the neck or abdomen. There are many causes, including recent surgery, penetrating trauma, asthma, tracheobronchial or esophageal injury, infection, and barotrauma. Blunt trauma to the chest may cause pneumomediastinum owing to alveolar rupture or tracheobronchial injury. In asthmatic patients, pneumomediastinum is a result of air trapping owing to mucus plugging. Barotrauma includes mechanical ventilation, vomiting, and coughing. With vomiting, pneumomediastinum is

the result of straining against a closed glottis. Extra-thoracic causes include dissection of air from an odontogenic infection or intra-abdominal air from abdominal surgery or bowel perforation.

Diagnosis

Radiographically, air is seen anterior to the pericardium and around the great vessels. In pediatric patients, air can elevate the thymus and cause the *sail sign*. The continuous diaphragm sign is created by air posterior to the pericardium. Diagnostic challenges include differentiating pneumomediastinum from medial pneumothorax and pneumopericardium.

Management

Generally, pneumomediastinum does not require treatment apart from treating the underlying cause. In this case, the foreign body should be removed. Close inspection and evaluation for intrinsic esophageal injury are recommended.

CASE 73

Pulmonary Contusion

1. **C, D.** Given the history, **C** and **D** are possibilities. Although **A** and **B** could occur, the location of the findings are not consistent with typical aspiration pneumonia nor atelectasis. Neoplasm would not be included in the differential of an otherwise healthy young patient.
2. **C.** CT chest study shows details of lung parenchyma and is a rapid imaging technique in the setting of trauma. **A** and **D** are utilized as screening tools in the trauma setting. VQ scan is not routinely employed in the acute traumatic setting.
3. **B.** Although each of these injuries can be life threatening, aortic injury is the most rapidly fatal.
4. **D.** Ideal endotracheal tube (ETT) placement is 2 to 6 cm above the carina on chest radiography. Repeat films should be acquired periodically because of periodic shifting.

Comment

Background

Pulmonary contusions are the most common potentially lethal chest injury and generally occur from blunt trauma, although high-energy projectiles may also cause significant contusion, as in this case. In the case of blunt trauma, contusions generally coincide with rib fractures. Children are more susceptible to contusions owing to greater chest wall pliability.

Diagnosis

Initial evaluation of a trauma patient generally involves coordinated care, including imaging in the secondary survey. This generally includes a chest and, if indicated, a pelvic x-ray. In the chest x-ray taken above, a bullet is clearly seen in the apex of the R chest with a chest tube in place. A CT scan further characterizes the injury and reveals a pulmonary contusion along with a small pneumothorax.

Irregular, nonlobular opacification seen on chest x-ray is the classic diagnostic appearance of pulmonary contusion. Most contusions develop over a 24-hour period and resolve over a week. Although many are diagnosed during initial radiographs, radiography is not a sensitive test for detecting contusions.

Management

Definitive treatment is to ensure adequate oxygenation, to administer fluids judiciously, and to provide analgesia. Respiratory failure can develop over time and requires close monitoring. Radiographic clearing is generally rapid and occurs over a few days.

CASE 74

Diaphragmatic Injury

1. **B, D.** Diaphragmatic injury and phrenic nerve palsy may both be included in the differential diagnosis in this case because the right hemidiaphragm is elevated compared with the left. Eventration typically refers to focal thinning and an abnormal contour of the dome of diaphragm, which is not seen in this case. A Bochdalek hernia is a congenital form of diaphragmatic hernia caused by a defect in the posterior attachment of the diaphragm.
2. **D.** Contiguous injury describes injuries that are present above and below the diaphragm (both sides). In this case, the liver, pleural, and lung parenchyma are injured. The other signs are herniation-related signs, not seen in this case.
3. **D.** Discontinuity of the diaphragm is most sensitive for the detection of diaphragmatic injury and is the only direct sign of diaphragmatic injury listed. The other signs are occasionally referred to as indirect signs related to herniation.
4. **C.** Left-sided injuries are most common and occur three times more commonly than right-sided injuries. Central tendon and bilateral diaphragmatic injuries are rare.

Comment

Background

Diaphragm injuries are uncommon but serious injuries, and appear to be more commonly associated with penetrating rather than blunt trauma. Diaphragm injuries are potentially serious injuries, because complications secondary to delayed herniation can result in respiratory compromise and lead to visceral strangulation or visceral perforation. Detection on imaging can be difficult because signs may be subtle. Diaphragmatic injury can mimic normal variants, including congenital posterolateral defects (Bochdalek's hernia) or focal thinning and contour abnormality (eventration).

Left-sided hemidiaphragm injuries occur three times more commonly than right-sided injuries. Central tendon and bilateral injuries are rare. Diaphragm injuries are thought to occur most frequently on the left side owing to a congenital weakness in the posterolateral diaphragm. Additionally, the liver is postulated to have a protective effect on the right side. Tears, usually 10 cm or greater in size, typically begin posterolaterally and extend medially toward the central tendon.

Diagnosis

A chest radiograph, which is often initially obtained, can detect left-sided injuries in up to two-thirds of cases. Specific signs of diaphragmatic rupture on a chest x-ray include intrathoracic herniation of a hollow viscus and detection of a gastric tube above the left hemidiaphragm. Elevation of the right hemidiaphragm by greater than 4 cm compared with the left should be considered suggestive of diaphragm injury. Adjacent pulmonary abnormalities, such as atelectasis, contusion, or hemothorax, can mask or mimic diaphragmatic injuries on radiography.

MDCT can evaluate the integrity of the diaphragm and herniation of intraabdominal contents. Injury to the diaphragm should be suspected with penetrating injuries when then trajectory of the missile traverses or extends to the diaphragm (Figure 74-2 and Figure 74-3). The finding of contiguous injuries on both sides of the diaphragm in thoracoabdominal injuries is another indicator of diaphragmatic injury (Figure 74-2), and peridiaphragmatic contrast extravasation should also alert the radiologist to the possibility of a diaphragmatic injury.

Other signs include herniation of intraabdominal contents into the thoracic cavity through a diaphragmatic defect. The *collar sign* describes focal constriction of herniated fat or viscera by the free edges of the diaphragm, and the *dependent-viscera sign* demonstrates upper abdominal viscera in direct contact with the posterior chest wall in a supine patient. The liver can also produce a hump or band-like contour in cases of right-sided diaphragmatic injury.

MRI can also be performed, and relies predominantly on T1-weighted sequences with coronal and sagittal reformats. MRI is not normally a primary tool for evaluation in the emergent setting.

Management
Surgical repair.

CASE 75

Esophageal Foreign Body

1. **B.** A foreign body is seen in the upper esophagus, posterior to the trachea. A Mallory-Weiss tear is a mucosal laceration that is likely to be radiographically occult. Esophagitis would show diffuse esophageal thickening and submucosal edema on CT.
2. **C.** Hypersalivation and the inability to swallow saliva are key features of severe esophageal obstruction, which requires emergent attention. Chest pain, nausea, vomiting, and dysphagia are all possible presentations of esophageal body impaction, but they do not generally indicate complete obstruction.
3. **A.** All of the mentioned options are common locations for esophageal foreign body impaction, but the most common is the upper esophagus, at the level of the cricopharyngeus muscle.
4. **B.** Coins are most frequently ingested in the pediatric population, whereas vinyl gloves are seen in the psychiatric population. Plastic bread bag clips pose a great diagnostic challenge because they have been reported to be invisible on both radiographs and CT.

Comment

Background
Once they manage to pass through the gastroesophageal junction, the majority of ingested foreign bodies make their way through the GI tract without complications. However, approximately 10% to 20% of foreign body ingestions require intervention. Most adults present with symptoms, including dysphagia, odynophagia, retrosternal fullness, chest pain, regurgitation, hiccups, and retching. The inability to swallow saliva should also raise suspicion for severe esophageal obstruction. In infants and children, foreign body ingestion could present as drooling, coughing, or refusal to eat.

Diagnosis
The initial evaluation of a patient with suspected foreign body ingestion includes 2-view radiography, which are generally sufficient to detect and localize a radiopaque foreign body, such as a tooth or stone. Many commonly swallowed bodies, such as plastic, thin bones, and wooden objects, may be radiolucent and radiographically occult. In the setting of negative radiographs and high clinical suspicion, further evaluation with a CT or endoscopy is necessary. The use of oral contrast examinations, such as barium swallow, are discouraged because they increase the patient's risk of aspiration and might impair subsequent endoscopic visualization.

Management
The urgency of an intervention is determined by the shape, size, and chemical composition of the ingested foreign object. Sharp foreign objects and button batteries in the esophagus require emergency endoscopic removal, whereas blunt objects (with the exception of coins) and magnets require at least urgent endoscopic removal. Any ingested foreign body causing symptoms of complete esophageal obstruction warrants emergency endoscopic removal regardless of its size or type. If esophageal perforation is suspected at any point, CT imaging and a surgical consultation should be sought immediately.

CASE 76

Esophageal Perforation

1. **B, D.** Pneumomediastinum is present. The distal esophagus mucosa is discontinuous and irregular. Ingested contrast is noted extraluminally adjacent to the esophagus and in the left pleural space.
2. **B.** Iatrogenic etiology accounts for approximately 70% of esophageal perforations.
3. **D.** All choices are true.
4. **D.** Left anterolateral distal esophagus.

Comment

Background
The most common cause of esophageal perforation is medical instrumentation and therapeutic endeavors, which account for 65% to 70% of cases. Other important causes of esophageal perforation include emesis and trauma. Other rare causes of esophageal perforation ($\approx$1%) include caustic ingestion, peptic ulcer disease, foreign body, aortic pathology, and disease of the esophagus. The distribution of perforation by location is as follows: cervical 27%, intrathoracic 54%, and intraabdominal 19%. The site of perforation varies depending on the cause. Instrumental perforation is common in the pharynx or distal esophagus. Spontaneous rupture from emesis may occur just above the diaphragm in the posterolateral wall of the esophagus; left side is more common than the right. The esophagus lacks a serosal layer and hence is more vulnerable to rupture or perforation. Full-thickness tear in the esophageal wall allows gastric contents, saliva, bile, and other substances to enter the mediastinum, causing mediastinitis. Boerhaave's syndrome describes perforation of the esophagus, usually owing to repeated vomiting, retching, or childbirth. The point of perforation is usually along the left anterolateral surface of the distal esophagus. Mallory-Weiss syndrome is a mucosal, not a transmural, tear and usually is not apparent on imaging.

Diagnosis
The diagnosis of esophageal injury requires a high index of suspicion. On radiography pneumomediastinum and subcutaneous gas can be seen. Bilateral pleural effusions and hydropneumothorax are other radiographic signs of perforation. CT findings of esophageal injury include esophageal wall thickening, periesophageal gas and fluid collections, contrast material extravasation, mediastinal fluid collection, mediastinal inflammation, focal esophageal wall defect, and pleural effusion.

Management
This is a rare but serious entity. The mortality rate can reach as high as 50%; mortality is significantly higher if diagnosis is delayed greater than 24 hours. Variation and controversy surround treatment. Some cases are treated conservatively with parenteral nutrition support, nasogastric suction, and broad-spectrum antibiotics. More serious cases warrant surgical intervention. Operative therapy depends on etiology, location/extension of the perforation, time elapsed since injury, and overall medical condition of the patient.

CASE 77

Cardiac Tamponade

1. **A, C.** There is a large pericardial effusion with compression of the cardiac chambers resulting in appearance of a small heart. Contrast bolus is seen in the right atrium.
2. **A, B, C, D.** Cardiac tamponade can occur from any etiology that allows accumulation of air or fluid between the pericardial layers.

3. **C.** The physiologic presentation of cardiac tamponade depends on the ratio of pressure in the pericardial space to pressure in the heart chambers. Slower accumulation of pericardial fluid increases pericardial compliance and shifts the curve relating filling volume to pressure. With slow accumulation for a given volume, the pericardial pressure rises less than it would in the setting of rapid increase in volume.

4. **C.** Although not specific to the diagnosis of pericardial tamponade, reflux of contrast material into the inferior vena cava, internal jugular, or azygos vein can be seen. This occurs owing to decreased diastolic filling of the ventricles and decreased stroke volume.

Comment

Background
Pericardial tamponade can occur owing to any etiology that expands the potential space between the visceral and parietal pericardium. This can include hemopericardium, such as from penetrating trauma or retrograde extension of aortic dissection; pericardial effusion associated with viral, uremic, or congestive cardiac disease; or air from tension pneumopericardium. The most important influence in the physiologic presentation of tamponade is the rate of accumulation of the fluid, followed by the volume accumulated. Rapid rate of accumulation is more precipitous because of the limited ability of the pericardium to accommodate the change in pressure. When this pericardial pressure meets or supersedes the right atrial or ventricular pressure, cardiac tamponade occurs.

Diagnosis
Radiographic diagnosis is difficult, but the diagnosis of pericardial effusion should be suspected if there is recent or rapid increase in heart size. Lateral radiographs can show apposition of the fluid in the pericardial space between the mediastinal and pericardial fat ("oreo cookie" sign), but radiographs do not provide adequate evidence for poor diastolic filling of the heart chambers. CT findings of tamponade demonstrate lack of cardiac filling, including enlargement of the superior or inferior vena cava, with a diameter greater than that of the adjacent aorta, periportal lymphedema, and excessive reflux of contrast material into the inferior vena cava or azygos vein. The flattened heart sign, in which poor end-diastolic filling leads to compression and flattening, or even inversion, of the free wall of the right ventricle, may be seen. Paradoxic bowing of the interventricular septum toward the left ventricle can be seen if intravenous contrast bolus has been given.

Management
In the setting of cardiac tamponade, urgent drainage of the pericardial collection is paramount. Percutaneous drainage or ultrasound-guided pericardiocentesis, via open sternotomy or, increasingly, with a balloon pericardiotomy, can be performed. Treat any underlying causes for pericardial effusion accumulation.

CASE 78

Acute Traumatic Thoracic Aortic Injury

1. **B, D.** The CT images demonstrate irregularity at the aortic isthmus with circumferential intimal flap along with focal outpouching representing a pseudoaneurysm. The irregular serpiginous bright areas of extraluminal contrast inferior to the pseudoaneurysm represent active vascular extravasation from the aortic injury. Also noted are bilateral pleural effusions and mediastinal hematoma. Transection, also called aortic rupture, involves all three layers of the aortic wall and is usually fatal. Pseudoaneurysm has an intact adventitial layer and has

to be differentiated from ductus diverticulum, which is a developmental outpouching at the aortic isthmus; it is usually smooth with obtuse margins with the aorta versus pseudoaneurysm, which has sharp, acute margins.

2. **C.** Aortic isthmus (90%), which is within 2 cm of the origin of the left subclavian artery where the aorta is relatively immobile, tethered by ligamentum arteriosum, is the most common site of aortic injury. Other areas where the aorta is relatively immobile—ascending aorta/aortic root (5% to 14%) and distal descending aorta at the diaphragmatic hiatus (5% to 12%)—account for the rest of the cases.

3. **A.** Mediastinal hematoma is an indirect sign of acute traumatic aortic injury (ATAI). Mediastinal hematoma with preserved fat planes with the thoracic aorta is not from ATAI and is usually from small mediastinal veins. Direct signs of ATAI include presence of an intimal flap, traumatic pseudoaneurysm, contained rupture, intraluminal mural thrombus, abnormal aortic contour, and sudden change in aortic caliber (aortic pseudocoarctation).

4. **C.** MDCT chest with contrast is the imaging modality of choice in the acute trauma setting. Although the role of conventional angiography is severely limited in the MDCT era, it remains an important problem-solving tool in the stable patient for planning prior to endovascular stent graft therapy and for detection of branch vessel injury. The other listed modalities have a limited role.

Comment

Background
A life-threatening injury, ATAI and can result from blunt or penetrating (stab, gunshot) trauma. Motor vehicle accidents (MVAs) are the most common (70% to 80%) cause of ATAI followed by falls from height, pedestrian-automobile collisions, and crush injuries. Blunt ATAI contributes to approximately 0.5% to 2% of all nonlethal MVCs and 10% to 20% of all high-speed deceleration fatalities. Pathophysiology of ATAI is complex, and proposed mechanisms include rapid deceleration, hydrostatic and shearing forces, and osseous pinching of the aorta between the anterior chest wall and the thoracic spine. Rapid deceleration causes cardiac displacement, resulting in torsion and shearing forces against the aorta at areas of relative immobility, mainly at the aortic isthmus (ligamentum arteriosum), aortic root, and diaphragmatic hiatus.

Diagnosis
One major role of supine chest radiography in the trauma setting is to evaluate for possible aortic injury apart from other life-threatening conditions such as tension pneumothorax and massive hemothorax. Although mediastinal widening greater than 8 cm or more than 25% of the width of the thorax is the most frequent observation, it is not the most sensitive finding. More discriminatory findings include abnormal contour of the aorta and loss of aortopulmonary window. Other findings include rightward tracheal, esophageal/nasogastric tube deviation, left apical cap, and depression of left mainstem bronchus. Chest x-ray may be normal in about 7% of ATAI cases.

Contrast MDCT is the modality of choice for evaluating ATAI with sensitivity about 98% and specificity, if direct signs alone are taken, approaching 100%. Direct signs of ATAI include presence of an intimal flap, traumatic pseudoaneurysm, contained rupture, intraluminal thrombus, abnormal aortic contour, and sudden change in aortic caliber (aortic pseudocoarctation). Mediastinal hematoma is an indirect sign. Mediastinal hematoma with preserved periaortic fat planes is not from ATAI but is usually from small mediastinal veins in the absence of other major vascular or overlying osseous injuries. Periaortic hematoma, which is hematoma in direct continuity with the aortic wall, could represent an occult intimal injury, and the source of hematoma is from vasa vasorum or small veins immediately adjacent to the aorta. This can be further evaluated with intravascular ultrasound or transesophageal echoaortography (TEA). Stable patients with low clinical suspicion can be followed up with a CTA in 48 to 72 hours.

Although MR angiography is good in evaluating the aorta, its use in the emergent setting is limited. It may have a role in follow up, particularly as a strategy to reduce radiation in young trauma victims. Endovascular ultrasound and TEA are used as adjunctive imaging modalities.

Management
Endovascular stent graft repair is currently preferred over open thoracotomy because it is less invasive and can be performed in an acutely injured patient with multiple comorbid injuries. Planning with multidetector CT is critical for technical success of endovascular repair. Dimensions to document on CT include (a) caliber of the aorta proximal and distal to the injury, (b) distance from the left subclavian artery to the injury, (c) length of the vascular injury, and (d) any anatomic variants.

CASE 79

Abdominal Aortic Aneurysm (AAA) With Impending Rupture

1. **D**.
2. **A, D**.
3. **A**.
4. **B, D**

Comment

Background
Abdominal aortic aneurysm is defined as focal dilatation of the abdominal aorta 50% greater than the proximal normal segment of greater than 3 cm. Rapid enlargement or diameter greater than 7 cm is considered high risk for rupture. The prevalence of AAA increases with age. Estimated 10% of individuals over 65 have AAA. Male-to-female ratio is 4:1. Most AAAs are asymptomatic until they begin to leak or rupture. Pulsatile abdominal masses may be detected on physical examination. Patients may complain of back or abdominal pain. In cases of rupture, hypotension and shock may be present.

Diagnosis
Radiographs are not optimal for detection or follow up. US is sensitive and specific for AAA and appropriate for monitoring of small aneurysms. CT can easily detect signs of frank rupture (contrast extravasation in the retroperitoneum, para-aortic fat stranding, retroperitoneal hematoma). Signs of impending/contained rupture (thrombus fissuration, high attenuation crescent sign [IMH], draped aorta, tangential calcium) are subtler and should not be overlooked.

Management
Surgical repair
Risk of rupture is related to size of aneurysm. AAAs greater than 5 cm in men and 5.5 cm in women carry a significant risk and warrant elective surgical repair.

Mortality rate from rupture is up to 83% in some series. Operative mortality rates are significantly lower (40%). Elective surgical mortality rates are below 5%.

CASE 80

Body Packing Rupture With Overdose

1. **A**. Multiple hyperattenuating ovoid foci are noted throughout the colon. No renal stones are noted. The gallbladder fossa has a normal postoperative appearance. Although there is increased stool in the colon, which may be seen in constipation or after a large meal, no complications are noted.
2. **A**. This patient with altered mental status was stopped by airport security entering the country and suspected of ingesting or concealing drugs. During interrogation, the patient expressed feeling "high" and was concerned that the drug packet may have "ruptured in his stomach."
3. **D**. Clinical examination (history, physical examination, and laboratory tests) is always helpful in evaluating patients. Although radiography is a good screening tool, low-dose CT has higher sensitivity for detecting ingested drugs in this setting.
4. **D**. All of the above.

Comment

Background
Body packing is the intentional concealment of drugs inside the body (GI tract or other orifices). Drugs may be packed in balloons, condoms, cellophane, foil, and so forth. Most patients are males and less than 40 years of age. By the time patients present, they have often encountered law enforcement, who ask for screening for internal drug concealment.

Diagnosis
Radiography and US can be used as screening tools; however, non-contrast CT is most effective at detection (accuracy, 97% to 100%). Radiography, US, and CT may demonstrate multiple 2- to 3-cm circumscribed foci. Surrounding air halos or air trapped in the tied ends of the packets may be noted. US may be considered useful screening in pregnant patients. CT can accurately determine size, number, and location of drugs and assess for complications (e.g., obstruction, perforation).

Management
The vast majority (95%) of cases are asymptomatic. Watchful waiting or laxative therapy may be employed. In symptomatic cases (as in this case where the pill packet ruptured, the contents are freely flowing into the GI track, and the patient is overdosing) may require intervention (Naloxone blockade, surgical intervention).

CASE 81

Choledocholithiasis

Choledocholithiasis and Cholelithiasis

1. **A, C, D**. The sonographic images demonstrate stones and sludge in the gallbladder and a dilated common bile duct with stones. The gallbladder wall is not thickened nor is there surrounding fluid.
2. **C**. Risk factors include cholangitis, anatomic abnormalities of the bile ducts, sphincter of Oddi dysfunction, cirrhosis, and hemolytic disease. The other choices are risk factors for secondary choledocholithiasis.
3. **D**. Magnetic resonance cholangiopancreatography (MRCP) images are heavily T2-weighted.
4. **B**. Stone impacted within the cystic duct or Hartmann's pouch of the gallbladder causing extrinsic compression on the common hepatic duct.

Comment

Background

Choledocholithiasis is the most common cause of bile duct obstruction. Biliary stones are classified according to their etiology. Secondary duct stones are the most common type and account for 95% cases. These stones, usually composed of cholesterol, arise in the gallbladder and move into the common bile duct (CBD), whereas primary duct stones form within the bile ducts and are commonly made up of pigment. The risk factors for primary stones include cholangitis, anatomic abnormalities of the bile ducts, sphincter of Oddi dysfunction, cirrhosis, and hemolytic disease. The risk factors for secondary stones include gender (female), obesity, Crohn's disease, elevated triglycerides, total parenteral nutrition, and genetics/ethnicity. Mirizzi syndrome refers to common hepatic duct obstruction caused by external compression from a stone or multiple stones impacted within the cystic duct or within Hartmann's pouch of the gallbladder (outpouching of the wall at the junction of the gallbladder neck and cystic duct). Predisposing risk factors for Mirizzi syndrome include a long cystic duct parallel to the common hepatic duct or a low insertion of the cystic duct into the common bile duct.

Diagnosis

Transabdominal US has a sensitivity of 21% to 63% for intrabiliary stones owing to limited acoustic window, absence of bile duct dilatation, and complex anatomy. Intraductal stones appear as echogenic foci with posterior acoustic shadowing along the course of the bile duct. With CT, stone detection depends on stone attenuation. Biliary stones may be heterogeneous in appearance—heavily calcified and radiopaque, less radiopaque than bile owing to cholesterol or gas attenuation owing to locules of nitrogen. The reported sensitivity of CT for choledocholithiasis is between 72% and 88%. MRCP is based on the acquisition of heavily T2-weighted images to provide visualization of stationary or slow-moving fluids with high signal intensity. MR cholangiography can demonstrate calculi as small as 2 mm despite its limited spatial resolution compared with ERCP. Most intraductal calculi appear as round or faceted low-signal intensity foci surrounded by high-signal intensity bile on heavily T2-weighted images. MRCP has a reported sensitivity and specificity of 89% to 100% and 83% to 100%, respectively. ERCP is the gold standard for CBD stone detection.

Management

Once the diagnosis of choledocholithiasis has been established, ERCP with attempted stone extraction is usually appropriate.

CASE 82

Renal Abscess

1. **A, D.** A mildly enhancing, rounded lesion in the upper pole of the asymmetrically enhanced left kidney. Differential diagnosis includes renal cell carcinoma and renal abscess. The history provides information to help narrow the possibilities.
2. **B.** Renal abscess is the best choice given the imaging findings and additional history.
3. **C.** Angiomyolipomas are hyperechoic on US.
4. **C.** Negative urine cultures may be seen in patients with renal abscess.

Comment

Background

Most urinary tract infections are confined to the bladder. Pyelonephritis, inflammation of renal pelvis and parenchyma, occurs when infection migrates to the upper urinary tract or is spread hematogenously. Renal abscess, localized collection of pus caused by suppurative necrosis, usually occurs as a sequel of acute pyelonephritis or focal bacterial nephritis. The most common presentation of renal abscess is with fever, flank or abdominal pain, chills, and dysuria. The risk factors for renal abscess include diabetes, immunosuppression, and urinary tract obstruction.

Diagnosis

Routine radiologic imaging is not required for diagnosis and treatment of uncomplicated cases of urinary tract infection in adult patients. CT is the modality of choice for evaluating acute pyelonephritis. The pathophysiologic disturbances within the renal parenchyma tend to decrease the flow of contrast agent through the tubule, causing delayed and persistent enhancement. CT is also the best modality for fully evaluating the secondary signs of renal inflammatory disease and its complications. These signs include focal or global enlargement of the kidney, perinephric stranding, thickening of Gerota's fascia, and abscess formation. At CT, abscesses are typically identified as round or geographic low-attenuation collections that do not enhance centrally, but that may have an enhancing rim. At ultrasound, the typical abscess appears as a hypoechoic mass with through transmission that lacks internal flow on Doppler interrogation. Occasionally mobile debris may be seen within the lesion. Other differential considerations for hypo-/isoechoic renal lesions on US are renal cell carcinoma, renal metastases, lymphoma, focal bacterial nephritis, tuberculosis, and xanthogranulomatous pyelonephritis.

Management

Between 15% and 20% of patients with renal abscess have negative urine cultures. This observation may reflect the fact that the infection has been relatively contained. Renal abscesses are generally treated with antibiotic therapy; percutaneous drainage via image guidance may be warranted. Surgery for renal abscess is rarely necessary.

CASE 83

Bowel Infarction

1. **C.** There are dilated loops of small bowel with poor wall enhancement, air in the bowel wall (pneumatosis), portal venous and superior mesenteric vein (SMV) air, mesenteric edema and fluid, compatible with bowel infarction.
2. **B.** In pneumobilia, air in the biliary radicals accumulate in the central hepatic parenchyma, whereas in portal venous gas, air in the portal veins are found in the periphery of hepatic parenchyma.
3. **B.** In cases of suspected ischemic bowel, IV and neutral oral contrast agents are preferred to enhance detection of mucosal enhancement patterns.
4. **C.** There is no role for endoscopic decompression in the management of ischemic and infarcted bowel.

Comment

Background

Ischemic bowel is associated with high mortality if not recognized and treated in a timely manner. Bowel ischemia may be classified based on several factors:

- Duration: acute or chronic
- Underlying cause: hypovolemia, thromboembolism, vascular occlusion, bowel obstruction
- Bowel involved: small bowel or colon

Any pathologic process that compromises vascular blood flow to the bowel may result in ischemic bowel. The spectrum of ischemic bowel ranges from mild mucosal changes to life-threatening infarct and necrosis. In pneumatosis intestinalis, the gas may extend through mesenteric vessels (mesenteric or portal vein gas). Systemic bacterial spread may result in sepsis, and bowel necrosis may result in perforation and peritonitis. This cascade of events is associated with high mortality.

Diagnosis
Computed tomography is the preferred imaging modality to assess bowel and vascularity with multiphasic imaging including arterial and portal venous phases. Intravenous contrast is administered. Instead of positive oral contrast, a neutral contrast agent is preferred to distend bowel without obscuring the mucosal enhancement pattern. In cases of suspected ischemic colitis of the distal colon or rectum, rectal contrast may be considered. CT signs of ischemic bowel include bowel wall thickening and dilatation. In advanced cases of bowel infarction, imaging features include pneumatosis intestinalis, pneumoperitoneum, and variable amounts of free fluid. It is important to note that bowel wall thickness is not increased in all causes and can be thinned in complete arterial occlusion or bowel obstruction.

Management
Bowel infarction is generally treated with surgical exploration and resection of necrotic bowel. In cases of mesenteric venous thrombosis, anticoagulation may be indicated. In some instances, endovascular thrombolysis or thrombectomy may be beneficial.

CASE 84

Penetrating Colonic Injury

1. **A, D.** In the setting of trauma, bowel contusion and perforation are diagnostic considerations. Although both bowel injury and shock bowel can have altered bowel wall enhancement, bowel trauma usually appears focal with high-attenuation submucosa (owing to hematoma). Shock bowel will appears diffuse with near-water attenuation submucosa. Unlike shock bowel, intense mucosal enhancement is typically not present in bowel trauma. Colitis is considered in the differential diagnosis of bowel wall thickening; however, history provides a clue.
2. **C.** More specific imaging features of bowel injury on CT include extraluminal contrast extravasation, extraluminal air, and bowel wall discontinuity. Hemoperitoneum can be helpful to assess for bowel injury; however, it is less specific as it can be seen in the solid organ injury.
3. **C.** Extraluminal contrast is a sensitive sign of colonic perforation.
4. **B.** Unlike MR (time consuming and low sensitivity for detection of free air) and US (low specificity for specific organ injury), CT is the test of choice to evaluate traumatic injury in hemodynamically stable patients owing to fast image acquisition and increased sensitivity and specificity. Radiography is not helpful in the evaluation of abdominal injuries.

Comment

Background
Historically, patients with suspected injury to abdominal organs and viscera underwent diagnostic peritoneal lavage and US. Although peritoneal lavage has a high sensitivity for the detection of hemoperitoneum, it is not specific for retroperitoneal injuries. Moreover, it may compromise the interpretation of the study owing to fluid and air introduced by lavage. US is not specific for organ and visceral injury despite high sensitivity and specificity for detection of free fluid. CT is the test of choice in the evaluation of traumatic injury in hemodynamically stable patients. It can help to significantly reduce time from diagnosis to treatment and confidently diagnose solid organ, vascular, and bowel injury.

Diagnosis
Injuries to the bowel and mesentery are difficult to diagnose both clinically and on imaging. Radiologists need to carefully inspect the images for direct and indirect signs. Direct imaging features of bowel injury on CT show bowel injury (enteric contrast extravasation, bowel wall discontinuity/transection, intramural gas, and extraluminal air). Indirect signs include bowel wall thickening and abnormal bowel wall enhancement. Fat stranding, free gas, hematoma, fluid, vascular beading, and contrast extravasation along the mesentery can be seen in mesenteric injuries. Secondary signs include hemoperitoneum, hemoretroperitoneum, and abdominal wall injury. Extraluminal contrast is an uncommon finding. The use of oral contrast has been questioned; there is a growing trend toward nonoral contrast CT.

Management
Delayed diagnosis of bowel or mesenteric injury is a leading cause of morbidity and mortality. Traumatic bowel and/or mesenteric injuries typically require surgical management.

CASE 85

Epiploic Appendagitis

1. **A, B.** In this case, the differential diagnosis for a localized, inflammatory focus adjacent to the colon includes omental infarction and epiploic appendagitis.
2. **D.** Oval fat attenuation lesion abutting the anterior colonic wall with thin enhancing rim, surrounded by inflammatory changes is a classic description of epiploic appendagitis.
3. **D.** Of epiploic appendagitis, 57% occurs in the sigmoid region followed by 26% in the ileocecal region.
4. **C.** Epiploic appendagitis is self-limited with most patients recovering with only conservative therapy.

Comment

Background
Acute epiploic appendagitis most commonly manifests with acute lower quadrant pain. Epiploic appendages are peritoneal pouches that arise from the serosal surface of the colon and are attached by vascular stalk. They frequently arise in association with colonic diverticula. Acute epiploic appendagitis most commonly results from torsion, with resultant vascular occlusion that leads to ischemia. Epiploic appendagitis is associated with obesity, hernia, and unaccustomed exercise. The condition most commonly manifests in the second to fifth decades of life, predominantly in women. The most common sites of epiploic appendagitis, in order of decreasing frequency, are sigmoid colon, the ileocecal region, ascending colon, transverse colon, and descending colon. Epiploic appendages are not found near the rectum.

Diagnosis
The CT features of acute epiploic appendagitis mainly include a fat density ovoid structure adjacent to the colon, usually 1.5 to 3 cm in diameter (<5 cm); thin high-density rim (1 to 3 mm thick); surrounding inflammatory fat stranding; thickening of the adjacent peritoneum; and central hyperdense dot (representing thrombosed vascular pedicle). The absence of a central dot sign does not preclude a diagnosis of epiploic appendagitis. The inflammatory change with epiploic appendagitis is very focal and limited to the inflamed pericolonic fat and rarely causes thickening of the colonic wall. The conditions that may mimic acute epiploic appendagitis on CT include acute omental infarction, mesenteric panniculitis, fat-containing tumor, and primary and secondary acute inflammatory process in the large bowel (e.g., diverticulitis and appendicitis). Omental infarction is most commonly located next to the cecum or the ascending colon. Although omental infarction

may have a CT appearance that resembles that of acute epiploic appendagitis, it lacks the thin high-density rim that is seen in epiploic appendagitis.

Management
Epiploic appendagitis is a self-limited condition to be treated conservatively with oral antiinflammatory medications.

CASE 86

Misplaced Urinary Catheter (Prostatic Urethra)

1. **A, B, C, D.** The prostate is enlarged and irregular. Soft tissue occupies the bladder base, and an irregular isoattenuating lesion is noted in the bladder lumen adjacent to the soft tissue.
2. **B.** The sagittal image best demonstrates the urinary catheter is the prostatic urethra, not in the bladder lumen as expected.
3. **C.**
4. **E.** No additional imaging is warranted in the acute setting. The urinary catheter should be appropriately placed in the bladder.

Comment

Background
Indwelling bladder catheters are one of the most universal medical devices encountered. These short-term devices are used to decompress a distended bladder, collect urine, and monitor urine output. The distal tip and the inflated balloon should be placed in the bladder.

Diagnosis
Adequate placement of the catheter is usually assessed clinically. Imaging is not routinely used. However, when encountered, the placement should be assessed.

Management
Misplaced catheters should be repositioned or removed. In this case, a catheter was unable pass the mass. A suprapubic tube was placed.

CASE 87

Splenic Lacerations

Splenic Laceration With Active Hemorrhage

1. **A, B, C, D.** Although all of the choices could conceivably be included in the differential diagnosis for hypodense splenic lesions, given the history of trauma with imaging findings including perisplenic fluid and irregular, linear hypodensities throughout the parenchyma, splenic laceration is the most correct answer.
2. **A, B, D.** Blunt traumatic injuries of the solid organs, such as the spleen and liver, can result in contained or noncontained vascular injuries within the parenchyma. The contained injuries can be either pseudoaneurysm or arteriovenous fistula formation. On the other hand, a noncontained vascular injury, active extravasation of contrast, can also be seen in blunt organ injuries. Contrast extravasation is characterized by high-density contrast material outside the expected location of a vessel. Generally, this contrast will have irregular, poorly defined margins, whereas pseudoaneurysm will usually have a more rounded appearance. Differentiating these lesions can be determined using the arterial phase imaging and either the portal venous or delayed phase of the study. During active extravasation of contrast, the amount and shape of the extraluminal contrast will change on the delayed study, whereas the pseudoaneurysm and arteriovenous fistula will follow the attenuation pattern of

vessels like the aorta, which will have decreased attenuation on portal venous or delayed phases.
3. **B.** All of the findings listed are used in determining the grade of injury according to the American Association for the Surgery of Trauma (AAST) trauma grading scale, except for active extravasation of contrast.
4. **B.** The AAST scale has been shown to be a poor predictor of success when using nonoperative, conservative management in splenic injuries. The reason for this failure is that the AAST grading scale does not account for vascular injuries, such as active extravasation of contrast and pseudoaneurysm formation. Low-grade injuries can still have these vascular lesions present and, as such, are a predictor of conservative management failure if not adequately treated via angiography and embolization.

Comment

Background
Splenic trauma can occur after blunt or penetrating trauma or iatrogenic intervention. It is the most common solid abdominal organ injured after blunt trauma. Up to 49% of abdominal organ injuries involve the spleen.

Diagnosis
Multidetector CT is vital in the assessment of patients with blunt abdominal trauma because it is highly sensitive and specific for identifying solid organ injuries. On portal venous phase imaging, splenic lacerations are linear, branching, irregular, or geographic hypodensities, often involving the lateral aspect of the spleen. Curvilinear, low-density perisplenic fluid or hemoperitoneum may also be seen. A blush of irregular contrast material outside the expected lumen of a blood vessel is consistent with active extravasation of contrast or active, noncontained bleeding. On the other hand, pseudoaneurysm and arteriovenous fistulas are contained vascular injuries. They may be detected when comparing the imaging findings on the arterial, portal venous, or delayed phases. These vascular injuries occur in about 20% of splenic injuries and should be considered in treatment algorithms.

Management
The AAST developed a grading scale that correlates the injuries visualized during laparotomy with the associated CT findings. Specifically, the imaging findings of splenic injury include subcapsular hematoma, splenic laceration, and splenic hilar vascular injuries. The more complex the injury, the higher the injury grade.

Multiple studies have demonstrated that the grade of active hemorrhage, pseudoaneurysm, and arteriovenous fistula formation is a poor predictor of successful conservative management because the MDCT findings are not included in the scale. Patients with any of these findings of active or contained hemorrhage with low-grade injuries are likely to fail nonoperative management. Reporting these findings is important for appropriate clinical management. In fact, Marmery et al. proposed modifying the grading scale such that these vascular injuries are included and would result in the highest grade of splenic injury noted by MDCT.

Although the grading scale is up for debate, blunt splenic trauma treatment has changed significantly over the past few decades. In hemodynamically stable patients, nonoperative management is the standard of care because it eliminates the morbidity associated with splenectomy while preventing a life-long susceptibility to certain infections. Nonetheless, in cases with active extravasation of contrast, pseudoaneurysm, or arteriovenous fistulae, embolization is generally considered the treatment of choice, while augmenting nonsurgical management.

CASE 88

Renal Laceration

1. **A, B, C, D.** Major renal injuries are often associated with other injured organs. Both renal and liver injuries are present on the current study. Urinoma is included in the differential consideration because the right perinephric fluid may be owing to combination perinephric hemorrhage and urine. Note the dissection flap in the left renal artery.
2. **A.** In cases when significant perirenal fluid is present or renal pedicle injury is suspected, delayed imaging through the abdomen and pelvis can help to assess renal collecting system involvement and urine extravasation.
3. **C.** Grade 4 renal laceration is a parenchymal laceration extending through the renal cortex, medulla, and collecting system with urinoma. Grade 2 and 3 lacerations are less than 1 cm and more than 1 cm in size, respectively, and do not extend into the renal collecting system (no urinoma).
4. **C.** Blunt abdominal trauma is the most common mechanism for renal injury. Penetrating trauma, including iatrogenic (renal biopsy or interventional procedure), is the cause in less than 10% of renal injuries.

Comment

Background
Urinary tract injuries occur in up to 10% of patients with blunt abdominal trauma, with the kidney injured most commonly. Significant renal trauma is often accompanied by injuries to other major organs. In contrast, isolated renal injuries are frequently minor and can be successfully managed conservatively. Penetrating trauma accounts for less than 10% of renal injuries.

The spectrum of renal injuries includes renal contusions, hematomas, lacerations, fractures, shattered kidney, and renal vascular and pedicle injuries.

Diagnosis
Contrast-enhanced CT is the preferred imaging modality in assessing renal injuries in patients who are hemodynamically stable owing to its high diagnostic accuracy. The main clinical finding in suspected cases of renal injury is hematuria. The kidneys are typically evaluated as part of a CT protocol for major trauma. Delayed phase imaging through the abdomen and pelvis, in selected cases, can help to evaluate for a urine leak in cases with significant perinephric or periureteric fluid or suspected renal pedicle injury. Extension into the renal collecting system can be difficult to assess without delayed phase imaging. In a full-thickness collecting system injury, the excreted urinary contrast will have a higher attenuation than the adjacent perinephric hematoma on delayed phase.

Ultrasound and focused assessment sonography for trauma (FAST) may detect free fluid and hemoperitoneum, but renal ultrasound has a low sensitivity in detecting renal injuries.

Management
Imaging findings as detected with CT are important predictors of outcome and determine management. The AAST has developed a grading system for renal injury that can be used to characterize renal injuries on CT. The classification system is based on surgical findings and is the one most widely used in classifying renal injuries. Renal injuries are graded 1 to 5 based on severity and involvement of the collecting system or renal vascular injuries. Minor injuries (grades 1–3) include contusion, small subcapsular hematoma, lacerations that spare the collecting system, or a small nonexpanding perinephric hematoma. Minor injuries can often be managed conservatively. Major injures (grades 4–5) include lacerations extending into the collecting system, injuries to the main renal artery or vein, segmental infarcts, and shattered or devascularized kidneys.

CASE 89

Pancreatic Transection

1. **A, D.** The axial image demonstrates pancreatic transection involving the entire depth of the gland. Although not the most salient finding, pancreatitis can develop in the setting of pancreatic injury and often shows an enlarged, inflamed pancreas with surrounding fluid. The visualized portal vein is patent. The heterogeneity in the left renal vein is mixing artifact from the inferior vena cava (IVC) at the confluence.
2. **B.** Pancreatic injury is rare, and it is even rarer as an isolated injury in the setting of blunt trauma.
3. **C.** The other three choices are more commonly associated with pancreatic injury.
4. **E.** Each choice may be a complication of a missed pancreatic injury.

Comment

Background
Pancreatic injury is rare, occurring in about 1% of patients with blunt abdominal trauma. The pancreas is the tenth most injured organ, whereas the brain, spleen, and liver are the most commonly injured organs. Injuries of the pancreas are usually associated with multiorgan injury, often involving the liver, duodenum, spleen, or stomach. There is a higher incidence associated with penetrating trauma, including gunshot wounds and stab wounds. Pancreatic injuries in adults are associated with MVCs, whereas in children, pancreatic injuries are associated with bicycle handlebar injury and child abuse.

Diagnosis
Symptoms are nonspecific and unreliable. There may be associated leukocytosis and elevated amylase levels. The majority of injuries occur at the pancreatic neck. Pancreatic head injuries are more likely to be lethal owing to associated vascular injury to the portal vein, IVC, or superior vena cava (SVC). Injuries that spare the pancreatic duct rarely result in morbidity. The main source of delayed morbidity is disruption of the pancreatic duct. Delay in diagnosis may result in pancreatitis, pseudocyst, abscess, and fistula. Treatment of pancreatic duct disruption includes stent placement or surgery.

Computed tomography sensitivity for detecting pancreatic injury is modest at 65% to 75%. CT findings include pancreatic edema or enlargement, peripancreatic fluid, fluid around the superior mesentaric vein (SMV), and fluid in the lesser sac. Contusions are low attenuation areas, whereas lacerations are linear. The depth of laceration is a useful indicator of main duct involvement. Involvement of greater than half the depth of the gland is more likely associated with duct transection. A CT grading system has been suggested by Moore: Grade A, pancreatitis or superficial laceration; Grade B1, deep laceration, more than half the depth of the tail; Grade B2, transection of the pancreatic tail; Grade C1, deep laceration of the head; and Grade C2, transection of the head.

One pitfall is misinterpretation of peripancreatic fluid without direct evidence of parenchymal injury. A repeat CT in 1 to 2 days will show resolution of retroperitoneal fluid in the setting of aggressive hydration, whereas true pancreatic injuries will demonstrate increasing fluid collections.

Management
Surgical Repair
Imaging findings as detected with CT are important predictors of outcome and determine management. The AAST has developed a grading system for renal injury that can be used to characterize pancreatic injuries on CT. The classification system is based on

surgical findings and is the most widely used in classifying traumatic pancreatic injuries. Injuries are graded 1 to 5 based on severity and involvement of the duct. Minor injuries (grades 1–3) include contusion, small subcapsular hematoma, and lacerations that spare the duct. Minor injuries can often be managed conservatively. Major injures (grades 4–5) include lacerations extending into the duct and full-thickness transections.

Endoscopic retrograde cholangiopancreatography (ERCP) is increasingly being used to diagnose the presence of pancreatic ductal injury and communication with a fluid collection. ERCP enables endoscopic intervention via stenting. MRCP is noninvasive and may assess parenchymal injury.

CASE 90

Adrenal Hemorrhage

1. **A, C.** The images demonstrate bilateral suprarenal heterogeneous lesions with evidence of active hemorrhage in the right adrenal hematoma. In addition, thrombus in noted in the portal vein.
2. **C.** Although all choices are associated with adrenal hemorrhage, it occurs most often in adults as a complication of anticoagulation therapy.
3. **D.** All choices are associated with spontaneous adrenal hemorrhage.
4. **D.** The majority of adrenal hemorrhages can be managed conservatively.

Comment

Background
Adrenal hemorrhage is a relatively uncommon condition, but potentially a catastrophic event seen in patients of all ages. Adrenal hemorrhage is more common in neonates than children and adults. Spontaneous or nontraumatic hemorrhage (often bilateral) can occur in stress (surgery, sepsis, burns, steroids), hemorrhagic diathesis or coagulopathy, and adrenal tumors. Anticoagulation therapy is the most common cause of spontaneous adrenal hemorrhage in the adult population. Spontaneous rupture of adrenal tumors can occur in pheochromocytoma, myelolipoma, adrenocortical carcinoma, and metastases. Waterhouse-Friderichsen syndrome represents hemorrhagic necrosis of several organs, including adrenal hemorrhage, in the setting of overwhelming sepsis. Spontaneous adrenal hemorrhage during pregnancy has rarely been described. Blunt trauma can also cause adrenal hemorrhage, which is mostly unilateral (often involves the right adrenal).

Diagnosis
On ultrasound, the acute hematoma can be seen as a hyperechoic mass-like lesion, and Doppler study reveals the avascular nature of the mass. CT plays a crucial role in evaluation of adrenal hemorrhage. CT has an additional advantage of illustrating associated adrenal or renal vein thrombosis (portal vein thrombosis was shown in our case). Acute or subacute adrenal hemorrhage can be seen as a round or oval mass of high attenuation (50–90 HU). Fluid-fluid level in the context of hematoma known as "hematocrit effect" can be visible. Thickening of the adjacent diaphragmatic crura can be seen. On MR examination, T1 and T2-weighted image show varied signal based on the age of hematoma.

Management
Patients with spontaneous adrenal hemorrhage are at risk of developing acute adrenal insufficiency. Medical therapies are used to replace adrenal function, to provide vital function support as needed, to treat the underlying conditions, and to correct fluid and electrolyte deficits. Surgery is not usually required in cases of spontaneous hemorrhage, except in patients with primary adrenal tumors or extensive retroperitoneal hemorrhage.

CASE 91

Bladder Perforation

1. **B.** The coronal image demonstrates interruption of the bladder dome with leakage of contrast, making the other diagnoses unlikely.
2. **A.** MVAs account for 90% of cases of bladder rupture.
3. **C.** On average, 80% of cases of bladder rupture are seen in patients with a pelvic fracture; 6% of patients with pelvic fractures have concurrent bladder injury.
4. **C.** Although extraperitoneal bladder rupture is highly associated with pelvic fractures, it can be seen in patients without pelvic fractures or on the side of the bladder contralateral to the pelvic fractures, leading to the belief that a shearing mechanism is the cause of bladder perforation.

Comment

Background
Urinary bladder injuries are classically divided into intraperitoneal and extraperitoneal injuries. Intraperitoneal injury, accounting for approximately 30% of rupture cases, is most commonly caused by a blow to the anterior pelvic or abdominal wall that causes a rapid pressure rise in the bladder and rupture at its weakest point, at the dome. Extraperitoneal bladder rupture, accounting for approximately 60% of rupture cases, is highly associated with pelvic fractures. Mechanism of injury is believed to be a shear injury from pelvic ring distortion, but can also be caused by a perforation from pelvic bone fracture fragments. Combined injuries occur in approximately 10% of patients.

Diagnosis
Bladder injury is seen in 29% of the patients presenting with combined gross hematuria and pelvic fracture; therefore, in these patients, a cystogram should be performed to rule out bladder injury. Diagnosis can be made using a conventional cystogram, but CT cystogram has replaced conventional cystography at most trauma centers because it can be performed as a part of the trauma CT protocol. After urethral continuity is confirmed (based on clinical examination and/or a retrograde urethrography), the bladder is catheterized. The bladder is distended with 300 to 350 mL of diluted iodinated contrast administered by gravity drip. Clamping the Foley catheter following contrast-enhanced CT and waiting for the bladder to fill with excreted contrast and urine will not allow for adequate bladder distention; retrograde filling is required.

The classic CT appearance of extraperitoneal bladder rupture is flame-shaped contrast extravasation around the base of the bladder, particularly in the perivesicular and prevesicular space (of Retzius). The bladder may be compressed into a "teardrop" or "pear" shaped configuration on coronal reformatted images owing to a combination of compression by pelvic hematoma and extravasated urine. In more severe cases, urine and contrast may dissect upward into the retroperitoneum or downward into the thighs and scrotum. For intraperitoneal bladder rupture, contrast extravasates into the peritoneum to surround loops of bowel, fill the rectouterine or rectovesical pouch, and layer in the paracolic gutters. The actual tear in the bladder dome may be visualized on axial images but can more easily be visualized on sagittal or coronal reformatted images.

Management
Surgical repair.

CASE 92

Retroperitoneal Hemorrhage

1. **A, B, C.** The CT images demonstrate fat stranding and fluid anterior to the IVC that tracks anterior to the right psoas representing retroperitoneal hemorrhage. Notice the midline bowel/mesenteric hematoma on the second axial image.
2. **A.** Zone I is the central zone associated with pancreaticoduodenal and major vessel (aorta/IVC) injury.
3. **A.** Infrarenal segment of the IVC is the most common segment injured by blunt trauma (39%). Retrohepatic is the second most common (19%). The infrarenal IVC is the segment affected most frequently with penetrating trauma.
4. **C.** Zone III encompasses the pelvic retroperitoneum and is the most common location of retroperitoneal hemorrhage usually associated with pelvic fractures.

Comment

Background
IVC injury in blunt trauma is rare and associated with high mortality. More than a third of patients with caval injuries die before they reach the hospital. Most IVC injuries (85% to 90%) are caused by penetrating trauma (gunshot and stab injuries). Only 3% to 10% of injuries are secondary to blunt trauma. Patterns of IVC injury include contusions, lacerations, and complete transections. Avulsion type injuries and lacerations greater than 5 cm are associated with the highest mortality rate.

Traumatic retroperitoneal hemorrhage can be the source of significant but clinically occult blood loss in the trauma patient. It can arise from major vascular structures, hollow viscera, solid organs, and/or musculoskeletal structures.

Diagnosis
The goals of imaging are to evaluate the retroperitoneal hemorrhage size/location and whether there is active extravasation. Whereas IV contrast is not necessary to identify the presence of retroperitoneal hemorrhage, it is useful in the traumatic setting and can assess active bleeding.

Management
From the surgical standpoint, the retroperitoneum is divided into three zones and the location of hematoma has therapeutic implications.

 Zone I: The central midline retroperitoneum extends from the aortic hiatus to the sacral promontory. It contains the abdominal aorta, the IVC, the root of the mesentery, and portions of the pancreas and duodenum. This zone caries the highest risk for vascular injury. Unless the hemorrhage is small and stable, Zone 1 hemorrhages are usually investigated by through a surgical approach.

 Zone II: The flank or lateral retroperitoneum includes the perirenal spaces. It contains the kidneys, adrenal glands, renal vasculature, and ascending and descending colon. This is the second most common site of retroperitoneal hemorrhage. Renal injuries account for the majority of the hemorrhages in this region. Most of these hemorrhages are managed conservatively by observation if the patient is hemodynamically stable with no evidence of active vascular extravasation.

 Zone III: The pelvic retroperitoneum is the most common site of retroperitoneal hemorrhage and is frequently associated with pelvic fractures. Surgical intervention is avoided in most cases of blunt pelvic trauma with external fixation and angiographic embolization being the preferred methods for addressing active bleeding.

CASE 93

Perched Facets

1. **A.** On both the cervical and thoracolumbar spine images, the salient finding is the perched facet, which is a hyperflexion-type injury. There is a compression deformity on the thoracolumbar spine CT images, but it is not a simple compression fracture because the facets are perched, which is consistent with a higher-grade spinal injury. A burst fracture of the vertebral body requires disruption of the posterior vertebral cortex with retropulsion into the spinal canal. These images do not demonstrate this fracture pattern.
2. **D.** Axial CT images will demonstrate the "naked facet sign," which shows an uncovered facet because the superior and inferior facets are dislocated and not anatomically aligned.
3. **B.** Posterior element integrity is not a component of the subaxial injury classification and severity score.
4. **B.** Bilateral interfacetal dislocation has, by definition, 50% or greater anterior translation of the vertebral body, whereas unilateral interfacetal dislocation has less than 50% anterior translation of the superior vertebral body.

Comment

Background
Approximately 150,000 people per year have a traumatic injury to the spinal column; 11,000 have concurrent cord injuries. Cervical spine injuries are common (55%). Missing a spine injury in polytrauma patients can have devastating consequences.

Traumatic spinal injuries can be classified by the mechanism of injury, including hyperflexion and hyperextension type injuries, rotational, axial loading, and lateral flexion, but they can often be diagnosed concurrently. Cervical spine fractures can be classified further by injuries of the craniocervical junction, the occipital condyles, C1, and C2. However, approximately 65% of cervical spine fractures and 75% of all cervical dislocations involve the subaxial cervical spine, C3-C7. A scoring system, called the Sub-Axial Injury Classification (SLIC) and Severity Scale, has been created to describe the structural integrity of the vertebral column using CT findings. The three components in the SLIC score are (1) morphologic findings of the spinal column injury; (2) integrity of the DLC; and (3) neurologic status. A higher score signifies a more severe injury, with a summed score of 10 being the maximum; a score of 5 or more indicates the need for surgery. A separate but similarly organized severity scale for the thoracolumbar spine is called the Thoraco-lumbar Injury Classification and Severity Score (TLICS).

Diagnosis
Cervical spine CT has become a mainstay in the evaluation of trauma patients, especially given the risk of undiagnosed injuries using conventional radiography. Cervical spine multidetector CT can be easily incorporated in routine traumatic CT protocols. Studies have found that CT has a sensitivity rate of almost 99% in identifying cervical spine fractures. In fact, the American College of Radiology recommends cervical spine CT as the standard of care for high-risk, polytrauma patients, especially those who are obtunded.

The current case images demonstrate a hyperflexion-type injury, known as perched facets. Facet subluxation is defined as when the articular surfaces between the superior and inferior facets have less than 50% overlap or more than 2 mm of diastasis. Posterior disk space widening is also often present with focal kyphosis. A more severe injury involves translation or a rotational injury from either unilateral or bilateral facet dislocations, which is also commonly known as locked facets. With unilateral locked facets, there is less than 50% anterior translation of the superior vertebral body; conversely, bilateral locked facets result in greater than 50% anterior translation of the superior vertebral body in relation to the inferior vertebral body. A common radiologic sign is the "naked facet" sign, in which an uncovered facet is noted on the axial CT images, which can be present in either perched or locked facets.

Management

Generally, these fracture patterns are highly suggestive of spinal instability. Recognizing the findings that suggest underlying ligamentous injury is essential for radiologists because it helps guide surgical management.

CASE 94

Pheochromocytoma

1. **A, B, C.** Although the history suggests pheochromocytoma, malignancy should be considered. The visualized kidney is normal.
2. **B.** Of cases, 10% are not associated with hypertension.
3. **C.** The majority of cases are sporadic.
4. **A.** Radiography is not helpful in diagnosis.

Comment

Background

Pheochromocytoma is a catecholamine-secreting tumor of the adrenal gland. The estimated prevalence in hypertensive adults ranges from 0.1 to 0.6%. The majority of cases are sporadic. In 5% to 10% of cases associations with multiple endocrine neoplasia (MEN II), von Hippel-Lindau, von Recklinghausen, Sturge-Weber, Carney triad, tuberous sclerosis, and familial clustering. Remember the 10% rule: Infrequently these tumors are extra-adrenal, bilateral, malignant, found in children, familial, not associated with hypertension, and contain calcification. Patients commonly present with uncontrolled secondary hypertension, but may also present with cardiac infarction, hemorrhagic stroke, pulmonary edema, headache, or visual changes.

Diagnosis

Tumors are usually more than 3 cm at time of imaging. Overall, 98% of tumors will be located in the abdomen and 90% will be located in the adrenal glands. When metastatic, lung, liver, and bone are common sites. CT is a first-line tool. Masses are usually heterogeneous and may contain areas of necrosis and cystic change. They typically enhance avidly. MR is highly sensitive. T1 hypointense/T2 hyperintense/in-out-of phase no signal loss/T1 C+ enhances. Octreotide scans can detect pheochromocytomas as can iodine-123 meta-iodobenzylguanidine (MIBG).

Management

Definitive treatment is surgical resection. Preoperative medical management is essential in reducing the risk of hypertensive crisis.

CASE 95

Gastrointestinal Track (Small Intestine) Lipomatosis

1. **B.** Multiple fat-attenuating foci within the lumen of several segments of the small bowel are noted, which is most consistent with intestinal lipomatosis.
2. **D.** These fatty lesions can pedunculate and act as lead points for intussusception. When large, they may ulcerate and slowly bleed. The completely fatty composition is not characteristic of adenocarcinoma.
3. **D.** Colon is the most common location and more often right sided. Esophageal lesions are rare.

4. **C.** Of these tumors, 95% are submucosal. Rarely subserosal, sessile, and pedunculated lesions are present. This lesion is not common and found frequently among patients 50 to 70 years. Of age Most are incidentally identified, uncomplicated, and warrant no intervention.

Comment

Background

Gastrointestinal track (GIT) lipomas are rarely encountered in autopsy series (<5%). They can occur anywhere along the tract but are most commonly encountered in the colon (right colon most commonly). GIT lipomas rarely occur in the esophagus. This entity is frequently encountered in individuals between 50 and 70 years of age. The majority are asymptomatic and incidentally noted. Submucosal location comprises the vast majority (95%) of locations. Lesion will rarely be sessile, pedunculated, or subserosal. Pedunculated lesions can act as lead points for intussusception. Large lesions may ulcerate and slowly bleed. Patients may present, in this context, with anemia. Brisk acute bleeding is uncommon.

Diagnosis

Well-circumscribed, fatty lesions (−80 to −120 HU) on CT. If solid components are present, consider including liposarcoma. Ulceration may result in stranding near the mucosal surface.

Management

No intervention if asymptomatic. Excise if symptomatic.

CASE 96

Pelvic Inflammatory Disease

1. **B.** Pelvic inflammatory disease (PID) is most commonly mistaken for ectopic pregnancy because the diagnosis of PID is primarily based on clinical and historical findings.
2. **D.** Pregnant women suspected to have PID are at high risk for maternal morbidity and preterm delivery. They should be hospitalized and treated with intravenous therapy. Parental antibiotics should be used for at least 24 to 48 hours after clinical improvement is observed. Transition can then be made to a 14-day course of oral antibiotics
3. **B.** There exists a high chance for potential *Neisseria gonorrhoeae* fluoroquinolone resistance, and quinolone monotherapy for PID is no longer routinely recommended.
4. **C.** Fitz-Hugh-Curtis syndrome is a potential complication of PID that presents as right upper quadrant pain secondary to inflammation and adhesion formation in the liver capsule. The pain can mimic cholecystitis or pyelonephritis.

Comment

Background

Pelvic inflammatory disease is a polymicrobial infection-induced inflammation of the female's upper reproductive tract. Microorganisms ascend from the cervix or vagina to the endometrium to cause endometriosis. This can then spread to the fallopian tubes and other surrounding structures. The most common sexually transmitted microorganisms include *Neisseria gonorrhoeae* and *Chlamydia trachomatis*. Other organisms include *Mycoplasma genitalium*, endogenous vaginal microflora, gram-negative organisms, and respiratory pathogens. PID predominantly affects sexually active women between 15 and 29 years of age. Untreated, PID can lead to infertility, ectopic pregnancy, and chronic pelvic pain. Risk factors for PID include sexually transmitted infection (STI), new or multiple sexual partners, prior STIs or PID.

Diagnosis

Pelvic inflammatory disease may be difficult to diagnose clinically owing to the fact that the signs and symptoms are increasingly non-specific and mild. Because of these mild symptoms, women often might not seek medical attention. On the other hand, PID may present atypically with presentations dyspareunia, vaginal bleeding, and dysuria in the setting of pelvic pain. It is important to consider PID as a differential diagnosis in young sexually active women presenting with lower abdominal or pelvic pain. Diagnosis can be made with clinical parameters, history, physical examination, and laboratory results. The role of imaging is limited in this context. Ultrasound or CT may help identify complications of PID.

Management

Treatment of PID must be empiric and provide broad coverage against *N. gonorrhoeae* and *C. trachomatis*. Patients with PID requiring hospitalization need parental antibiotics, whereas outpatient treatment includes a combination of oral and intramuscular regimens.

CASE 97

Frontal Lobe Trauma

1. **D.** The bifrontal encephalomalacia pattern in an otherwise healthy patient should raise the possibility of prior traumatic brain injury. Parafalcine calcifications are noted; however, no hemorrhage is noted. The parenchymal changes are not characteristic of acute injury (volume loss—no swelling). The frontal bone is intact, but the inner table demonstrates hyperostosis.
2. **A.**
3. **C.**
4. **D.**

Comment

Background

Cerebral contusion is a form of traumatic brain injury. Contusion primarily affects the cortical tissue. The tissues under the areas of bony protuberances are more commonly injured in closed head trauma. The protuberances are located in the frontal and temporal lobes and the rooves of the orbits. Attention, emotional, and memory problems are associated with damage to the frontal and temporal lobes. In the acute setting, edema and hemorrhage with herniation are noted. Remote contusions are associated with areas of encephalomalacia.

Diagnosis

Characteristic pattern of focal parenchymal volume loss are shown on CT/MR. An injury in classic locations or patterns should raise the question of traumatic brain injury.

Management

In the acute setting avoidance of edema can be medically and surgically managed. The long-term sequel of this injury includes the changes in cognition as noted above.

CASE 98

Uvulitis and Tonsillitis With Abscess

1. **D.** Extensive soft-tissue swelling in the pharyngeal space. Close inspection shows diffuse edema and enlargement of the uvula. The bilateral tonsils are enlarged and obstruct the airway. A small right peritonsillar abscess is noted. No foreign body is noted.

2. **A, B.** Uvulitis can be caused by a number factors including bacteria, viruses, fungus, allergic reactions, and acid reflux. Tonsillitis is commonly caused by viruses and bacteria.
3. **A.** The diagnosis can be made on clinical examination. CT may be helpful for evaluating complications.
4. **A.** Unknown airway compromise should be immediately relayed to the clinical team. The abscess is small and not likely easily drained. No retropharyngeal extension is noted. The epiglottis is normal.

Comment

Background

Patients can present with uvulitis, an inflamed uvula, for many reasons, such as infection (viral, bacterial, fungal), allergies, direct irritants (alcohol, smoking, acid reflux), and genetics. They may present with difficulty breathing, sore throat, swollen tonsils, excessive secretions, gagging, fever, or pain with swallowing.

See also the discussion on tonsillitis for additional details.

Diagnosis

The uvula can easily be visualized on physical examination. CT may help to evaluate complications, such as degree of extension, abscess formation, or airway obstruction.

Management

Conservative supportive therapy, medical management, or surgical intervention, depending on the severity and complexity.

CASE 99

Pelvic Disruption

Pelvic Fracture: Disruption of the Pelvic Ring

1. **A, B, C.** Pubic symphysis diastasis can be seen with trauma, pregnancy, and bladder extrophy. Hypothyroidism, not hyperthyroidism, is also a known cause of widening at the symphysis pubis.
2. **D.** Pelvic hemorrhage is the main concern in patients with pelvic ring disruption. Application of a pelvic binder is the next step in managing this patient to decrease the risk of hemorrhage and to tamponade, the source of potential bleeding. Further evaluation with CT and angiography may be performed to identify (and treat) potential sources of bleeding.
3. **C.** The most commonly applied classification system of pelvic ring disruption is the Young-Burgess classification, which classifies pelvic ring disruption into four types based on the direction of the applied forces. The main radiographic abnormality in this case is widening at the symphysis pubis and of the sacroiliac joints bilaterally, resulting in an "open book" appearance, secondary to an anteroposterior compression injury.
4. **A,B.** Urinary tract injuries can occur in patients with pelvic ring disruption. Gross hematuria is the most obvious clinical sign of potential injury to the urinary tract. In the initial setting, evaluation for suspected urinary tract injury should include CT with contrast, including delayed images during the excretory phase and CT cystogram.

Comment

Background

Blunt trauma to the pelvis can produce complex injuries and fractures resulting in severe, life-threatening hemorrhage. The most common mechanisms of pelvic ring disruption are MVCs, followed by falls from height and crush injuries to the pelvis.

The strength and stability of the pelvis is dependent on strong ligaments that connect the sacrum to the other pelvic bones. Disruption of one part of the pelvic ring should raise suspicion for disruption at a second location; disruption at two or more sites is a marker of a potential biomechanically unstable injury.

Mortality from pelvic ring disruption can reach up to 50% in hemodynamically unstable patients, predominantly owing to the risk of life-threatening hemorrhage secondary to direct injury to the pelvic vasculature. Hemorrhage may occur from the venous plexus of the pelvis, branches of the iliac arteries, or fracture fragments.

There are several classification systems of pelvic ring disruption. Young-Burgess classification system is widely used. It classifies pelvic injuries according to the mechanism of injury and the major direction of the involved force—lateral compression, anteroposterior compression (APC), vertical shear (VS), or combined/complex mechanism. Each category can further be subclassified into types 1 to 3 (less to more severe) based on the degree of ligamentous injury, bony injury, or overall displacement of the hemipelvis.

Determining and classifying the fracture pattern may help identify those patients at increased risk of hemorrhage and guide subsequent intervention. Higher grade injuries, especially APC and VS injuries, can be more commonly associated with hemodynamic instability, and they need further intervention.

Diagnosis

As part of the initial evaluation in the trauma bay, pelvic disruption may be detected on radiography. Follow-up CT evaluation is warranted. IV contrast, delayed images, and cystogram will aid in comprehensive evaluation.

Management

An injury to the pelvis is an indicator of high-energy trauma, and patients with fractures of the pelvis will frequently have associated injuries. Vascular injury and bleeding can occur, which are more commonly associated with higher grade pelvic injuries. Venous injury occurs most commonly, and patients frequently require blood transfusion. In hemodynamically unstable patients, angiographic embolization or surgical pelvic packing may be required for definitive management.

Injury to the urinary tract is more commonly associated with pelvic fractures that include fractures of the pubic rami and pubic symphysis diastasis. Gross hematuria is the most evident clinical sign of injury to the urinary tract. Further investigation with CT during the excretory phase and cystogram should be performed as clinically indicated. Bony pelvic injuries can result in direct trauma to the rectum, anus, vagina, and perineum. Neurologic deficit from pelvic ring disruption is more frequently associated with higher grade and more unstable pelvic injuries, and with central (zone 3) sacral fractures.

CASE 100

Anomalous Coronary Artery

Anomalous Origin of the Left Coronary Artery With Intramural Segment

1. **C.** The left coronary artery arises from a separate ostia adjacent to the right coronary artery. It courses between the aorta and pulmonary artery with short intramural segment.
2. **C.** The origin of a coronary artery from the contralateral coronary sinus with passage between the aorta and pulmonary artery is called an interarterial course that can lead to myocardial ischemia and sudden death. Other courses—

retroaortic, prepulmonary, subpulmonary, and septal—are considered less often to be symptomatic or cause for sudden cardiac death.

3. **A.** Although coronary artery anomalies are rare, anomalous course of the right coronary artery is the most frequent.
4. **C, D.** Bypass grafting or reimplantation is the preferred treatment. Unroofing may be a part of the procedure if the artery takes an intramuscular course.

Comment

Background

Congenital coronary artery anomalies are uncommon, with a reported incidence of 0.3% to 1.6%. Among the subtypes, anomalous origin of the left coronary artery (LCA) from the right sinus of Valsalva is less common. The anomalous LCA can take different routes, including septal (through the crista supraventricularis portion of the septum), retroaortic, anterior (coursing in front of the right ventricular outflow tract), and interarterial (between the aorta and right ventricular outflow tract).

The interarterial course has the poorest prognosis; it is associated with a higher risk of sudden cardiac death, which can occur in up to 50% of affected individuals. Mortality is often seen during exercise, possibly owing to impaired flow or compression impeding the ability to meet the increased myocardial demand. Approximately 13% of sudden cardiac deaths in young athletes are secondary to coronary anomalies.

Diagnosis

Careful attention should be paid to the origin of coronary vessels on chest CT imaging in young patients presenting with collapse to identify anomalous origins or course. CT coronary angiography excels at providing visualization of the coronary vessels with respect to the coronary cusps, main pulmonary artery, and aorta.

Management

Surgery is frequently performed for asymptomatic patients with anomalous left coronary artery. Unroofing of the vessel, if it takes a myocardial course, is insufficient but may be performed with reimplantation or reconstruction of the more proximal artery.

CASE 101

Calcaneal Fracture

1. **C.** On lateral radiographs, a calcaneal spur is seen as an inferomedial bony projection, whereas a Haglund deformity is a prominence of the superior aspect of the posterior calcaneus. Os calcaneus secundarius is an accessory ossicle of the anterior calcaneal process.
2. **B.** Most of the calcaneal spurs are identified in asymptomatic patients, but an association between plantar fasciitis and calcaneal spurs has been described. On radiography Achilles tendinopathy may demonstrate spurring at the Achilles tendon insertion site or intratendinous calcifications. Tarsal tunnel syndrome and Sever disease are usually radiographically occult.
3. **D.** The calcaneal inclination angle is drawn between the calcaneal inclination axis and the supporting surface, whereas the lateral talocalcaneal angle is formed by the calcaneal inclination axis and the mid-talar axis. The Gissane angle is the angular measurement formed by the downward and upward slopes of the calcaneal superior surface.
4. **B.** All of the mentioned options could occur in the setting of a fall from a height, but around 10% of patients with calcaneal fractures have an associated lumbar spine injury.

Comment

Background

The calcaneus is the most commonly fractured tarsal bone, with up to 75% of calcaneal fractures defined as intraarticular. Calcaneal fractures usually occur in the setting of a high axial load to the hindfoot, such as a fall from height or a high-impact situation, such as an MVC. A smaller percentage of these fractures occur as a result of a twisting injury or an avulsion fracture.

Diagnosis

Patients usually complain of heel pain with swelling and ecchymosis evident on physical examination. When a calcaneal fracture is suspected, initial radiographic evaluation includes the foot and ankle. Typically, the lateral view of the hindfoot allows the visualization of a calcaneal fracture. This view also allows angular measurements, such as the tuber angle of Bohler and the crucial angle of Gissane. Bohler's angle usually varies between 20 and 40 degrees, whereas the angle of Gissane is an obtuse angle of 120 to 145 degrees. A decreased angle of Bohler indicates a calcaneal fracture, and both angles are commonly used to evaluate the severity of the fracture. In the event of a normal plain radiograph and a high clinical suspicion, a CT scan should be obtained. An MRI should also be considered if the foot is unstable. Although most calcaneal fractures occur in isolation, associated injuries, including lumbar spine fractures and other lower extremity fractures, have been reported. Recent studies have suggested the occurrence of a lumbar spine fracture in up to 10% of patients with calcaneal fractures. Physicians should thus have a high suspicion for such concomitant injuries, especially in the setting of high-energy trauma or bilateral calcaneal fractures.

Management

Treatment of calcaneal fractures generally depends on the type of fracture and the presence or absence of displacement. High-energy fractures could also lead to severe soft-tissue disruption with complications such as acute compartment syndrome and skin blisters.

CASE 102

Retained Products of Conception (RPOC)

1. **B, C.** Heterogeneously echogenic, vascular, and thickened endometrium is noted. Blood clots would not demonstrate vascularity. Ectopic pregnancy evaluation should include interrogation of the adnexal region and ovaries. Beta human chorionic gonadotropin (BHCG) values to confirm pregnancy are also helpful.
2. **B.** Combined gray-scale/Doppler US is the first-line imaging modality for suspected RPOC.
3. **D.** The reported incidence of RPOC seems to depend on the gestational age of the pregnancy, with RPOC occurring most frequently after a second trimester delivery or termination of pregnancy.
4. **A.** The most sensitive finding of RPOC with gray-scale US is a thickened endometrial echo complex. The exact definition of "thickened" varies in the literature, ranging from 8 to 13 mm.

Comment

Background

The term RPOC refers to intrauterine tissue—including placental and/or fetal tissue—remaining in the uterus following delivery, pregnancy termination, or miscarriage. One of the most common causes of primary and secondary postpartum hemorrhage is RPOC. The reported incidence of RPOC depends on the

gestational age of the pregnancy, occurring most frequently after second trimester delivery or termination of pregnancy.

Diagnosis

Risk factors for RPOC include failure to progress during delivery, placenta accreta, and instrument delivery. Patients often present with bleeding in addition to lower abdominal pain and fever. The first-line imaging study for RPOC is gray scale and color Doppler ultrasound, which will demonstrate a thickened endometrial echo complex. Microscopic diagnosis notes the presence of chorionic villi, which indicates the presence of placental tissue.

Management

Early diagnosis is key to guiding patient management and limiting further complications. Treatment options include expectant management, prostaglandin E1 analogs, dilation and curettage, or hysteroscopic removal.

CASE 103

Le Fort Type III Fracture

1. **D.** Le Fort type III fracture. To simplify the Le Fort classification, think of type I as floating palate, type II as floating maxilla, and type III as floating face.
2. **B.** Approximately half of midfacial fractures are isolated to the nasal bones. The zygoma are the second most commonly fractured bones of the midface.
3. **C.** There is considerable variability in the presentation of tripod fractures. These fractures most commonly result from a combination of sutural separation and fractures, but can occur with separation at suture lines or fracture of the adjacent bones alone. The four major articulations of the zygoma are formed with the maxilla, greater wing of the sphenoid, temporal, and frontal bones.
4. **A.** Although B, C, and D are all weak areas of the mandible susceptible to fracture, A is the most common.

Comment

Background

Le Fort fractures are facial fractures that occur in a recognizable pattern divided between types I, II, and III. Accurate diagnosis can often be difficult, but recognizing fracture patterns can aid in identification and communicating complex fractures.

Le Fort I (Guerin fracture) is transverse and transects the inferior part of the maxilla above the dentition line, the nasal septum, and the inferior portions of the pterygoid plates. This results in a mobile/floating palate. Le Fort II produces a pyramid-shaped fracture involving the nasal bones, medial portions of the orbits to the lateral walls of the maxillae. Le Fort III results in craniofacial separation from the nasal frontal suture, the orbital walls, zygomatic arches, to the pterygoid bases.

Diagnosis

Computed tomography is the imaging modality of choice with reconstruction in orthogonal planes or three-dimensional reconstruction.

Management

As with any trauma, stabilizing and maintaining an airway is the first priority in these patients. Clinicians should follow advanced cardiovascular life support (ACLS) procedures. Once stabilized, specialists will need to be consulted for further care. This may include an ophthalmologist for orbit injuries; a maxillofacial surgeon; an ear, nose, and throat specialist; and/or a plastic surgeon.

CASE 104

Hyperdense MCA (Thrombus)

1. **B.** Asymmetric and focal hyperattenuation in the middle cerebral artery (MCA) is noted. Elevated hematocrit and contrast administration would result in symmetric hyperattenuation of the MCA. No calcified plaques are noted.
2. **C.** The hyperdense MCA sign is seen prior to any brain parenchymal changes that progress with increasing ischemic time.
3. **D.** According to the updated 2015 American Heart Association/American Stroke Association guidelines, endovascular clot retrieval should be attempted for a proximal MCA thrombus as long as other criteria (delineated in the guidelines) are met.
4. **A.** A dot sign is a hyperdense MCA sign of a more distal MCA branch, which appears as a hyperdense dot in the sylvian fissure.

Comment

Background

Whereas flowing blood has attenuation of 40 HU, a clot has attenuation of approximately 80 HU. The hyperdense vessel should have higher attenuation than the contralateral side. This may require scrolling superiorly or inferiorly to find the comparable vessel. Hyperdense vessels have been reported for all of the major intracranial vessels including the MCA, anterior cerebral artery (ACA), posterior cerebral artery (PCA), and basilar artery. The dot sign is owing to a clot within an M2 branch travelling in the sylvian fissure as it courses over the insula. Detection of a dense MCA is important as it portends a poorer prognosis with IV TPA treatment alone. According to a recent meta-analysis a hyperdense MCA sign has a sensitivity of 52% and specificity of 95%.

Diagnosis

Initial stroke imaging is most commonly with noncontrast CT where a hyperdense MCA may be seen prior to parenchymal changes. It is more easily seen when the contralateral MCA is on the same image so that the MCA vessels can be compared. Diagnosis is sometimes compromised by atherosclerotic disease. The presence of a clot can be confirmed using CTA or MRA.

Management

According to the updated 2015 American Heart Association/American Stroke Association guidelines, when there is a proximal MCA clot (initially detected with a hyperdense MCA sign), endovascular clot retrieval should be attempted. The patient should receive IV TPA if the patient is within the eligibility time window (generally 4.5 hours). Clinical criteria include having a modified Rankin score of 0 to 1 and having a National Institutes of Health stroke score of 6 or greater. The guidelines strongly recommend vascular imaging, such as CTA or magnetic resonance angiography (MRA), be performed prior to intervention, but it considers advanced imaging, such as collateral vessel imaging, diffusion imaging, and perfusion imaging, as techniques that need more investigation on whether they are beneficial for patient selection for intervention.

CASE 105

Urethral Injury

1. **A, C, D, E.** The CT images demonstrate a malpositioned Foley bulb in the posterior urethra resulting in injury to the prostatic position of the urethra. The extraperitoneal urinary contrast extravasation into the prevesical space is from the associated bladder neck injury at its junction with the posterior urethra (extraperitoneal). The sagittal image clearly depicts the discontinuity between the bladder neck and posterior urethra with the prostatic urethra (Foley bulb) positioned more anteriorly relative to the bladder neck.
2. **C.** Retrograde urethrography (RUG) image demonstrates complete disruption of the prostatic portion of the posterior urethra with contrast extravasation above the urogenital diaphragm.
3. **C.** Posterior urethral injuries are more common than anterior urethral injuries due to the relative mobility of the anterior urethra.
4. **D.** RUG findings demonstrate disruption of the posterior urethra (prostatic urethra) at its junction with bladder neck, with contrast extravasation above the urogenital diaphragm. Associated bladder neck injury contributes to the extraperitoneal extravasation of contrast into the prevesical space visualized on the sagittal CT image. This represents type IV injury according to Goldman classification.

Comment

Background

Urethral injuries are commonly associated with blunt or penetrating pelvic trauma. Iatrogenic injuries to the urethra are not uncommon and occur when difficult urethral catheterization leads to mucosal injury with subsequent scarring and stricture formation. Transurethral procedures, such as prostate and tumor resections and ureteroscopy, can also lead to urethral injury.

Posterior urethral injuries (membranous and prostatic portions) are more common than anterior urethral injuries (penile and bulbar portions) and are most commonly associated with pelvic fractures. Most common mechanisms are road traffic accidents and a fall from a height. About 20% of these patients have an associated bladder injury.

Anterior urethral injuries are less common than posterior urethral injuries owing to relative mobility of the anterior urethra. Straddling injury, which results in compression of the urethra against the pubis, is the most common mechanism.

Female urethral injuries are rarer than those to the male urethra because of shorter length, internal location, increased elasticity, and less rigid attachment of the urethra to the adjacent pubic bones.

Diagnosis

Blood at the meatus or a high-riding prostate gland found on rectal examination is the usual physical finding. RUG is the imaging study of choice to evaluate urethral injury and should be performed prior to the insertion of urethral catheter when urethral injury is suspected.

Management

Goldman system for classification of urethral injuries at urethrography:

- Type I: Stretching or elongation of the otherwise intact posterior urethra.
- Type II: Urethral disruption above the urogenital diaphragm. Urogenital diaphragm forms the external sphincter and surrounds the membranous urethra. The membranous segment remains intact. Contrast extravasation is seen above the urogenital diaphragm.
- Type III: Disruption of the membranous urethra extending below the urogenital diaphragm and involving the anterior urethra. Contrast extravasation is seen below the urogenital diaphragm, possibly extending to the pelvis or perineum; bladder neck is intact.
- Type IV: Bladder neck injury extending into the proximal urethra. Extraperitoneal contrast extravasation; bladder neck disruption.
- Type V: Isolated anterior urethral injury. Contrast agent extravasation below the urogenital diaphragm, confined to the anterior urethra.

REFERENCES

Case 53

Emergency Radiology: The Requisites, 1st ed, Ch 1.
Wasserman JR, Koenigsberg, RA, Feldman JS, et al. Diffuse axonal injury imaging. *Medscape*. Web. 2014. http://emedicine.medscape.com/article/339912-overview.

Case 54

Emergency Radiology: The Requisites, 1st ed, Ch 1.
Parizel PM, van der Zijden T, Gaudino S, et al. Trauma of the spine and spinal cord: imaging strategies. *Eur Spine J*. 2010;19(Suppl 1):S8–S17.
Shuman WP, Rogers JV, Sickler ME, et al. Thoracolumbar burst fractures: CT dimensions of the spinal canal relative to postsurgical improvement. *AJR Am J Roentgenol*. 1985;145(2):337–341.

Case 55

Emergency Radiology: The Requisites, 1st ed, Ch 9.
Moore CJ, Corl FM, Fishman EK. CT of cecal volvulus: unraveling the image. *AJR*. 2001;177:95–98.
Peterson CM, Anderson JS, Hara AK, et al. Volvulus of the gastrointestinal tract: appearances at multimodality imaging. *Radiographics*. 2009;29:1281–1293.

Case 56

Bulakbasi N, Kocaoglu M. Central nervous system infections of herpesvirus family. *Neuroimaging Clin N Am*. 2008;18(1):53–84.
Emergency Radiology: The Requisites, 1st ed, Ch 1.
Solbrig MV, Hasso AN, Jay CA. CNS viruses—diagnostic approach. *Neuroimaging Clin N Am*. 2008;18(1):1–18.

Case 57

Emergency Radiology: The Requisites, 1st ed, Ch 1.
LeBedis CA, Sakai O. Nontraumatic orbital conditions: diagnosis with CT and MR imaging in the emergent setting. *Radiographics*. 28(6):1741–53.

Case 58

Bishop JY, Kaeding C. Treatment of the acute traumatic acromioclavicular separation. *Sports Medicine Arthroscopy*. 2006;14(4):237–245.
Emergency Radiology: The Requisites, 1st ed, Ch 4.
Marincek B, Dondelinger RF. *Emergency Radiology, Imaging and Intervention*. Springer Berlin; 2006.

Case 59

Emergency Radiology: The Requisites, 1st ed, Ch 7.
Hong SH, Choi JY, Lee JW, et al. MR imaging assessment of the spine: infection or an imitation? *Radiographics*. 2009;29(2):599–612.

Case 60

Emergency Radiology: The Requisites, 1st ed, Ch 6.
Hedge S, Hui P, Lee E. Tracheobronchial foreign bodies in children: imaging assessment. *Seminars in Ultrasound CT and MRI*. 2014;36:8–20.
Kim M, Lee K, Lee K, et al. MDCT evaluation of foreign bodies and liquid aspiration pneumonia in adults. *AJR*. 2008;190:907–915.
Tseng H, Hanna T, Shuaib W, et al. Imaging foreign bodies: ingested, aspirated and inserted. *Ann Emerg Med*. 2008;66:570–582.

Case 61

Bord SP, Linden J. Trauma to the globe and orbit. *Emerg Med Clin North Am*. 2008;26:97–123.
Emergency Radiology: The Requisites, 1st ed, Ch 1.
Kubal WS. Imaging of orbital trauma. *Radiographics*. 2008;28:1729–1739.
Kuhn F, Morris R, Mester V, et al. Epidemiology and socioeconomics. *Ophthalmology Clinics of North America*. 2002;15:145–151.

Case 62

Bord SP, Linden J. Trauma to the globe and orbit. *Emergency Medicine Clinics of North America*. 2008;26:97–123.
Emergency Radiology: The Requisites, 1st ed, Ch 1.
Kubal WS. Imaging of orbital trauma. *Radiographics*. 2008;28:1729–1739.
Kuhn F, Morris R, Mester V, et al. Epidemiology and socioeconomics. *Ophthalmology Clinics of North America*. 2002;15:145–151.

Case 63

Emergency Radiology: The Requisites, 1st ed, Ch 5.

Pineda C, Espinosa R, Pena A. Radiographic imaging in osteomyelitis: the role of plain radiography, computed tomography, ultrasonography, magnetic resonance imaging, and scintigraphy. *Seminars in Plastic Surgery*. 2009;23(02):80–89.

Case 64

Benedetti BS, Desser T, Jeffrey RB. Imaging of hepatic infections. *Ultrasound Quarterly*. 2008;24:267–278.
Emergency Radiology: The Requisites, 1st ed, Ch 9.
Hernandez JL, Ramos C. Pyogenic hepatic abscess: clues for diagnosis in the emergency room. *Clin Microbiol Infect*. 2001;7:567–570.
Huang CJ, Pitt HA, Lipsett PA, et al. Pyogenic hepatic abscess. Changing trends over 42 years. *Ann Surg*. 1996;223:600–609.
Johannsen EC, Sifri CD, Madoff LC. Pyogenic liver abscesses. *Infect Dis Clin North Am*. 2000;14(3):547Y563.
Lin AC, Yeh DY, Hsu YH, et al. Diagnosis of pyogenic liver abscess by abdominal ultrasonography in the emergency department. *Emerg Med J*. 2009;26:273–275.
Ochsner A, DeBakey M, Murray S. Pyogenic abscess of the liver. *I*. 1938;40:292–319.

Case 65

Cooper MN, Abrishamian LK, Newton KI. Odontogenic abscess. *J Emerg Med*. 2013;45(1):86–87.
Emergency Radiology: The Requisites, 1st ed, Ch 1.

Case 66

Emergency Radiology: The Requisites, 1st ed, Ch 11.
Hiratzka L, Bakris G, Beckman J, et al. Guidelines for the diagnosis and management of patients with thoracic aortic disease. *J Am Coll Cardiol*. 2010;55(14):127–129.
Maddu KK, Shuaib W, Telleria J, Johnson JO, Khosa F. Nontraumatic acute aortic emergencies: part 1, acute aortic syndrome. *AJR Am J Roentgenol*. 2014;202:656–665.

Case 67

Emergency Radiology: The Requisites, 1st ed, Ch 7.
Kasliwal MK, Fontes RB, Traynelis VC. Occipitocervical dissociation—incidence, evaluation, and treatment. *Current Review of Musculoskeletal Medicine*. 2016;9(3):247–254.

Case 68

Emergency Radiology: The Requisites, 1st ed, Ch 7.
Tarantino R, Donnarumma P, Marotta N, et al. Atlanto axial rotatory dislocation in adults: a rare complication of an epileptic seizure–case report. *J Pediatric Orthop B*. 2014;54(5):413–416.
Tauchi R, Imagama S, Ito Z, et al. Surgical treatment for chronic atlantoaxial rotatory fixation in children. *J Pediatr Orthop B*. 2013;22(5):404–408. https://doi.org/10.1097/BPB.0b013e3283633064.

Case 69

Emergency Radiology: The Requisites, 1st ed, Ch 7.
Giauque AP, Bittle MM, Braman JP. Type I hangman's fracture. *Curr Probl Diagn Radiol*. 2012;41(4):116–117.

Case 70

Costa DN, Cavalcanti CF, Sernik RA. Sonographic and CT findings in lipohemarthrosis. *AJR Am J Roentgenol*. 2007;188(4):W389.
Emergency Radiology: The Requisites, 1st ed, Ch 4.

Case 71

Emergency Radiology: The Requisites, 1st ed, Ch 7.
O'Shaughnessy J, Grenier JM, Stern PJ. A delayed diagnosis of bilateral facet dislocation of the cervical spine: a case report. *Journal of the Canadian Chiropractic Association*. 2014;58(1):45–51.
Vaccaro AR, Hulbert RJ, Patel AA, et al. The subaxial cervical spine injury classification system: a novel approach to recognize the importance of morphology, neurology, and integrity of the disco-ligamentous complex. Spine Trauma Study Group. *Spine*. 2007;32(21):2365–2374.

Case 72

Emergency Radiology: The Requisites, 1st ed, Ch 7.
O'Shaughnessy J, Grenier JM, Stern PJ. A delayed diagnosis of bilateral facet dislocation of the cervical spine: a case report. *Journal of the Canadian Chiropractic Association*. 2014;58(1):45–51.

Vaccaro AR, Hulbert RJ, Patel AA, et al. The subaxial cervical spine injury classification system: a novel approach to recognize the importance of morphology, neurology, and integrity of the disco-ligamentous complex. Spine Trauma Study Group; *Spine*. 2007;32(21):2365–2374.

Case 73

Emergency Radiology: The Requisites, 1st ed, Ch 7.
O'Shaughnessy J, Grenier JM, Stern PJ. A delayed diagnosis of bilateral facet dislocation of the cervical spine: a case report. *Journal of the Canadian Chiropractic Association*. 2014;58(1):45–51.
Vaccaro AR, Hulbert RJ, Patel AA, et al. The subaxial cervical spine injury classification system: a novel approach to recognize the importance of morphology, neurology, and integrity of the disco-ligamentous complex. Spine Trauma Study Group; Spine (Philadelphia, PA 1976). *Spine*. 2007;32(21): 2365–2374.

Case 74

Emergency Radiology: The Requisites, 1st ed, Ch 8.
Hammer MH, Flagg E, Mellnick VM, Cummings KW, Bhalla S, Raptis CA. Computed tomography of blunt and penetrating diaphragmatic injury: sensitivity and inter-observer agreement of CT signs. *Emerg Radiol*. 2014;21:143–149. https://doi.org/10.1007/s10140-013-1166.
Iochum S, Ludig T, Walter F, Sebbag H, Grosdidier G, Blum AG. Imaging of diaphragmatic injury: a diagnostic challenge? *Radiographics*. 2002;22. Oct. Spec No:S103–16, https://doi.org/10.1148/radiographics.22.suppl_1.g02oc14s103.

Case 75

Emergency Radiology: The Requisites, 1st ed, Ch 8.
Triadafilopoulos G, Roorda A, Akiyama J. Update on foreign bodies in the esophagus: diagnosis and management. *Curr Gastroenterol Rep*. 2013; 15(4):317. https://doi.org/10.1007/s11894-013-0317-5.
Tseng HJ, Hanna TN, Shuaib W, Aized M, Khosa F, Linnau KF. Imaging foreign bodies: ingested, aspirated, and inserted. *Ann Emerg Med*. 2015;66(6):570–582. e5, https://doi.org/10.1016/j.annemergmed.2015.07.499.

Case 76

Emergency Radiology: The Requisites, 1st ed, Ch 8.
Soreide JA, Viste A. Esophageal perforation: diagnostic work-up and clinical decision making in the first 24 hours. *Scandinavian Journal of Trauma Resuscitation and Emergency Medicine*. 2011;19:66. https://doi.org/10.1186/1757-7241-19-66.

Case 77

Emergency Radiology: The Requisites, 1st ed, Ch 8.
Restrepo CS, Lemos DF, Lemos JA, et al. Imaging findings in cardiac tamponade with emphasis on CT. *Radiographics*. 2007;27(6):1595–1610. https://doi.org/10.1148/rg.276065002.
Spodick DH. Acute cardiac tamponade. *New Engl J Med*. 2003;349(7): 684–690. https://doi.org/10.1056/NEJMra022643.

Case 78

Emergency Radiology: The Requisites, 1st ed, Ch.
Steenburg SD, Ravenel JG, Ikonomidis JS, et al. Acute traumatic aortic injury: imaging evaluation and management. *Radiology*. 2008;248(3): 748–762.

Case 79

Emergency Radiology: The Requisites, 1st ed, Ch 11.
Rakita D, Newatia A, Hines JJ, et al. Spectrum of CT findings in rupture and impending rupture of abdominal aortic aneurysms. *Radiographics*. 2007;27(2):497–507.
Schwartz SA, Taljanovic MS, Smyth S, et al. CT findings of rupture, impending rupture, and contained rupture of abdominal aortic aneurysms. *AJR Am J Roentgenol*. 2007;188(1):W57–W62.

Case 80

Bulakci M, Kalelioglu T, Bulakci BB, et al. Comparison of diagnostic value of multidetector computed tomography and x-ray in the detection of body packing. *Eur J Radiol*. 2013;82(8):1248–1254.
Emergency Radiology: The Requisites, 1st ed, Ch 9.
Mehrpour O, Sezavar SV. Diagnostic imaging in body packers. *Mayo Clin Proc*. 2012;87(7):e53–e54.

Case 81

Emergency Radiology: The Requisites, 1st ed, Ch 9.
Yeh BM, Liu PS, Soto JA, et al. MR imaging and CT of the biliary tract. *Radiographics*. 2009;29(6):1669–1688.

Case 82

Craig WD, Wagner BJ, Travis MD. Pyelonephritis: radiologic-pathologic review. *Radiographics*. 2008;28(1):255–277.
Emergency Radiology: The Requisites, 1st ed, Ch 9.

Case 83

Emergency Radiology: The Requisites, 1st ed, Ch 9.
Weiner W, Bharti K, Hoon J, et al. CT of acute bowel ischemia. *Radiographics*. 2003;226:635–650.

Case 84

Brody J, Leighton D, Murphy B, et al. CT of blunt trauma bowel and mesenteric injury: typical findings and pitfalls in diagnosis. *Radiographics*. 2000;20(6):1525–1536.
Brofman N, Atri M, Epid D, et al. Evaluation of bowel and mesenteric blunt trauma with multidetector CT. *Radiographics*. 2006;26(4):1119–1131.
Emergency Radiology: The Requisites, 1st ed, Ch 9.
Tsang B, Panacek E, Brant W, Wisner D. Effect of oral contrast administration for abdominal computed tomography in the evaluation of acute blunt trauma. *Ann Emerg Med*. 1997;30:7–13.

Case 85

Emergency Radiology: The Requisites, 1st ed, Ch 9.
Singh AK, Gervais DA, Hahn PF, Sagar P, Mueller PR, Novelline RA. Acute epiploic appendagitis and its mimics. *Radiographics*. 2005;25 (6):1521–1534.

Case 86

Emergency Radiology: The Requisites, 1st ed, Ch 9.
Hunter TB, Taljanovic MS. Medical devices of the abdomen and pelvis. *Radiographics*. 2005;25(2):503–523.

Case 87

Emergency Radiology: The Requisites, 1st ed, Ch 3.
Marmery H, et al. Optimization of selection for nonoperative management of blunt splenic injury: comparison of MDCT grading systems. *AJR Am J Roentgenol*. 2007;189(6):1421–1427.
Soto JA, Anderson SW. Multidetector CT of blunt abdominal trauma. *Radiology*. 2012;265(3):678–693.
Steenburg S, Whitesell R. MDCT imaging of abdominal solid organ injuries: what the surgeon wants to know. *Contemporary Diagnostic Radiology*. 2013;36(13):1–5.

Case 88

Alonso RC, Nacenta SB, Martinez PD, Guerrero AS, Fuentes CG. Kidney in danger: CT findings of blunt and penetrating renal trauma. *Radiographics*. 2009;29(7):2033–2053. https://doi.org/10.1148/rg.297095071.
Emergency Radiology: The Requisites, 1st ed, Ch 9.
Gross JA, Lehnert BE, Linnau KF, Voelzke BB, Sandstrom CK. Imaging of urinary system trauma. *Radiol Clin North Am*. 2015;53(4):773–788. https://doi.org/10.1016/j.rcl.2015.02.005.

Case 89

Emergency Radiology: The Requisites, 1st ed, Ch 9.
Gupta A, Stuhlfaut J, Fleming K, et al. Blunt trauma of the pancreas and biliary tract: a multimodality imaging approach to diagnosis. *Radiographics*. 2004;24:1381–1395.

Case 90

Caleo O, Bocchini G, Paoletta S, et al. Spontaneous non-aortic retroperitoneal hemorrhage: etiology, imaging characterization and impact of MDCT on management. A multicentric study. *Radiol Med*. 2015;120 (1):133–148.
Emergency Radiology: The Requisites, 1st ed, Ch 9.

Case 91

Chan DP, Abujudeh HH, Cushing Jr GL, Novelline RA. CT cystography with multiplanar reformation for suspected bladder rupture: experience in 234 cases. *AJR Am J Roentgenol*. 2006;187(5):1296–1302.
Emergency Radiology: The Requisites, 1st ed, Ch 9.

Gomez RG, Ceballos L, Coburn M, et al. Consensus statement on bladder injuries. *British Journal of Urology International.* 2004;94(1):27–32.
Morey AF, Brandes S, Dugi 3rd DD, et al. Urotrauma: AUA guideline. *J Urol.* 2014;192(2):327–335.

Case 92

Daly KP, Ho CP, Persson DL, Gay SB. Traumatic retroperitoneal injuries: review of multidetector CT findings. *Radiographics.* 2008;28:1571–1590.
Emergency Radiology: The Requisites, 1st ed, Ch 9.
Vaidya SS, Bhargava P, Marder CP, Dighe MK. Inferior vena cava dissection following blunt abdominal trauma. *Emergency Radiology.* 2010;17 (4):339–342.

Case 93

Dreizin D, Letzing M, Sliker CW, et al. Multidetector CT of blunt cervical spine trauma in adults. *Radiographics.* 2014;34(7):1842–1865.
Emergency Radiology: The Requisites, 1st ed, Ch 7.
Vaccaro AR, Hulbert RJ, Patel AA, et al. The subaxial cervical spine injury classification system: a novel approach to recognize the importance of morphology, neurology, and integrity of the disco-ligamentous complex. *Spine.* 2007;32(21):2365–2374.

Case 94

Blake MA, Kalra MK, Maher MM, et al. Pheochromocytoma: an imaging chameleon. *Radiographics.* 2004;24(Suppl 1):S87–S99.
Emergency Radiology: The Requisites, 1st ed, Ch 9.
Leung K, Stamm M, Raja A, et al. Pheochromocytoma: the range of appearances on ultrasound, CT, MRI, and functional imaging. *AJR Am J Roentgenol.* 2013;200(2):370–378.

Case 95

Emergency Radiology: The Requisites, 1st ed, Ch 9.
Thompson WM. Imaging and findings of lipomas of the gastrointestinal tract. *AJR Am J Roentgenol.* 2005;184(4):1163–1171.

Case 96

Brunham RC, Gottlieb SL, Paavonen J. Pelvic inflammatory disease. *N Engl J Med.* 2015;372(21):2039–2048.
Emergency Radiology: The Requisites, 1st ed, Ch 10.

Case 97

Emergency Radiology: The Requisites, 1st ed, Ch 1.
Hardman JM, Manoukian A. Pathology of head trauma. *Neuroimaging Clin N Am.* 2002;12(2):175–187.
Rehman T, Ali R, Tawil I, Yonas H. Rapid progression of traumatic bifrontal contusions to transtentorial herniation: a case report. *Cases Journal.* 2008;1(1):203.

Case 98

Cohen M, Chhetri DK, Head C. Isolated uvulitis. *Ear Nose Throat J.* 2007;86:462–464.
Emergency Radiology: The Requisites, 1st ed, Ch 1.
Huang CJ. Isolated uvular angioedema in a teenage boy. *Internet Journal of Emergency Medicine.* 2007;3(2).

Case 99

Emergency Radiology: The Requisites, 1st ed, Ch 4.
Khurana B, Sheehan SE, Sodickson AD, Weaver MJ. Pelvic ring fractures: what the orthopedic surgeon wants to know. *Radiographics.* 2014;34(5): 1317–1333. https://doi.org/10.1148/rg.345135113.

Case 100

Emergency Radiology: The Requisites, 1st ed, Ch 11.
Hauser M. Congenital anomalies of the coronary arteries. *Heart.* 2005;91:1240–1245. https://doi.org/10.1136/hrt.2004.057299.

Case 101

Emergency Radiology: The Requisites, 1st ed, Ch 4.
Sanders RW, Rammelt S. Fractures of the calcaneus. In: Coughlin MJ, Saltzman C, Anderson RB, eds. *Mann's Surgery of the Foot and Ankle.* Philadelphia, PA: Saunders Elsevier; 2014:2041–2100.
Tu P, Bytomski JR. Diagnosis of heel pain. *Am Fam Physician.* 2011;84(8): 909–916.

Case 102

Emergency Radiology: The Requisites, 1st ed, Ch 10.
Sellmyer MA, Desser TS, Maturen KE, Jeffrey RB, Kamaya A. Physiologic, histologic, and imaging features of retained products of conception. *Radiographics.* 2013;33(3):781–796.

Case 103

Emergency Radiology: The Requisites, 1st ed, Ch 1.
Imai T, Sukegawa S, Kanno T, et al. Mandibular fracture patterns consistent with posterior maxillary fractures involving the posterior maxillary sinus, pterygoid plate or both: CT characteristics. *Dentomaxillofacial Radiology.* 2014;43(2):21030355.
Juhl JH, Crummy AB. *Paul and Juhl's Essentials of Radiologic Imaging.* 6th ed. Philadelphia: Lippincott; 1993.

Case 104

Emergency Radiology: The Requisites, 1st ed, Ch 1.
Mair G, Boyd EV, Chappell FM, et al. IST-3 Collaborative Group. Sensitivity and specificity of the hyperdense artery sign for arterial obstruction in acute ischemic stroke. *Stroke.* 2015;46(1):102–107.
Powers WJ, Derdeyn CP, Biller J, et al. American Heart Association Stroke Council. 2015 American Heart Association/American Stroke Association Focused Update of the 2013 Guidelines for the early management of patients with acute ischemic stroke regarding endovascular treatment: a guideline for healthcare professionals from the American Heart Association/American Stroke Association. *Stroke.* 2015;46 (10):3020–3035.
Shetty SK. The MCA dot sign. *Radiology.* 2006;241(1):315–318.

Case 105

Emergency Radiology: The Requisites, 1st ed, Ch 9.
Ingram MD, Watson SG, Skippage PL, et al. Urethral injuries after pelvic trauma: evaluation with urethrography. *Radiographics.* 2008;28: 1631–1643.

Challenge

CASE 106

Ranula

1. **A, B, C.** The differential diagnosis for this neck mass includes necrotic lymph node, ranula, and abscess. Further interrogation revealed no pain or fever. Thyroglossal duct cysts are generally midline structures.
2. **C.** Simple ranulas originate in and occupy the sublingual space. Diving or plunging ranulas extend into the submandibular space.
3. **B.** Simple ranulas are thin-walled with low-attenuating centers. When infected, they can become thick-walled with hyperattenuating centers and may resemble soft-tissue masses. They result from obstruction of the sublingual gland. Incision and drainage are associated with 70% recurrence.
4. **A.** Ranula walls may demonstrate some wall enhancement after gadolinium administration.

Comment

Background
Ranulas are benign acquired retention cysts with origins at the floor of the mouth. They result from obstruction of the sublingual gland or adjacent minor salivary glands. They arise spontaneously or as a result of trauma or surgery to the floor of the mouth. Ranulas can be classified as simple (confined to the sublingual space) or plunging (extending to the submandibular space). The fluid contained within the ranula resembles normal sublingual secretions. Rarely ranulas may be associated with infection or hemorrhage.

Diagnosis
The key to diagnosing a ranula is tracing its origin to the sublingual space. Plunging ranulas will connect to this space even if only by a thin, fluid tail. Transdermal or transoral sonography can be performed; however, they are usually evaluated in the emergency department (ED) setting with computed tomography (CT). Thin-walled cystic lesions with simple fluid centers are noted in the sublingual or submandibular space. Infected or hemorrhagic ranulas may resemble nonenhancing soft-tissue masses and may be mistaken for abscesses or necrotic lymph nodes. Magnetic resonance (MR) evaluation demonstrates T1 low signal and T2 high signal. Gadolinium administration may evoke some wall enhancement.

Management
Surgical resection is definitive but should include excision of the associated sublingual gland. Other surgical methods such as I&D and marsupialization are associated with 50% to 70% recurrence. Sclerotherapy has been used with good outcomes.

CASE 107

Obstructive Sialadenitis

1. **D.** Each choice may present with enlarged salivary glands. However, the presence of an obstructing stone in the salivary duct associated with gland inflammation is most consistent with sialadenitis.

2. **B, C.** Both *Staphylococcus aureus* and *Streptococcus viridans* are common pathogens responsible for bacterial sialadenitis.
3. **C.** Submandibular stone are noted five times more often than parotid stones.
4. **D.** Bilateral parotitis is associated with the mumps virus and usually seen in children.

Comment

Background
Sialadenitis refers to inflammation of the salivary gland. It is differentiated from sialadenosis, the noninflammatory, non-neoplastic enlargement of the salivary gland. Sialadenitis has broad-ranging etiologies: bacterial (*S. aureus* and *S. viridans* are most common), obstructive sialadenitis (salivary colic may be present; associated with obstructing stone in duct; most commonly affects the submandibular gland), virus (mumps), immunosuppression, iodine 131 administration, Sjögren's syndrome, dehydration, and radiation.

Diagnosis
Patients usually present with painful swelling of the gland. Symptoms may be heightened after eating. In the acute setting, CT demonstrates an enlarged salivary gland with abnormal hyperattenuation and adjacent fat stranding. Sialoliths may be present.

Management
Conservative medical management of sialoliths may include hydration, warm compresses, and nonsteroidal antiinflammatory drugs (NSAIDs). Failure of conservative therapy may be followed by lithotripsy, endoscopic removal, or surgery.

CASE 108

Ludwig angina

1. **A, B.** Although salivary gland infection can lead to Ludwig angina, the lesion does not include the salivary glands.
2. **B, C, D.** *Escherichia coli* is not a pathogen associated with Ludwig angina.
3. **A, B, C.** The retropharyngeal space is not included.
4. **D.** Each of the choices listed can be associated with Ludwig angina; however, the most often cause is odontogenic.

Comment

Background
Ludwig angina is a rapidly progressive inflammation of the floor of the mouth. This infection can involve the submandibular, sublingual, and submental spaces. It can rapidly progress to airway compromise. If left unchecked, it can spread to the neck and mediastinum. Trismus, odynophagia, and dysphagia may be present. Immunocompromised patients are at increased risk of developing Ludwig angina. The majority of cases are thought to originate from *Staphylococcus*, *Streptococcus*, and *Bacteroides sp*. Other causes include penetrating trauma, peritonsillar abscess, epiglottitis, and sialadenitis.

Diagnosis
Although Ludwig angina is primarily a clinical diagnosis, CT may be helpful to evaluate for abscess.

Management
Airway protection is paramount. Intravenous (IV) antibiotics and steroids are the mainstay. Abscess drainage as needed.

CASE 109

Lemierre Syndrome (Septic Jugular Thrombophlebitis)

1. **A, B, C, D**. Extensive unilateral inflammation in this region may represent a number of entities.
2. **A.** The lungs are the most common site of septic emboli. Septic arthritis is also common. Meningitis can rarely occur.
3. **A, B, C.** Polymicrobial bacteremia is often noted in patients with Lemierre syndrome.
4. **A.** An initial oropharyngeal infection with or without abscess may precipitate Lemierre syndrome.

Comment

Background
First described by Andre Lemierre in 1936, Lemierre syndrome refers to thrombophlebitis of the jugular vein with septic emboli. Emboli are most often noted in the lungs but can be seen in any organ. There is a predilection for joint spaces manifesting septic arthritis. Polymicrobial bacteremia is common with *Streptococcus sp*, gram-negative anaerobes, and methicillin-resistant staphylococcus aureus (MRSA).

Diagnosis
Computed tomography is considered the gold standard for detecting jugular vein thrombophlebitis. In addition, CT can detect sites of septic emboli. Ultrasound (US) may show thrombus in the jugular vein; however, the site of infection is not frequently depicted.

Management
Systemic dissemination can occur if not properly treated. Mortality rate is as high as 18%.

CASE 110

Orbital Pseudotumor

1. **A, B**, and **C**. Glaucoma is a condition that causes damage to the optic nerve. **A, B**, and **C** are all possible and must be considered.
2. **C.** A, B, C, and D are possible, but **C** best describes indicates an orbital pseudotumor.
3. **A.** A, B, C, and D are possible and have been recorded. However, **A** is the most common presentation.
4. **B.** Proptosis, which is defined as the bulging of an eye anteriorly, is common with orbital pseudotumor. This may cause A or C. Refractive errors are not generally seen.

Comment

Background
Orbital pseudotumor, also known as idiopathic orbital inflammatory disease (IOI), is the most common orbital mass found in the adult population. IOI is associated with retinal detachment, uveitis, Tolosa-Hunt syndrome, proptosis, sarcoidosis, systemic lupus erythematosus, and other inflammatory and autoimmune conditions. Orbital pseudotumor, the third most common orbital disorder following thyroid orbitopathy and lymphoproliferative disease,

is found in middle-aged individuals but can be seen in the young as well. Patients typically present with unilateral, painful proptosis and diplopia.

Diagnosis
An enlarged muscle of one or more of the ocular muscles is characteristic of IOI. The best imaging technique is contrast-enhanced MRI. Diffuse irregularity and enhancement of other structures is indicative of IOI and can be seen on CT and MR imaging.

Management
Most cases respond to steroid therapy; however, chemotherapy or radiotherapy may be required to treat refractory cases.

CASE 111

Peripheral Arterial Disease

1. **A, B.** CTA demonstrates a high-grade stenosis of the [x] artery. Diffuse atherosclerosis is noted.
2. **D.** 12 %.
3. **E. A, B, C,** and **D** are all risk factors for peripheral artery disease (PAD).
4. **A.** Of the modalities listed, radiography is the least likely to yield significant results in evaluating PAD in the emergent setting.

Comment

Background
Peripheral artery disease is a common entity with age-adjusted prevalence of 12%. Atherosclerosis is a leading cause of PAD involving the extremities in patients over age 40. The peak incidence of disease is among patients in the sixth and seventh decades. Risk factors include: diabetes, smoking, hypercholesterolemia hypertension, obesity, and advanced age.

Diagnosis
Ultrasound may be used to assess the ankle-brachial index. B-mode can evaluate the arterial wall and degree of luminal stenosis. Atherosclerosis (hyperechoic foci in the wall and lumen) can be noted. CTA can assess vessels, stenosis, and collateral circulation. MIP, volume rendered techniques, and multiplanar reconstructions are helpful in the assessment. Magnetic resonance angiography (MRA) can be acquired without contrast administration; however, it can overestimate stenosis. Angiography is invasive, but it is the gold-standard. In the emergent setting is may not be as readily available as CT; however, it can be both diagnostic and therapeutic.

Management
Endovascular therapy.

CASE 112

Intestinal Angioedema

Peripheral Arterial Disease

1. **A, B, C, D.** Each entity could be considered in the differential diagnosis. Further history, physical examination, and laboratory analysis could help narrow the field.
2. **A.** Intestinal angioedema is associated with hereditary or acquired deficiency of C1 enzyme. Medications such as angiotension-converting enzyme (ACE) inhibitors and calcium channel blockers can also be contributory.

3. **C.** Nonspecific abdominal pain, nausea, and vomiting are common presenting findings.
4. **B.** Intestinal angioedema can affect small and large bowel but is most commonly seen in jejunum.

Comment

Background
Edema in the intestinal submucosal space following protein extravasation and leaky vessels characterizes this entity. It can affect the small and large bowel; however, the jejunum is most commonly impacted. Hereditary or acquired C1 inhibitor enzyme deficiency or medication (ACE inhibitor/calcium channel blockers) are noted.

Diagnosis
Patients often present with nonspecific abdominal pain, nausea, and vomiting. CT may show long segment submucosal thickening, mild edema without lymphadenopathy, or obstruction.

Management
Avoid provoking factors, inhibit histamine-provoking reactions, and treat C1 inhibitor deficiency.

CASE 113

Tracheobronchial Injury

1. **A, B.** Although tracheobronchial injury is suggested by history, diverticulum can be included in the differential. The esophagus is normal. No ingested foreign body.
2. **D.**
3. **B.**
4. **D.**

Comment

Background
Tracheobronchial injury is a manifestation of chest trauma. Usually fatal, few patients make it to the hospital and are imaged. The force required to injure the airway and the associated injuries are usually fatal. Penetrating injuries most commonly impact the cervical trachea. Blunt injuries tend to impact the distal trachea.

Diagnosis
Computed tomography is considered the gold standard for detecting these injuries in the emergent setting. Disruption of the airway, focal thickening, laryngeal disruption, fallen lung, pneumomediastinum, pneumothorax, and subcutaneous emphysema may be present. If left untreated, bronchiectasis, airway stenosis, and recurrent infections may occur.

Management
Surgical repair.

CASE 114

Esophageal Rupture

Tracheobronchial injury

1. **B.**
2. **D. A, B**, and **C** are associated with esophageal perforation.
3. **B.** Fluoroscopic evaluation within the first 24 hours is most sensitive.
4. **C.** 80% of cases are iatrogenic.

Comment

Background
A rare entity with a high mortality rate (25% to 50%), esophageal perforation is a medical emergency. Most patients are older and male. Patients may present with neck, chest, epigastric pain, dysphagia, or dyspnea. Chest pain is the most consistent symptom. Iatrogenic causes—post instrumentation—are the most common cause; however, trauma—blunt or penetrating—ingestions (foreign bodies or corrosive materials), malignancy, and post emesis (Boerhaave syndrome) can all precipitate rupture.

Diagnosis
Radiographs may demonstrate pneumomediastinum, irregular cardiac silhouette, pneumothorax, and left pleural effusion. Fluoroscopic evaluation within the first 24 hours is most sensitive. CT can detect extraluminal gas, pleural fluid, and effusions. Water-soluble contrast can be administered to evaluate the esophagus. CT is also helpful to evaluate complications such as acute mediastinitis, empyema, pneumonia, or fistula formation.

Management
Conservative management versus endoscopic or surgical repair.

CASE 115

Myocardial Infarction

1. **A.** CT demonstrates a regional area of myocardial hypoperfusion involving the left ventricle.
2. **A.** Anemia is not strongly associated with myocardial ischemia.
3. **B.** Electrocardiogram (ECG) and cardiac enzymes are more appropriate and cost-effective.
4. **C.** Patients with poor visceral sensation are more likely to experience silent ischemia—void of the classic radiating chest pain symptomatology.

Comment

Background
Myocardial infarction results from myocardial ischemia—myocardial blood flow less than myocardial metabolic needs. This is the leading cause of death worldwide. Risk factors include male gender and advancing age. Smoking, hypertension, hypercholesterolemia, obesity, and diabetes are contributing risk factors. Patients classically present with radiating chest pain.

Diagnosis
Imaging is not the first pass tool for evaluation—ECG, cardiac enzymes. Radiography may explain other causes of chest pain. CTA of the coronary arteries is a promising tool to clear patients with low risk in the emergent setting. Nuclear medicine may aid in diagnosis and evaluation of some patients.

Management
Includes emergent, in-patient, out-patient, and long-term multi-pronged therapeutics.

CASE 116

Myocardial Laceration

1. **A, B, C.** A gunshot wound to the chest with a bullet is seen at the interventricular septum. There is hemopericardium and a sternal fracture. There is no compression of the heart chambers to suggest tamponade physiology based on imaging.
2. **A, B, C, D.** Myocardial injury can occur in blunt or penetrating trauma and also secondary to iatrogenic causes, such as during

cardiopulmonary resuscitation or as a result of hemodynamic collapse and traumatic myocardial infarction.

3. **A, B, C, D, E.** Myocardial injury can be detected by ECG changes, troponin elevation, CT or MR imaging, and in the setting of ischemia by nuclear scintigraphy.

4. **D.** Myocardial injuries are commonly expectantly managed, especially in the setting of blunt trauma. Laceration injury or frank rupture of the free wall, however, is often fatal and requires emergent repair. With concern for subsequent formation of underlying fistula to the coronary vasculature, angiography can be performed. Revascularization is considered if there is resultant ischemia.

Comment

Background
Injury to the heart, including the pericardium and myocardium, can be seen in both blunt and penetrating trauma, which includes contusion, laceration, and ischemic injury. Laceration injury to the myocardium can occur from penetrating trauma, sheering during blunt trauma, from cardiopulmonary resuscitation, or from pericardiocentesis. The right ventricle, owing to its anterior position, is most frequently injured.

Diagnosis
Often the diagnosis of myocardial injury is based on a high index of clinical suspicion. Sensitivity of portable technologies–chest radiography or bedside ultrasound–is low, but the presence of cardiomegaly or pericardial fluid is suspicious. CT, often performed in these patients given concern for significant thoracic trauma, can show hemopericardium, contusion of the pericardial fat, or frank rupture of the pericardium and myocardium. In penetrating trauma, CT best demonstrates the tract of injury and any retained objects. Contrast-enhanced MR imaging does not play a role in emergent imaging of these patients but can be used in stable patients for whom distinction of contusion injury from traumatic myocardial ischemia needs to be made.

Management
Laceration of the myocardium is a critical injury, and rupture of a cardiac chamber requires urgent surgical repair. If the injury involves the coronary vessels, stenting or bypass may also be necessary. Larger pericardial lacerations can allow for herniation and strangulation of a cardiac chamber. Such a complication necessitates surgical repair. Myocardial contusion injuries are often expectantly managed with consideration for the patient's hemodynamic status and monitoring for rhythmic abnormalities.

CASE 117

Sialolith Obstruction

Obstructive Sialoadenitis With Abscess

1. **C.** A large collection with associated inflammation is noted at the left floor of the mouth. A large sialoliths is noted in the left submandibular duct. The duct is obstructed. The left submandibular gland is heterogeneously enhancing. Although a radiopaque density is noted in the floor of the mouth, it does not localize to the oral cavity or airway. The inflammation and collection are focal and localized to the region of the left submandibular duct. The tonsils are not involved.

2. **B.** 80% to 90% of all ducts are noted in the submandibular duct/gland.

3. **C, D.** Sialoliths are the most common disease of the parotid glands and ducts and most commonly affect the submandibular

glands/ducts. Submandibular secretions are more viscous than the parotid gland secretions.

4. **A, B, C, D.** Complications of sialolithiasis include all the choices listed.

Comment

Background
Sialolithiasis, or salivary stones, form within the salivary ducts or parenchyma of the glands. It comprises over 50% of salivary gland disease. The submandibular gland is most commonly affected (80% to 90%). It is hypothesized that the increased viscosity of submandibular gland secretions increases the likelihood of stone formation. Sialolithiasis affects males in the 30- to 60-year-old range most often. Patients will present with pain and swelling in the involved gland. Pain associated with eating may occur when the duct is obstructed. Obstruction can lead to bacterial infection, abscess formation, widespread inflammation and swelling, and airway compromise.

Diagnosis
Not all stones are radiopaque. Radiography may not detect small or radiolucent stones, but some series have detected up to 90% of submandibular and 60% of parotid stones. Sialography identifies the location and size of the obstructing stone; however, it is not commonly performed or available in the emergent settings. Ultrasound is readily available and can detect both radiopaque and radiolucent stones greater than 2 mm. CT/MR can detect stones and evaluate the gland and surrounding region for complications.

Management
Conservative supportive therapy (hydration, heat, pain relief), medical management (sialolithotripsy, duct dilatation, and extraction), or intervention (surgical excision), depending on the severity and complexity.

CASE 118

Lower Gastrointestinal Hemorrhage (LGIB)

1. **A, C.** Although each of the choices could appear as intraluminal hyperattenuating foci, the configuration of the density and the relative attenuation help to limit the differential choices

2. **A, B, C.**

3. **B.** The detection rate for bleeding on CTA is >0.35mL/min.

4. **D.** Patients with impaired renal function are at increased risk for developing contrast-induced nephropathy.

Comment

Background
Lower gastrointestinal bleeding (LGIB) anatomically occurs between the ligament of Treitz to the anus. LGIB is five times less common than upper gastrointestinal bleeding (UGIB). LGIB can occur at any age; however, certain entities are more common based on age. In the young (<30 years of age), inflammatory bowel disease, Meckel diverticulum, and polyps may be considered. In older adults, diverticular disease, angiodysplasia, bowel malignancy, polyps, and hemorrhoids are considerations. Other etiological precipitators include medications, such as warfarin or NSAIDs; surgical interventions, such as polypectomies; radiation; colitis; alcoholism; and chronic liver disease.

Diagnosis
Patients may present with hematochezia or melena. Depending on the time course and rate of hemorrhage, patients may be

chronically anemic or acutely hypotensive. Colonoscopy is a first-line modality in the evaluation of LGIB. Other modalities include CTA, tagged red blood cell scans, and conventional angiography.

CTA can detect bleeds greater than 0.35 mL/min and provides a noninvasive method for localizing the source of bleeding. It is particularly attractive in the emergent setting but is most effective in patients with continuous bleeding. Adequate renal function and allergy screening are requisite.

Tagged red blood cell scans are labelled with technetium-99m and can detect bleeds less than 0.1 mL/min. This modality helps to localize the general anatomic area of bleeding as a precursor to endoscopic, angiographic, or surgical therapy. Rapid bleeding can create false–positive localization.

Angiography can be both diagnostic and therapeutic; however, the detection rate is less than 0.5 mL/min. Renal function and allergic reactions should be assessed.

Management
Fluid resuscitation. Address underlying etiological or contributing factors. Surgery, endoscopy, and angiography can provide therapeutic options.

CASE 119

Hypovolemic Shock

1. **B.** Although each of the choices can have bowel manifestations, hypotension complex has findings associated with the vasculature and other solid organs.
2. **D.** Each choice can precipitate hypoperfusion complex; however, posttraumatic shock is the most common cause.
3. **A.** Each of the choices may demonstrate changes in the setting of hypoperfusion complex; however, the bowel changes are more commonly seen.
4. **C.** All of the statements are accurate, except **C.** Low-density fluid surrounding the aorta is associated with hypoperfusion complex.

Comment

Background
Primarily noted on CT abdominal imaging, hypoperfusion complex is a constellation of findings noted in the setting of extensive hypoperfusion. Most commonly seen in the setting of post-traumatic hypovolemic shock, hypoperfusion complex can be seen in the setting of severe systemic infection/shock, cardiac arrest, and severe head/spine injury.

Diagnosis
CT findings can include:

- Bowel: thickened loops with enhancing walls and mucosa, *shock bowel*; findings of hypoperfusion most commonly found in the anatomic location
- Small caliber IVC: <9 mm; surrounding low-density fluid, *halo sign*
- Small caliber aorta: <13 mm (as measured in the perirenal aorta)
- Liver: 25 HU hypoattenuated when compared with spleen
- Spleen: subjective hypoattenuation
- Adrenal glands: bilateral hyperenhancement; more common in pediatric populations
- Pancreas: heterogeneous hyperattenuation with low-density peripancreatic fluid
- Kidneys: homogeneous hyperattenuation

Management
Fluid resuscitation. Address underlying etiological or contributing factors.

CASE 120

Endometritis

1. **A, B.** Although each of the choices may result in endometrial contents, the history and demographics can help to narrow the differential diagnosis.
2. **A, C.** Thickened, heterogeneous, and hypervascular endometrium are commonly identified on US in the setting of endometritis. Gas in the endometrium or fluid in the endometrium or cul-de-sac may be present.
3. **A, B, C.** Misoprostol causes the uterus to contract and expel its contents; it is not a risk factor in the development of endometritis.
4. **D.** The complication rates of endometritis after C-section is as high as 85% in some series.

Comment

Background
Endometritis can be acute or chronic: it can be seen in the gynecologic setting (pelvic inflammatory disease or endometrial instrumentation) or obstetric setting (vaginal or C-section, abortion, or miscarriage). It is associated with 2% to 3% of vaginal deliveries, but in as many as 85% of C-sections.

Diagnosis
Patients typically present with pelvic pain and fever. Obstetric history may include retained products of conception or intrauterine clots, premature rupture of membranes, or prolonged labor. Endometritis is a clinical diagnosis. Notwithstanding, US may be used for evaluation. It may be normal in the early stages. In the later stages, thickened and heterogeneous endometrium, increased vascularity, intracavitary/cul-de-sac fluid, and intrauterine air may be noted. MR may demonstrate increased T2 signal with intense enhancement post contrast.

Management
If not adequately treated, endometritis may progress to pyometrium or septic thrombophlebitis.

CASE 121

Placental Abruption

1. **C.**
2. **D.** Placental abruption—premature separation of placenta after the 20th week of gestation and before the third stage of labor.
3. **A, B, C, D.** Each choice is a risk factor associated with placental abruption.
4. **A, B, C.**

Comment

Background
Placental abruption is the premature separation of the normally implanted placenta after the 20th week of gestation and before the third stage of labor. It affects 1% of all pregnancies and is a potentially fatal complication of pregnancy. Risk factors associated with this condition include preeclampsia, prolonged rupture of membranes, increased parity, cigarette/cocaine use, trauma, advanced maternal age, and prior placental abruption (6% to 17% recurrence).

Diagnosis
Patients typically present with bleeding and cramping. Fetal monitoring may show signs of fetal distress. Abruption is classified by location—marginal (most common), retroplacental, and preplacental.

Ultrasound is the first-line imaging modality; however, it is relatively insensitive for the diagnosis. Sonographic signs include retroplacental hematoma, separation and rounding of the placental edges, thickened placenta (>5.5 cm), and thickening of the retroplacental myometrium. The echogenicity of the hematoma is age dependent.

Management
Fetal morbidity is proportional to the size of the abruption. Fetal distress in the setting of abruption is associated with a poorer prognosis. Small abruptions may be managed conservatively—serial US to monitor interval growth, heart rate monitoring, and maternal symptoms.

CASE 122

Placental Previa

1. **B.**
2. **D.** Placenta previa is not usually diagnosed on US before 20 weeks gestation.
3. **D.** Although US is likely to be most often used in the emergent setting to evaluate pregnant patients, MR is the gold standard for imaging the placenta and its relationship to the cervix.
4. **A, B, C, D.**

Comment

Background
Placenta previa (abnormally low positioning of the placenta) can partially or completely cover the cervical os.

Risk factors include previous placenta previa, placenta accrete, previous C-section, increased parity, increased maternal age, large placenta, and smoking.

Diagnosis
This potentially life-threatening entity. Although MRI is the gold standard for evaluating the placenta and its orientation to the cervix, US is much more likely to be used. Distance between placenta and internal cervical os should be noted during the second- and third-trimester examinations. Previa can be graded based on positioning in the lower uterine segment (LUS).

- Grade I: placenta in LUS, but does not abut the internal cervical os
- Grade II: placenta reaches the margin of the internal os, but does not cover it
- Grade III: placenta partially covers the internal cervical os
- Grade IV: placenta completely covers the internal cervical os

Management
Placenta previa is potentially a maternal and fetal life-threatening condition. In the case of high-grade previa, C-section should be anticipated.

CASE 123

Necrotizing Fasciitis (Fournier's Gangrene)

1. **D.** No discrete collection or abscess is present. The gas does not collect in the intraperitoneal space. The gas is more extensive than the superficial tissues.
2. **A.**
3. **A, B, C, D.** This is a polymicrobial infection.
4. **C.** Outpatient antibiotics is not an initial therapeutic approach.

Comment

Background
First described by French scientist Jean Alfred Fournier in 1883, Fournier gangrene is a necrotizing fasciitis of the perineum. This urologic emergency carries up to 33% mortality. Typically it has an impact on older diabetic men, but can be seen in women. Diabetes, sedentary nature, alcoholism, and immunosuppression are risk factors. The infection is polymicrobial often involving *E. coli, Klebsiella, Proteus, Streptococcus, and Staphylococcus.* The nidus is usually anorectal in origin, but genitourinary, perineal, or cryptogenic etiology can occur. The infection begins as a cellulitis but advances through the fascial planes causing a necrotizing reaction (often producing gas).

Diagnosis
Computed tomography demonstrates soft-tissue inflammation and facial thickening, and soft-tissue gas. The cause of the infection may be present. US may demonstrate thickening of the scrotum or echogenic gas in the scrotum or perineum.

Management
This is a life-threatening condition. Immediate surgical debridement of necrotic tissue, IV antibiotics, and hyperbaric therapy can be used.

CASE 124

Urethral Foreign Bodies

1. **B, C.** Lateral views of the pelvis would help to localize the nail. Physical examination would also help narrow the differential.
2. **A, B, C.**
3. **A.** A retrograde urethrogram will evaluate the urethra for injury.
4. **A, B, C, D.**

Comment

Background
Patients engaging in urethral foreign body insertion may present to the emergency department. Although often related to autoerotic stimulation, psychiatric illness and intoxication may also be noted.

Diagnosis
Radiography can easily confirm the presence of a radiopaque foreign body. Small radiolucent items may not be easily identified. Retrograde urethrogram is helpful to identify any radiolucent intraluminal objects and evaluate mucosal integrity, narrowing, or false passages.

Management
Removal of foreign body.

CASE 125

Scrotal Trauma

Testicular Fracture

1. **A, B, C.** The testicle is focally heterogeneous and its contour is disrupted (tunica albuginea). There is vascularity in the testicle. Complex peritesticular fluid is noted.
2. **A.** The disruption of the tunica albuginea supports the diagnosis of testicular fracture in this case. Hematoceles may be seen in traumatic injuries other than testicular fractures. Heterogeneity may be seen in the setting of hematoma, torsion, cancer, or fracture.

3. **B.** Posttraumatic infarct is caused by increased intratesticular pressure resulting in venous obstruction and venous infarction.
4. **E.** All of the choices are expected findings of testicular fracture.

Comment

Background
Testicular trauma is a common cause for acute scrotal pain. Trauma can result in varying degrees of injury from no imaging findings to testicular rupture. Extratesticular injuries are likely to occur in the setting of moderate to severe trauma and include scrotal hematoma/swelling, hematoceles, reactive epididymitis, or epididymal fracture.

Diagnosis
Ultrasound is appropriate for detecting these injuries in the emergent setting. Disruption of the tunica albuginea, normally a smooth echogenic rim around the testicle, may include loss of continuity or buckling. In the setting of rupture, the seminiferous tubules are noted outside the testicle. Doppler may help distinguish tubules from hematocele. Hematocele should be devoid of Doppler signal.

Management
Depending on the degree of injury, management may be conservative or surgical repair may be warranted in higher level injuries.

REFERENCES

Case 106
Coit WE, Harnsberger HR, Osborn AG, et al. Ranulas and their mimics: CT evaluation. *Radiology.* 1987;163.
Emergency Radiology: The Requisites, 1st ed, Ch 1.
Rho MH, Kim DW, Kwon JS, et al. OK-432 sclerotherapy of plunging ranula in 21 patients: it can be a substitute for surgery. *AJNR Am J Neuroradiol.* 2006;27(5):1090–1095.

Case 107
Capps EF, Kinsella JJ, Gupta M, et al. Emergency imaging assessment of acute, nontraumatic conditions of the head and neck. *Radiographics.* 2010;30 (5):1335–1352.
Emergency Radiology: The Requisites, 1st edition, Ch 1.
Yousem DM, Kraut MA, Chalian AA. Major salivary gland imaging. *Radiology.* 2000;216(1):19–29.

Case 108
Emergency Radiology: The Requisites, 1st edition, Ch 1.
Nguyen VD, Potter JL, Hersh-Schick MR. Ludwig angina: an uncommon and potentially lethal neck infection. AJNR. *Am J Neuroradiol.* 1992;13(1): 215–219.

Case 109
Emergency Radiology: The Requisites, 1st edition, Ch 1.
O'Brien WT, Lattin GE, Thompson AK. Lemierre syndrome: an all-but-forgotten disease. *AJR Am J Roentgenol.* 2006;187(3):W324. https://doi.org/10.2214/AJR.06.0096.

Case 110
Emergency Radiology: The Requisites, 1st edition, Ch 1.
Jacobs D, Galetta S. Diagnosis and management of orbital pseudotumor. *Curr Opin Ophthalmol.* 2002;13(6):347–351.
Mombaerts I, Goldschmeding R, Schlingemann R, Koornneff L. What is orbital pseudotumor? *Surv Ophthalmol.* 1996;41(1):66–78.

Case 111
Emergency Radiology: The Requisites, 1st edition, Ch 11.
Norgren L, Hiatt WR, Dormandy JA, et al. Inter-Society Consensus for the Management of Peripheral Arterial Disease (TASC II). *Eur J Vasc Endovasc Surg.* 2007;33(Suppl 1):S1–S75.

Case 112
Scheirey CD, Scholz FJ, Shortsleeve MJ, et al. Angiotensin-converting enzyme inhibitor-induced small-bowel angioedema: clinical and imaging findings in 20 patients. *AJR Am J Roentgenol.* 2011;197(2):393–398. https://doi.org/10.2214/AJR.10.4451.

Case 113
Emergency Radiology: The Requisites, 1st edition, Ch 2.
Kaewlai R, Avery LL, Asrani AV, et al. Multidetector CT of blunt thoracic trauma. *Radiographics.* 2008;28(6):1555–1570.

Case 114
Emergency Radiology: The Requisites, 1st edition, Ch 8.
Søreide JA, Viste A. Esophageal perforation: diagnostic work-up and clinical decision-making in the first 24 hours. *Scandanavian Journal of Trauma, Resuscitation and Emergency Medicine.* 2011;19(1):66.

Case 115
Bastarrika G, Lee YS, Huda W, et al. CT of coronary artery disease. *Radiology.* 2009;253(2):317–338. https://doi.org/10.1148/radiol.2532081738.
Emergency Radiology: The Requisites, 1st edition, Ch 11.
Gosalia A, Haramati LB, Sheth MP, et al. CT detection of acute myocardial infarction. *AJR Am J Roentgenol.* 2004;182(6):1563–1566. https://doi.org/10.2214/ajr.182.6.1821563.

Case 116
Emergency Radiology: The Requisites, 1st edition, Ch 2.
Olsovsky MR, Wechsler AS, Topaz O. Cardiac trauma diagnosis, management, and current therapy. *Angiology.* 1997;48:423–432. https://doi.org/10.1177/000331979704800506.

Case 117
Emergency Radiology: The Requisites, 1st edition, Ch 1.
Kraaij S, Karagozoglu KH, Forouzanfar T, et al. Salivary stones: symptoms, aetiology, biochemical composition and treatment. *Br Dent J.* 2014;217(11):E23.
Witt RL. *Salivary Gland Diseases: Surgical and Medical Management.* Thieme Medical Publishers; Philadelphia: PA; 2006.

Case 118
Emergency Radiology: The Requisites, 1st ed, Ch 12.
Feuerstein JD, Ketwaroo G, Tewani SK, et al. Localizing acute lower gastrointestinal hemorrhage: CT angiography versus tagged RBC scintigraphy. *AJR Am J Roentgenol.* 2016;1–7. https://doi.org/10.2214/AJR.15.15714.
Geffroy Y, Rodallec MH, Boulay-Coletta I, et al. Multidetector CT angiography in acute gastrointestinal bleeding: why, when, and how. *Radiographics.* 2011;31(3):E35–E46. https://doi.org/10.1148/rg.313105206.

Case 119
Ames JT, Federle MP. CT hypotension complex (shock bowel) is not always due to traumatic hypovolemic shock. *AJR Am J Roentgenol.* 2009;192(5):W230–W235. https://doi.org/10.2214/AJR.08.1474.
Emergency Radiology: The Requisites, 1st ed, Ch 3.
Tarrant AM, Ryan MF, Hamilton PA, et al. A pictorial review of hypovolaemic shock in adults. *Br J Radiol.* 2008;81(963):252–257. https://doi.org/10.1259/bjr/40962054.

Case 120
Emergency Radiology: The Requisites, 1st ed, Ch 10.
Nalaboff KM, Pellerito JS, Ben-Levi E. Imaging the endometrium: disease and normal variants. *Radiographics.* 2001;21(6):1409–1424.

Case 121
Emergency Radiology: The Requisites, 1st ed, Ch 10.
Glantz C, Purnell L. Clinical utility of sonography in the diagnosis and treatment of placental abruption. *J Ultrasound Med.* 2002;21(8):837–840.
Kaakaji Y, Nghiem HV, Nodell C, et al. Sonography of obstetric and gynecologic emergencies: part I, obstetric emergencies. *AJR Am J Roentgenol.* 2000;174(3):641–649.

Case 122
Elsayes KM, Trout AT, Friedkin AM et al. Imaging of the placenta: a multimodality pictorial review. *Radiographics.* 2009;29(5):1371–1391.
Emergency Radiology: The Requisites, 1st ed, Ch 10.

Case 123

Emergency Radiology: The Requisites, 1st ed, Ch 10.
Rajan DK, Scharer KA. Radiology of Fournier's gangrene. *AJR Am J Roentgenol*. 1998;170(1):163–168.

Case 124

Emergency Radiology: The Requisites, 1st ed, Ch 2.
Hunter TB, Taljanovic MS. Foreign bodies. *Radiographics*. 2003;23(3): 731–757. https://doi.org/10.1148/rg.233025137.

Case 125

Bhatt S, Dogra VS. Role of US in testicular and scrotal trauma. *Radiographics*. 2008;28(6):1617–1629.
Emergency Radiology: The Requisites, 1st ed, Ch 10.

Index of Cases

Index

Note: Page numbers followed by *t* indicate tables.